STEP-UP to
FAMILY
MEDICINE

STEP-UP to FAMILY MEDICINE

Robert V. Ellis, MD
Assistant Professor of Family Medicine
Department of Family and Community
  Medicine
University of Cincinnati
Cincinnati, Ohio

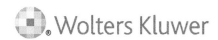 Wolters Kluwer

Philadelphia • Baltimore • New York • London
Buenos Aires • Hong Kong • Sydney • Tokyo

Acquisitions Editor: Matt Hauber
Development Editor: Andrea Vosburgh
Editorial Coordinator: Tim Rinehart
Editorial Assistant: Brooks Phelps
Marketing Manager: Mike McMahon
Production Project Manager: Linda Van Pelt
Design Coordinator: Holly McLaughlin
Manufacturing Coordinator: Margie Orzech
Prepress Vendor: Command Digital

9 8 7 6 5 4 3

Printed in the United States of America

Library of Congress Cataloging-in-Publication Data
Names: Ellis, Robert V., author.
Title: Step-up to family medicine / Robert V. Ellis, MD, Assistant Professor
   of Family Medicine, Department of Family and Community Medicine,
   University of Cincinnati, Cincinnati, OH.
Description: First edition. | Philadelphia: Wolters Kluwer Health, [2018] |
   Series: Step-up series
Identifiers: LCCN 2017045014 | ISBN 9781469864211 (paperback)
Subjects: LCSH: Family medicine. | BISAC: MEDICAL / Family & General Practice.
Classification: LCC RC46 .E466 2018 | DDC 610—dc23
LC record available at https://lccn.loc.gov/2017045014

LWW.com

CD082024

DEDICATION

To Bear, A, and Little Voldy, you are my inspiration and truly make me a better person.

ORSON J. AUSTIN, MD
Associate Professor of Clinical Family
Medicine
Department of Family and Community
Medicine
University of Cincinnati
Cincinnati, Ohio

SEAN BOYLE, DO
Volunteer Assistant Professor
Department of Family and Community
Medicine
University of Cincinnati
Cincinnati, Ohio

SUSAN SCHRIMPF DAVIS, DO
Associate Clinical Professor
Department of Family and Community
Medicine
Division of Geriatric Medicine
University of Cincinnati College of
Medicine
Cincinnati, Ohio

PHILIP M. DILLER, MD, PhD
Fred Lazarus, Jr. Professor and Chair
Department of Family and Community
Medicine
University of Cincinnati
Cincinnati, Ohio

KATHLEEN DOWNEY, MD
Associate Professor of Clinical Family
Medicine
Department of Family and Community
Medicine
University of Cincinnati
Cincinnati, Ohio

ROBERT V. ELLIS, MD
Assistant Professor of Family Medicine
Department of Family and Community
Medicine
University of Cincinnati
Cincinnati, Ohio

JERRY A. FRIEMOTH, MD
Emeritus Associate Professor
Family and Community Medicine
University of Cincinnati
Cincinnati, Ohio

MICHAEL B. HOLLIDAY, MD
Assistant Professor
Vice Chair, Clinical Operations
Department of Family and Community
Medicine
University of Cincinnati
Cincinnati, Ohio

CHRISTOPHER LEWIS, MD
Assistant Dean of Diversity and Inclusion
Associate Professor of Family Medicine
Department of Family and Community
Medicine
University of Cincinnati
Cincinnati, Ohio

HILLARY MOUNT, MD
Assistant Professor of Family Medicine
Director of Inpatient Family Medicine
Services
The Christ Hospital/University of
Cincinnati
Family Medicine Residency Program
Cincinnati, Ohio

SOUMYA NADELLA, MD
Outpatient Physician
Sycamore Internal Medicine
Kettering Physician Network
Miamisburg, Ohio

LAURI E. NANDYAL, MD, NCMP
Adjunct Associate Professor of Family Medicine
Department of Family and Community
Medicine
University of Cincinnati
Cincinnati, Ohio

EDWARD ONUSKO, MD
Program Director
Adena Family Medicine Residency
Program
Adena Health System
Chillicothe, Ohio

RONALD REYNOLDS, MD, FAAFP
Professor of Family Medicine
Department of Family and Community
Medicine
University of Cincinnati
Cincinnati, Ohio

RICK RICER, MD
Professor Emeritus
Family and Community Medicine
University of Cincinnati
Cincinnati, Ohio

MEGAN RICH, MD
Associate Program Director
The Christ Hospital/University of Cincinnati
   Family Medicine Residency Program
Associate Professor
Department of Family and Community
   Medicine
University of Cincinnati
Cincinnati, Ohio

MONTIEL T. ROSENTHAL, PhD
Associate Clinical Professor
Department of Family and Community
   Medicine
Directory of Maternity Services
University of Cincinnati
Cincinnati, Ohio

LEILA J. SAXENA, MD
Adjunct Assistant Professor
Department of Family and Community
   Medicine
University of Cincinnati
Cincinnati, Ohio

RACHEL SNEED, MD
Physician, Family Medicine
Healthsource of Ohio Wilmington
Wilmington, Ohio

ZACHARY THURMAN, MD
Assistant Professor
Family Medicine
University of Cincinnati
Cincinnati, Ohio

BARBARA B. TOBIAS, MD
Robert and Myfanwy Smith Professor
Vice Chair
Department of Family and Community
   Medicine
University of Cincinnati College of
   Medicine
Cincinnati, Ohio

ELIZABETH WEAGE, MD
Physician
Family Medicine
Southwestern Medical Clinic
Niles, Michigan

When creating *Step-Up to Family Medicine*, we set out to write a review book to aid students on their family medicine clerkship and to study for the NBME Family Medicine Shelf Exam as well as to study for the ambulatory component of Step 2 CK. As a clerkship director, I found a lack of study material that was complete enough to help students do well on the clerkship and shelf exam yet succinct enough for students to get through in a 4- to-6-week clerkship. This book fills that gap. The outline format makes it a quick, easy read that is efficient and high yield. As with most family medicine clerkship curricula, there is a strong ambulatory focus to this book.

Chapters and topics were chosen on the basis of the Society of Teachers of Family Medicine National Clerkship Curriculum as well as content areas of the NBME Family Medicine Shelf Exam. We focused on the information that is important to know without getting into extraneous details. The "Quick Hits" in the margins reinforce key facts and give helpful pearls. There are a series of questions at the end of each chapter for a quick self-assessment of important topics.

I thank all of the chapter authors for their work and expertise. This could not have been accomplished without them. I especially thank Dr. Rick Ricer for his years of mentorship as well as stepping in whenever I needed him to review or write a chapter.

Robert V. Ellis, MD

CONTENTS ● ● ●

FAMILY MEDICINE IN CONTEXT

1

Philip M. Diller • Barbara B. Tobias

I. Definition and Principles of Family Medicine

A. Definition of primary care

1. Primary care is the provision of *integrated*, *accessible* health care services by clinicians who are *accountable* for addressing a *large majority* of personal health care needs, developing a sustained *partnership* with patients, and practicing in the context of *family* and *community* (emphasis added).[1]

2. "At its best, primary care supports individuals and families in pursuing what matters most to them." (Cory B. Sevin, RN, MSN, NP, Director at the Institute for Healthcare Improvement.)

B. **Definition of family medicine:** Family medicine is the medical specialty that provides continuing, comprehensive health care for the individual and family. It is a specialty in breadth that integrates the biologic, clinical, and behavioral sciences. The scope of family medicine encompasses all ages, both sexes, each organ system, and every disease entity.[2]

C. Core principles of family medicine

1. Patient-centered, whole person care: An approach to patient care that conceptualizes the patient as a human being with multiple dimensions (physical, psychological, spiritual, social, chronologic) and places the patient's problems into one or more contexts to create care that is tailored to the individual patient

2. Continuity of care: Create and manage continuous relationships between the doctor and the patient from infancy to old age, in health and disease, with special emphasis on the family

3. Comprehensive care: Provide a broad spectrum or scope of primary care services

4. Coordination of care: Organizing and orchestrating health care services to meet the unique health care needs of each patient in any setting

5. Access to care: Commitment to providing/promoting access to health care (obtain health services when needed) to all patients

6. Management of care: Providing health services in the practice in an efficient and fiscally responsible manner in multiple settings—ambulatory office, nursing home, hospital, and home

7. Population-based care: Utilizing systems to analyze and deliver appropriate health services to defined subpopulations of patients

II. Historical Context

A. **The 1960s saw widespread dissatisfaction with the state of medicine, for reasons including:**

1. The high cost of health care

2. The shortage of physicians

3. The inaccessibility of health care in rural areas and the urban core

4. The increased depersonalization of medicine

5. The fragmentation of care

B. **Family medicine was created in 1969 as a terminal training discipline to respond to the national need for increased primary care access and health care.**

1. The Folsom Report (1966),[3] sponsored by national public health authorities, stated that every American should have their own personal physician.
2. The Millis Report (1966),[4] sponsored by the American Medical Association (AMA), recommended increasing the number of physicians who could replace the dwindling reserve of general practitioners. It emphasized clinical competence, continuity, and prevention.
3. The Willard Report (1966),[5] also sponsored by the AMA, recommended creating a separate training track in family practice and a specialty board to oversee certification in family practice. It stated, "The American public does want and need large numbers of qualified Family Physicians."

III. Illness in the Community and Initial Approach to the Patient

A. **Ecology of medical care model:** The human illness experience is a foundation for understanding health services in a community.
   1. Experience of symptoms and where patients seek care in the health system (Figure 1-1): In a month, 75% of individuals will experience some health-related symptoms.
   2. Patients exercise considerable discretion in seeking care:
      a. In a month, 25% actually seek care from a health care provider.
      b. In a month, 1% are seen in a large academic health center; thus, a majority of symptoms are cared for in the community.

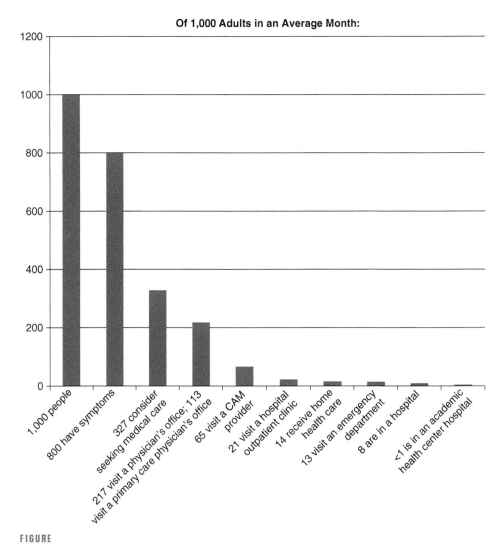

Of 1,000 Adults in an Average Month:

- 1,000 people
- 800 have symptoms
- 327 consider seeking medical care
- 217 visit a physician's office; 113 visit a primary care physician's office
- 65 visit a CAM provider
- 21 visit a hospital outpatient clinic
- 14 receive home health care
- 13 visit an emergency department
- 8 are in a hospital
- <1 is in an academic health center hospital

FIGURE

1-1 The ecology of medical care. (Green, et al. The ecology of medical care revisited. *N Engl J Med.* 2001;344[26]).

3. Care-seeking behavior moves through three stages and is influenced by multiple factors:
   a. *Illness perception stage*: The patient pays attention to or ignores symptoms.
   b. *Deliberation stage*: This includes the response to self-care, persistence or worsening of symptoms, and seeking advice from others; it is influenced by worry or concern and beliefs about when to access care.
   c. *Access stage*: Barriers to access include availability of providers and health facilities, costs/payment coverage, transportation, time availability, dependence on others, and work limitations.
4. Responsibility of the costs of care is shifting. Patients limit care-seeking behavior because they take on more responsibility for costs.
B. **The undifferentiated patient**
   1. Definition: An undifferentiated patient is one with a health-related problem or set of symptoms that are poorly defined, organized, and/or not yet diagnosed.
   2. Approach to the undifferentiated patient:
      a. The family physician's role is to help the patient define, describe, and organize the illness.
      b. To effectively perform this role, the family physician needs a broad understanding of a myriad of processes that can cause a patient's health-related problem(s) as well as being able to recognize the multitude of problems.
      c. **Common problems seen in family medicine are listed in** Table 1-1.

IV. Functional Roles of a Family Physician

A. The functional roles of the family physician are set by the principles and scope of primary care and the patients' complaints.
B. The nine functional roles of a family physician are to:
   1. Seek to understand a patient in any season of life as a whole person and use this understanding to create care
   2. Establish continuity relationships with patients, using and managing multiple types of physician–patient relationships
   3. Provide primary care that includes a "comprehensive set of health services" in multiple settings, accounting for both the individual patient and the physician's population of patients according to their health care risks and needs
   4. Create individualized care for each patient
   5. Coordinate care in the local health system
   6. Advocate for access to care for all patients in a community
   7. Provide high-quality health services to a community population in a safe, efficient, and fiscally responsible manner
   8. Seek to understand the determinants of health in the population and actively support and create population interventions to solve "upstream problems"
   9. Carry out professional responsibilities, adhere to ethical principles, and continue to stay current and competent as a physician.

V. Scope of Services Provided by Family Physicians

A. Family medicine sees patients from birth to death (seasons of life perspective).
B. Scope of services that are potentially addressed by family physicians:
   1. Well care and preventive care
   2. Maternity care
   3. Mental health care
   4. Care of acute health problems
   5. Care of chronic health problems
   6. Nursing home care
   7. End of life care and home care
   8. Administrative patient services
   9. Procedural care

Family Medicine in Context

Family Medicine in Context

TABLE 1-1	Common Problems (Symptoms and Diagnoses) Seen in Family Medicine Ambulatory Office

Rank Order of Conditions

1. Essential hypertension	39. Acute sinusitis
2. Routine infant or child health check	40. Insomnia
3. Diabetes mellitus	41. Acute gastroenteritis
4. Depression	42. Malaise and fatigue
5. Hyperlipidemia	43. Attention deficit disorder
6. Acute upper respiratory infection (URI)	44. Dermatitis not otherwise specified
7. Normal pregnancy supervision	45. Acute pharyngitis
8. Routine general medical examination	46. Preoperative examination
9. Asthma	47. Bipolar disorder
10. Prophylactic vaccination	48. Chest pain
11. Otitis media	49. Arthropathy
12. Congestive heart failure	50. Cough
13. Gynecologic examination	51. Pain in limb
14. Nonspecific abdominal pain	52. Psychosexual dysfunction
15. Allergic rhinitis	53. Cellulitis
16. Chronic obstructive pulmonary disease (COPD)	54. Vertigo
17. Coronary atherosclerotic disease	55. Pneumonia
18. Hypothyroidism	56. Constipation
19. Bronchitis	57. Drug monitoring
20. Gastroesophageal reflux	58. Joint pain—shoulder
21. Urinary tract infection	59. Atrial fibrillation
22. Nonspecific backache	60. Acne
23. Unspecified sinusitis	61. Seizure disorder
24. Influenza	62. Wound care
25. Anemia	63. Renal disease
26. Myalgia	64. Edema
27. Conjunctivitis	65. Weight loss
28. Counseling for contraception	66. Nausea
29. Headache	67. Amenorrhea
30. Anxiety state	68. Sensory examination
31. Osteoarthritis	69. Otitis externa
32. Viral syndrome	70. Neck pain
33. Tobacco use disorder	71. Viral warts
34. Obesity	72. Cervical dysplasia
35. Migraine headache	73. Irritable bowel syndrome
36. Vulvovaginitis	74. Hair diseases
37. Newborn examination	75. Obstructive sleep apnea
38. Diarrhea	

VI. Emergence of the Patient-Centered Medical Home as a Superior Model of Primary Care Delivery

A. Definition of Patient-Centered Medical Home (PCMH) as recognized by the National Committee for Quality Assurance (NCQA):

1. A model of care that replaces episodic care with coordinated care and a long-term healing relationship
2. Nine categories of specific care elements must be met to qualify as a PCMH:
   a. Access and communication
   b. Patient tracking and registry functions
   c. Care management
   d. Patient self-management and support
   e. Electronic prescribing
   f. Test tracking
   g. Referral tracking
   h. Performance reporting and improvement
   i. Advanced electronic communication
3. Each patient has an ongoing relationship with a personal physician who leads a team at a single location that takes collective responsibility for patient care, providing for the patient's health care needs and arranging for appropriate care with other qualified clinicians working to the fullest extent of their licenses. The medical home is intended to result in more personalized, coordinated, effective, and efficient care.
4. A PCMH achieves these goals through a high level of accessibility, providing excellent communication among patients, physicians, and staff and taking full advantage of the latest information technology to prescribe, communicate, track test results, obtain clinical support information, and monitor performance.

B. Challenges to transforming a practice to the PCMH model[6]

1. Changing models of care while delivering care is similar to building a plane as you are flying it
2. Examples of challenges to transformation:
   a. Functional electronic health record (EHR)
   b. Effective operations management processes
   c. Previous experience with team-based activities
   d. Financial resources and organizational support
   e. Data measurement and feedback processes
   f. Effective leadership and communication strategies
   g. Readiness to change
   h. Cultural characteristics of collaboration, respect, accountability, and commitment

VII. Evidence for Primary Care Leading to Desirable Outcomes

A. Adopting and implementing the principles of primary care in a health system lead to desirable outcomes. There is strong consistent evidence for the following (Starfield review):

1. Access: Primary care *increases access to health care services* for relatively deprived population groups.
2. Quality of care: Primary care physicians do as well as specialists in caring for common problems and do better when compared with generic measures. For less common conditions, comanagement with a specialist offers a more optimal care model.
3. Prevention: Primary care physicians benefit a community *by offering preventive services.* A greater supply of family physicians is associated with earlier detection of breast cancer, colon cancer, cervical cancer, and melanoma.
4. Utilization: Having a regular source of primary care *leads to fewer hospitalizations and emergency room visits.*
5. Overtreatment/appropriate treatment: Having a regular source of primary care (patient continuity with a specific provider) prevents overtreatment.

B. When a primary care PCMH model is adopted into practice:
1. Quality of care and patient experiences improve.
2. There are reductions in hospitalization and preventable emergency department utilization.
3. There are net savings in total health care expenditures.
4. Physician burnout decreases.
5. Staff turnover decreases (Grundy and Grumbach review).

VIII. Career Paths for Family Physicians and Possible Subspecialization

A. There are many diverse career paths for family physicians. Family physicians have multiple practice communities to choose from, including rural, urban, and inner city and, in turn, different scopes of practice and patient populations. Family physicians can focus on ambulatory practice, including hospital and/or nursing home care, maternity care, or select academic or public health and public policy careers.

B. The following are fellowship opportunities that family physicians, certified by the American Board of Family Medicine as a Certificate of Added Qualifications, can pursue after completing residency training (https://www.theabfm.org/caq/index.aspx):
1. Geriatrics (1- to 2-year fellowship in an American Council for Graduate Medication Education [ACGME]–accredited program)
2. Palliative care and hospice care (12-month fellowship in a program related to an ACGME-accredited program)
3. Sports medicine (a minimum of 1 year in an ACGME-fellowship program associated with an ACGME-accredited residency in family medicine, emergency medicine, internal medicine, or pediatrics)
4. Adolescent medicine (2-year fellowship in an ACGME-accredited program)
5. Sleep medicine (12-month fellowship in an ACGME-accredited program)
6. Integrative medicine (1- to 2-year programs; nonaccredited programs are available for additional training in integrative medicine, not yet recognized by the American Board of Family Medicine)
7. Additional fellowship/educational experiences also exist for pursuing careers in academic medicine, public policy, or global health as examples

IX. What the Future Holds for Family Medicine

A. **The Triple Aim**
1. The Triple Aim, as coined by Don Berwick, Tom Nolan, and John Whittington in 2008, describes the fundamental goals of improving population health, improving the patient experience of care, and reducing per capita cost. Developed by the Institute for Healthcare Improvement (IHI), this statement of purpose captures the key areas that the future of health care must address. The Triple Aim is the organizing framework for the US National Quality Strategy as well as the strategic foundation for public and private health improvement organizations around the world.
2. Family medicine, as the cornerstone of patient-centered, comprehensive, continuous primary care, is uniquely aligned to support the goals of the Triple Aim.

B. **Trends in health care that will shape the future of family medicine**
1. *Team-based care models* are being designed and piloted all across the world.
   a. Family physician office practice, hospital-based medicine, and nursing home care are all redefining roles of various members of a care team.
   b. The role of the family physician will likely shift to overseeing care provided by midlevel providers for self-limited conditions, leading team-based care to support patient self-management for chronic conditions, and continuing to provide direct patient care for complex or poorly differentiated disease processes.
   c. Process and quality improvement activities are embedded in these future care models.

2. *Population-based management* is a growing need for health systems that complements the personal, individualized care offered in traditional family physician offices.

   a. Population-based medicine requires defining and managing the care needs of subsets of identifiable groups of patients who are part of a larger defined targeted population. For example, a subset might be all patients with diabetes who are poorly controlled from a specific geographic area.

   b. Population management also utilizes the physician's risk-stratified practice population to identify subgroups of patients who may benefit from enhanced care management support.

   c. Family physicians are involved in designing primary care and complex chronic disease care, applying their unique knowledge of the social fabric of the community to supporting the patients' own health agenda.

3. *Hospital medicine* is moving toward a hospitalist model in many major urban centers, although in rural community hospitals, family physicians are the primary providers of hospital-based care.

   a. The role of the family physician in hospital care in urban hospitals or in collaboration with a hospitalist is often to communicate key information at the time of admission and increasingly to facilitate and support care after discharge.

   b. The family physician is often the single provider who can support the patient's care with the knowledge of the patient as a person, such as the values the patient holds, the unique fears and concerns, and the patient's personality, which alters how information is delivered.

   c. When care is fragmented by disease-centric accountability, the bonding between family physician and patient through serious illness can become more limited. Family physicians are often the patient's most trusted source of information and are uniquely positioned to coordinate care among providers and settings. Family physicians must be skilled and able to help initiate crucial discussions with appropriate patients before health care crises and work interprofessionally with colleagues to support the patient's agenda in advanced care planning.

   d. The value of the human element related to hospital, palliative, and end of life care as provided by family physicians is a fertile area for future research.

4. *Integration of information technology into medical practice:* Introduction of the EHR is a technological innovation in the practice of medicine that has already had a significant impact on care delivery and physician satisfaction.

   a. In the present format, EHR benefits include reduced prescription errors, better monitoring of care quality, improvement in care coordination within and across health systems, and increased patient engagement.

   b. At the same time, EHRs have created some negatives, such as altering practice workflows in the care of the patient, challenging communication with the patient during the encounter, and adding physician time to the care of the patient for documentation.

   c. The EHR will continue to be refined to improve efficiency while improving quality of care, lowering cost, and drive toward improved physician and patient satisfaction.

   d. The clinical work of today's family physicians requires leadership, time, attention, and effort to improve the EHR experience.

5. *Payment models:* Although the current payment model is predominantly volume-driven fee-for-service, it is increasingly recognized that for our healthcare system to be sustainable, reimbursement must be based on quality and health outcomes.

   a. New models of payment are being introduced that will alter family physician reimbursement.

    b. The four most common new payment models currently piloted include pay-for-care coordination, pay-for-performance, episode or bundled payment, and comprehensive care or total cost of care payment.

    c. Whenever payment models shift, physician behavior will in turn be incentivized toward maintaining or further enhancing payment. Family physicians will need to continue to pay attention to these new models so that they can respond appropriately to the new incentives and retain the ability to provide high-quality care to meet the needs of the patient and the community.

    d. Team-based care and population health care management implementation will be a key component of successful pay-for-performance payment models in primary care.

6. *Gender shift and part-time practice*: One of the most significant social trends in medicine is the feminization of the physician workforce.

    a. Over the past 40 years, the number of female medical graduates has grown from 10% to nearly 50%. Many of these individuals are choosing primary care specialties, including family medicine.

    b. Increased attention to work–life balance and the increased need to learn how to integrate professional and personal roles have accompanied the feminization of American medicine.

    c. A common experience is part-time practice during the child-bearing and -rearing years. Workforce projections have not considered this social change.

    d. In addition, the new physician work environment will continue to evolve to meet the career expectations of both male and female physicians who are prioritizing personal and professional life balance.

QUESTIONS

1. Core principles of family medicine include:
   A. high-volume care
   B. access to care
   C. high-value care
   D. need-based care

2. Based on the Ecology of Medical Care Model in a month:
   A. 80% of patients seek care in an academic health center
   B. 50% of patients seek care in an academic health center
   C. 10% of patients seek care in an academic health center
   D. 1% of patients seek care in an academic health center

3. The Patient-Centered Medical Home (PCMH) is a model of care that
   A. replaces episodic care with longitudinal coordinated care
   B. increases access to care for the uninsured
   C. incentivizes home-based clinical care
   D. decreases reliance on the electronic health record (EHR)

4. Having a regular source of primary care has been shown to
   A. lead to better detection of prostate cancer
   B. lead to fewer hospitalizations
   C. lead to fewer specialty visits
   D. lead to decreased smoking rates

5. The Triple Aim includes
   A. increasing access for the uninsured
   B. decreasing costs of screening measures
   C. improving patient experience of care
   D. improving access to technology

6. The purpose of team-based care is to
   A. enhance the clinical priorities in chronic disease management
   B. limit ED and hospitalization utilization
   C. promote patient goals of self-management across the care team
   D. decrease episodic costs of care for separate providers

ANSWERS

1. **Answer: B.** "Access to care" is included in the seven Core Principles of Family Medicine: patient-centered, whole person care; continuity of care; comprehensive care; coordination of care; access to care; management of care; and population-based care. High-volume, high-value, and need-based care are not included in the core principles.

2. **Answer: D.** The Ecology of Medical Care Model suggests that in 1 month in a population of 1,000, almost 25% visit a physician's office, and approximately one-third visit a complementary or alternative medical care provider. The number of people who receive professional care at home is similar to the number of people who receive care in an emergency department (ED). Less than 1 person in 1,000 is admitted to an academic health center. The model highlights the need for comprehensive medical training, research, and care in the community, outside the traditional academic health center.

3. **Answer: A.** The PCMH is a model of care that replaces episodic care with longitudinal coordinated care. The PCMH model supports comprehensive care, care coordination, and better overall access. It requires a supportive payment model for value over volume and increased reliance on the EHR to be sustainable. Care for the underserved and incentives for home-based care may be a part of some practice models but not part of the guiding principles.

4. **Answer: B.** Having a regular source of primary care leads to improved utilization rates, including unnecessary hospitalizations and ED visits. Although a greater supply of primary care physicians in a community can lead to earlier detection of breast, colon, cervical cancers, and melanoma, it has not been associated with better detection of prostate cancer, decreased smoking rates, or fewer specialty visits.

5. **Answer: C.** The Triple Aim describes the fundamental goals of improving population health, the patient experience of care, and reducing per capita cost.

6. **Answer: C.** The purpose of team-based care is to primarily support patients' self-management goals across the practice team, enabling all members to work at the top of their licenses. Although patients' goals are aligned with clinical priorities, team-based care enables the patients' goals to be prioritized in a care plan. Team-based care must also include improved access to have an impact on costs and unnecessary ED and hospitalization rates.

References

1. Institute of Medicine. *Primary Care: America's Health in a New Era*. Washington, DC: The National Academies Press; 1996. https://doi.org/10.17226/5152.
2. AAFP definition of family medicine: http://www.aafp.org/about/policies/all/family-medicine-definition.html.
3. NCCHS. *Health is a Community Affair—Report of the National Commission on Community Health Services (NCCHS)*. Cambridge, MA: Harvard University Press; 1967.
4. American Medical Education. *The Graduate Education of Physicians: The report of the Citizens Commission on Graduate Medical Education*. Chicago, IL: American Medical Education; 1966.
5. Willard WR. Report of the National Commission on Community Health Services—next steps. *Am J Public Health Nations Health*. 1966;56(11):1828–1836.
6. McNellis RJ, Genevro JL, Meyers DS. Lessons learned from the study of primary care transformation. *Ann Fam Med*. 2013;11 (Suppl 1):S1–S5.

2

PREVENTIVE CARE

Orson J. Austin

I. Pediatric Preventive Care Guidelines

A. Recommendations for routine pediatric preventive healthcare assume that children have no known significant health problems and are being parented in an appropriate manner. Recommendations will differ for children with medical issues or concerns. **Appendix 3 has the United States Preventive Services Task Force (USPSTF) recommendations as well as recommendations from other organizations.** *Refer to Bright Futures web site for comprehensive information regarding Pediatric Preventive Care* (**https://brightfutures.aap.org/materials-and-tools/PerfPrevServ/Pages/default.aspx**).

B. **Care of the newborn**
   1. General:
      a. A newborn evaluation is mandatory for all infants after birth.
      b. Breastfeeding should be promoted, instructed, and otherwise supported.
   2. Important elements of newborn evaluation:
      a. History: Obtain a comprehensive initial history from parents, including a prenatal care history. *Important components of the prenatal medical history include parental past, prior* and *present/recent pregnancy history, and labor and delivery history* (Table 2-1).
      b. Growth measurements:
         i. Record length, height, and weight.
         ii. Head circumference and weight for length should also be recorded using standard growth charts. Blood pressure should be measured if certain risk conditions such as prematurity, very low birth weight, congenital heart disease, and urinary or renal problems are present.
      c. Sensory screening:
         i. Assess vision if newborn is at risk of developing ophthalmologic problems.
         ii. Hearing screening assessment should be performed on all newborns (usually done prior to hospital discharge).

TABLE 2-1 Labor and Delivery History

Labor and delivery history should include:

- Duration of labor
- Type of delivery (vaginal or Cesarean section)
- Spontaneous or induced labor
- Nonforceps or forceps delivery
- Maternal complications (eg, maternal fever or amnionitis)
- Apgar score
- Growth status (ie, gestational age information)

d. Developmental and behavioral assessment:
  i. Developmental surveillance should be performed during the newborn period (Table 2-2).
  ii. Psychosocial/behavioral assessment should also be performed during this period.
e. Physical exam:
  i. Apgar scoring assigned at 1 and 5 minutes of age, respectively (Table 2-3)
    (a) 1-minute Apgar is indicative of both the intrauterine environment and the birth process.
    (b) 5-minute Apgar reflects the neonate's success at transitioning.
    (c) No further intervention is usually required for neonates with a score ≥7.
  ii. Comprehensive physical exam is recommended for all newborns within the first 24 hours of life.
  iii. Evaluate for signs of birth trauma, such as cephalohematoma or caput succedaneum, fractured clavicle.
  iv. Check birth weight, cardiopulmonary exam, evidence of jaundice.
f. Procedures: Newborn blood screening for a multitude of congenital, genetic, and metabolic conditions is routinely performed on all newborns in the United States. Phenylketonuria (PKU), congenital hypothyroidism, hemoglobinopathies, and galactosemia are common disorders targeted for universal screening.
g. Critical congenital heart defect screening: Using pulse oximetry to screen for critical congenital heart defect is recommended in all newborns, after 24 hours of life and prior to hospital discharge.
h. Immunizations: First dose of hepatitis B should be administered at birth prior to hospital discharge.
i. Anticipatory guidance should be performed during the newborn period. Important components of anticipatory guidance include: injury prevention, violence prevention, sleep positioning counseling, and nutrition counseling.

C. **Infancy and childhood**
1. History:
  a. An interval history should be performed during infancy at ages 1 to 2 weeks and at ages 1, 2, 4, 6, and 9 months.
  b. During childhood, interval histories should be performed at ages 12, 15, 18, and 24 months; then annually from age 3 through middle childhood (age 10).
2. Growth measurements:
  a. Length/height, weight, weight for length, and head circumference should be assessed at ages 1 to 2 weeks; and at ages 1, 2, 4, 6, 9, 12, 15, and 18 months.
  b. Growth assessment using height and weight should continue annually.
  c. Head circumference measurements should cease at age 2.
  d. Annual screening to assess healthy weight via body-mass index (BMI) should start at age 2 during childhood.
3. Sensory screening:
  a. Routine visual acuity testing is recommended at ages 3, 4, 5, 6, 8, and 10 years.
  b. Hearing screening should occur at ages 4, 5, 6, 8, and 10 years.
4. Developmental and behavioral assessment should be performed at most well visits during infancy; then annually during childhood.
5. Autism screening: recommended at ages 18 and 24 months by several organizations, USPSTF I rating; use validated instruments (e.g., *M-CHAT-R– available for free educational use download at http://mchatscreen.com/*; Table 2-4).
6. Physical exam:
  a. A comprehensive physical exam should be performed at all well visits.
  b. Gross/fine motor and sexual development should be evaluated.

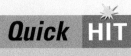

Quick HIT

Approximately 90% of newborns have Apgar scores in the 7-to-10 range.

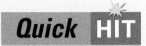

Quick HIT

The number and types of newborn blood screening will vary based on state laws.

TABLE 2-2	Developmental Milestones			
Age	**Gross Motor**	**Fine (Visual) Motor**	**Language**	**Social**
2 wk	Side-to-side head movement	May follow with eyes to midline only; tightly fisted hands	Startles with noise	Fixes on face
2 mo	Able to lift shoulder/head from prone position	Follows object or tracks past midline	Coos	Smiles; parental recognition
4 mo	Lifts up on hands in prone position; Rolls front to back; Good head control (no lag)	Reaches for and grasps object	Laughs; squeals	Looks at hands; Begins to interact socially
6 mo	Sits alone but may need support	Transfers objects from hand to hand; feeds self	Babbles	Recognizes unfamiliar persons
9 mo	Sits without support; crawls; pulls to stand	Pincer grasp	Nonspecific "mama" and "dada"	Waves bye-bye; Stranger anxiety
12 mo	Cruises; stands alone; may begin walking	Can release items (eg, places blocks in cup); Drinks from cup	Specific use of "mama" and "dada;" one to four other words	Imitates; cooperates (eg, getting dressed)
15 mo	Walks well including backward	Stacks two blocks; uses spoon	Up to six words	Follows commands
18 mo	Runs	Stacks four blocks	10–25 words usually (at least six)	Removes garment; uses words to communicate needs
2 yr	Walks up and down stairs without assistance; kicks ball	Stacks six blocks; copies a straight line	Two- and three-word phrases (ie, able to put two words together); 50% of speech understandable to stranger	Parallel play
3 yr	Pedals tricycle and broad jumps	Copies a circle; stacks eight blocks	75% of speech understandable to stranger	Group play; knows age/gender
4 yr	Balances and hops on one foot	Copies cross; draws person with three parts	Speech understandable to strangers	Brushes teeth without help; dresses self
5 yr	Skips (alternating feet)	Draws a person with six body parts	Counts; asks meaning of words	Names four colors; understands rules
6 yr	Rides a bike; balances on each foot for 6 s	Writes name	Defines words	Knows colors; knows right from left

TABLE 2-3 Apgar Scoring			
Physical Exam at 1 and 5 min	**0 Points**	**1 Point**	**2 Points**
Heart rate	Absent	<100	>100
Respiratory effort	Absent	Weak, irregular cry	Strong/vigorous cry
Color	Pale or cyanotic	Extremities cyanotic	Pink (generalized)
Muscle tone	Absent	Weak, slightly flexed extremities	Active
Reflex irritability	Absent	Grimace	Active cry and avoidance

TABLE 2-4 Selected Examples of Autism Spectrum Disorder Characteristics		
Social Interaction	**Communication**	**Behaviors**
Limited eye contact	Reciprocal communication impaired	Stereotyped and restrictive behavior patterns
Difficulty developing relationships with peers	Delayed and abnormal functioning language used in social communication	Repetitive motor activities/behaviors (eg, rocking, complex body movements)
Does not engage in pretend play activities	Echolalia (meaningless, repetitive speech pattern)	Preoccupation with a single object or parts of objects

    c. Blood pressure screening should be initiated at every well visit, beginning at age 3 years.

7. Immunizations: per Centers for Disease Control and Prevention (CDC's) guidelines. http://www.cdc.gov/vaccines/schedules/index.html

8. Anemia screening: Hemoglobin or hematocrit should be checked at 12 months and at clinical discretion for high-risk infants and children. USPSTF: I rating

9. Lead screening:
    a. Performed at 12 months or as dictated by risk assessment evaluation.
    b. Universal screening recommendations for Medicaid patients or patients in high-prevalence zip codes.
    c. Required by law in some states for high-risk patients
    d. The CDC and American Academy of Pediatrics are supportive of lead screening for high-risk children; the USPSTF gives a D rating for average-risk children and an I rating for children at increased risk.

10. Tuberculosis screening:
    a. Recommended periodically for patients at high risk during the first 12 months of life and annually during childhood for said high-risk patients
    b. Risk factors include contact with TB known or suspected person(s), HIV infection, illicit drug use, and living in high tuberculosis-prevalent area.

11. Oral health:
    a. During infancy, counsel against bottle-propping feeding and bottles to bed.
    b. Refer to dental home if possible. Risk-assessment should be performed if referral not possible or feasible.
    c. Assess for fluoride supplementation at 6 months. If main source of water is fluoride deficient, oral fluoride should be considered. For the high-risk, fluoride varnishes should be considered for prevention of caries.

    d. Brushing teeth with soft toothbrush or cloth and water should be encouraged beginning at age 6 months.

    e. Stress importance of bottle weaning by first birthday; wean to cup by age 12 months.

12. Anticipatory guidance should be performed at all well visits during infancy and childhood. **https://brightfutures.aap.org/materials-and-tools/PerfPrevServ/Pages/default.aspx**

D. **Adolescence**

1. History should be performed annually during the adolescent years.
2. Growth measurements:
    a. Height, weight, and BMI should be monitored during adolescence.
    b. Adolescents should be counseled regarding the importance of physical activity and healthy dietary practices.
    c. Focused counseling and evaluation should be provided for BMIs at or above the 85th percentile.
    d. In addition, screening for eating disorders should occur annually starting in the middle childhood years.
3. Sensory screening:
    a. Visual acuity screening should occur at ages 12, 15, and 18.
    b. Hearing screening should be performed only if risk assessment indicates need for such screening.
4. Developmental and behavioral assessment: Perform annually starting at age 11.
5. Alcohol and drug use assessment:
    a. Should be performed annually during the teenage years
    b. Parents should be asked about their family histories of alcohol and substance abuse.
    c. History should be obtained from adolescents as it relates to use of alcohol, drugs, and other illicit or over-the-counter drugs of potential abuse (eg, inhalants and anabolic steroids).
    d. Adolescents should be counseled regarding the deleterious effects of alcohol and substance use.
    e. Adolescents should also be counseled to avoid all driving when alcohol or drug use occurs.
6. Depression screening:
    a. Should occur annually during the adolescent years
    b. Screening tools such as the Patient Health Questionnaire (PHQ)-2 are recommended for screening evaluation (Table 2-5).
7. Physical exam:
    a. Recommended annually during adolescence
    b. Annual blood pressure measurements should be included as part of the physical exam.
8. Immunizations: per CDC's guidelines. http://www.cdc.gov/vaccines/schedules/index.html
9. Anemia screening: Check hemoglobin or hematocrit counts annually if risk assessment indicates high risk for anemia (eg, heavy menstrual bleeding).

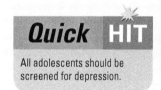

Quick **HIT**

All adolescents should be screened for depression.

| TABLE **2-5** | PHQ-2 Depression Screen |

Over the Past 2 Wks, How Often Have You Been Bothered by Any of the Following Problems?	Not at All	Several Days	More Than Half the Days	Nearly Every Day
Little interest or pleasure in doing things	0	1	2	3
Feeling down, depressed, or hopeless	0	1	2	3

A score ≥3 requires further evaluation.

10. Tuberculosis testing:
    a. Screen annually if risk assessment indicates high risk for tuberculosis.
    b. Risk factors include contact with TB known or suspected person(s), HIV infection, illicit drug use, and living in high tuberculosis-prevalent area.
11. Lipid screening: once between ages of 18 and 21, if not previously screened per the American Academy of Pediatrics (AAP); USPSTF: I rating.
12. STD/HIV screening:
    a. All adolescents should be confidentially screened once for HIV, ages 16 to 18.
    b. Adolescents participating in risky behavior (eg, intravenous drug use) or who are sexually active should be screened annually.
    c. Chlamydia and gonorrhea screening should occur annually for sexually active adolescents.
    d. Syphilis screening should be initiated for those at high risk.
    e. Physicians should counsel all adolescent patients regarding sexually transmitted infection prevention. In addition, counseling regarding the human papilloma virus (HPV) vaccine should also occur.
13. Anticipatory guidance should be performed annually at well visits during this period. **https://brightfutures.aap.org/materials-and-tools/PerfPrevServ/Pages/default.aspx**

II. Adult Preventive Service Recommendations

A. What follows is a summary discussion of clinical preventive services per the USPSTF. A more detailed discussion of these summary recommendations can be found at http://www.uspreventiveservicestaskforce.org/ (see Appendix 3). While there is a myriad of other recommendations from a multitude of organizations, the USPSTF is felt to be a conveyor of impartial evidence-based assessment of screening, counseling, and other preventive service recommendations. The **AHRQ ePPS app** is an excellent point-of-care clinical tool to see USPSTF recommendations for a given patient.

B. **Immunizations:** See CDC recommendations for details. http://www.cdc.gov/vaccines/schedules/index.html
    1. Tetanus: Td every 10 years; replace one adult Td with a Tdap booster
    2. Pneumococcal
       a. 23-valent (Pneumovax): one at ≥65 year old; earlier for certain high-risk populations.
       b. 13-valent conjugated (Prevnar): one at ≥65 year old; earlier for certain high-risk populations
       c. Separate the two shots by 1 year. The 13-valent ideally is given first.
    3. Shingles (Zostavax): one at ≥60 year old
    4. Influenza: yearly for all adults
    5. Others based on risk factors: See CDC recommendations.

C. **Abdominal aortic aneurysm (AAA) screening:** once by ultrasonography (US) for men aged 65 to 75 years who have ever smoked

D. **Alcohol misuse screening:** all adults; and provide counseling intervention

E. **Behavior counseling, healthful diet, and physical activity** for cardiovascular disease (CVD) recommended for overweight or obese adults and others with CVD risk factors

F. **Behavior counseling to prevent sexually transmitted infections (STIs):** adults at high risk of STIs

G. **Breast cancer screening:**
    1. Mammography every 2 years for women aged 50 to 74 years
    2. Breast cancer (BRCA) mutation testing
       a. Women whose family members include those with breast, ovarian, tubal, or peritoneal cancer in an attempt to identify those with an increased risk of possible harmful mutations in breast cancer susceptibility genes (*BRCA1* or *BRCA2*)
       b. Offer genetic counseling and BRCA testing to those who desire after counseling.

H. **Cardiovascular disease prevention**
   1. Aspirin for those 50 to 59 years and a 10-year CVD risk ≥10% is a B recommendation; 60 to 69 years is a C recommendation; younger or older, an I recommendation
   2. Statin therapy for those without a history of CVD and one or more CVD risk factors
      a. 40 to 75 year old and a 10-year CVD risk ≥10% is a B recommendation
      b. 40 to 75 year old and a 10-year CVD risk 7.5% to 10% is a C recommendation
      c. <75 year old is an I recommendation
I. **Carotid artery stenosis screening** for asymptomatic carotid artery stenosis is not recommended.
J. **Cervical cancer screening**
   1. Women aged 21 to 65: cytology every 3 years
   2. Alternatively, for women aged 30 to 65 wishing to lengthen the screening interval, screen with both cytology and HPV testing every 5 years.
K. **Chlamydia screening**
   1. All sexually active nonpregnant women, aged 24 and younger, and for older nonpregnant women deemed to be at high risk
   2. Pregnant women, aged 24 and younger, and for older pregnant women deemed to be at high risk
   3. Insufficient evidence to assess benefits versus harms of screening in men
L. **Colorectal cancer screening**: fecal occult blood testing yearly, sigmoidoscopy every 5 years, or colonoscopy every 10 years, in adults aged 50 to 75
M. **Diabetes, type 2 screening**: recommended in adults with persistent blood pressure elevations higher than 135/80 mm Hg per the adults 40–70 who are overweight or obese. The American Diabetes Association recommends screening for overweight and obese adults.
N. **Fall prevention**: Exercise or physical therapy and vitamin D supplements are recommended for adults ≥65 deemed to be at increased fall risk.
O. **Gonorrhea screening**
   1. All sexually active women, regardless of pregnancy status, deemed to be at high risk of infection
   2. Insufficient evidence to recommend for or against screening in men
P. **Human immunodeficiency virus (HIV) screening**
   1. All adolescents and adults, aged 18 to 65
   2. All pregnant women
Q. **Hypertension**: Blood pressure screening is recommended for adults aged 18 and older.
R. **Lipid disorders screening**: All adults 40-75 with 1 or more CVD risk factors such as dyslipidemia, DM, HTN, or smoking
S. **Lung cancer screening**
   1. Annually with low-dose computed tomography (CT) in adults aged 55 to 80 with a 30-pack year smoking history and are current smokers, or if they had quit smoking within the past 15 years
   2. Screening should be stopped once one has not smoked for 15 years and when other health problems limit life expectancy or the ability to undergo curative lung surgery.
T. **Osteoporosis screening**
   1. Women aged 65 or older
   2. Younger women with a fracture risk ≥ that of a 65-year-old white woman
   3. Insufficient evidence to recommend routine osteoporosis screening in men
U. **Ovarian cancer screening**: not recommended
V. **Prostate cancer prostate-specific antigen (PSA) screening**: not recommended
W. **Chronic obstructive pulmonary disease (COPD) screening**: not recommended for asymptomatic adults
X. **Syphilis screening**: strongly recommended for individuals at increased risk

Preventive Care

III. Preparticipation Physical Examination (PPE)

A. Recommendations regarding the preparticipation sports examination noted below are based primarily on expert opinion. There is generally a lack of randomized control trial evidence in this area and thus screening PPE recommendations are often cited as having "insufficient evidence" and/or being "controversial." Safe participation in sports by athletes (from childhood to adulthood) and identification of potential life-threatening or disabling conditions are the main goals of the PPE.

B. **History**
   1. The single most crucial part of the PPE is the medical history.
   2. It is recommended that athletes complete as much of the history portion of the PPE as is feasible.
   3. General:
      a. An athlete's past medical history should include history related to past and current medical problems, including previous hospitalizations.
      b. Attention should be paid to a previous history of sports participation restriction, and the rationale for such restriction.
      c. Medication lists including prescriptions, over-the-counter medications, and supplements should be reviewed.
      d. Immunizations should be reviewed and drug and alcohol history should be explored.
   4. Cardiovascular:
      a. Cardiac pathology accounts for most cases of sudden cardiac death (SCD) during sporting activities. Particular attention should be paid to the cardiac history. Specifically, history regarding chest pain, exercise-related syncope, shortness of breath, lightheadedness, and seizures require further investigation to aid in evaluation of potential arrhythmia, hypertrophic cardiomyopathy, and valvular disease.
      b. Historical data gathering should make note of hypertension, hyperlipidemia, Kawasaki disease, heart murmurs, or other heart-related pathology. Hereditary forms of cardiac pathology, such as Marfan syndrome, should be noted.
   5. Central nervous system:
      a. History should include questions related to a prior history of concussions and its long-term complications.
      b. History regarding head and neck injuries including headaches should also be obtained.
      c. Questions relating to past history of seizures should be explored.
   6. Pulmonary:
      a. The most common pulmonary problems faced by athletes are asthma and exercise-related bronchospasm. History in this area should focus on shortness of breath, wheezing, coughing, and inhaler use.
      b. Athletes should also be questioned about respiratory symptoms during and/or after exercise.
   7. Dermatology: Athletes can be restricted from play because of skin infections or other skin conditions (eg, herpes simplex virus [HSV] in contact sports such as wrestling).
   8. Musculoskeletal:
      a. A history of prior musculoskeletal injury should be noted.
      b. Athletic histories should make note of previous fractures, joint pain, or swelling, and use of orthotics/assistive devices.
      c. Female athletes should be questioned about previous histories of stress fractures and other injuries. Questions regarding eating habits and a past history of eating disorders should be explored.

C. **Physical examination**
   1. Special attention should be paid to the parts of the physical exam that most directly impact safe sports participation.

2. Vital signs:
   a. Blood pressure, pulse, weight, and height should all be recorded.
   b. Elevated blood pressure is the most common abnormality seen during the PPE.
   c. PPE blood pressure evaluation should be performed via brachial artery measurement in the sitting position. Appropriate cuff size is important in the evaluation of blood pressure and if elevated, should be repeated after a 5- to 10-minute rest period.
3. Cardiovascular:
   a. Auscultation for heart murmurs is a very important part of the physical examination of athletes. Auscultation should occur during both the supine and standing positions. During supine examination, athletes should be asked to perform the Valsalva maneuver. Murmurs that change with positional variations should be given careful attention.
   b. Radial and femoral pulses should be examined at the same time to aid in ruling out aortic coarctation. Athletes should also be evaluated for arrhythmias. Wolff–Parkinson–White syndrome, long-QT syndrome, and ventricular tachycardia are but some of the syndromes known to cause sudden death in athletes. Cardiac consultation should be initiated, prior to sports clearance, if there is concern about a possible arrhythmia.
4. Marfan syndrome:
   a. Athletes should be evaluated for the possible classic stigmata of Marfan syndrome.
   b. Arm span greater than height, arachnodactyly, pectus excavatum or carinatum, and a high-arched palate are all important elements of this syndrome.
   c. Mitral valve prolapse and aortic root dilatation or dissection are associated with Marfan syndrome.
5. Musculoskeletal:
   a. A history of previous musculoskeletal injury should prompt an evaluation of the involved area.
   b. Perform joint range of motion and strength evaluation.
6. Vision:
   a. Evaluate via use of the Snellen chart.
   b. Perform eye exam with corrective eyewear in place, if usually used by the examined athlete.
7. Respiratory: Evaluate lungs for the presence of wheezes.
8. Male genitalia:
   a. Evaluation of the testes and inguinal canal should be performed in the standing position.
   b. Abnormalities, such as inguinal hernias, should lead to further investigation.
9. Skin: Look for rashes, evidence of infections, and signs indicating possible illicit drug use.
10. Neurologic: History of previous head trauma or injury should prompt a detailed neurologic physical exam.

D. **Clearance**
1. When making a clearance determination, risk of harm to the athlete or others should be considered.
2. The sport type should be a factor in clearance decisions based on the amount of contact. Sports contact classification includes the following:
   a. Contact sports: basketball, boxing, soccer, tackle-football, and wrestling
   b. Limited-contact sports: baseball, flag football, martial arts, softball, and volleyball
   c. Noncontact sports: bowling, golf, running, swimming, and tennis
3. Clearance for sports participation is usually classified in one of four ways:
   a. Cleared for all activities without restriction
   b. Cleared with recommendations for further evaluation/treatment
   c. Not cleared, status to be determined after further evaluation or treatment
   d. Not cleared for any sports or certain types of sports

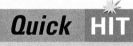

Quick **HIT**

A hypertrophic cardiomyopathy murmur is louder in standing position and softer in squatting position. Innocent murmurs increase with squatting but decrease with standing and Valsalva.

Preventive Care

IV. Preoperative Physical

A. The rationale for preoperative testing is determined by information obtained from a thorough history, physical examination, and subsequent perioperative risk assessment.

B. **Goal:** Identify and act upon conditions that may increase perioperative mortality and morbidity.

C. **Surgical risk estimate:** estimates the risk of cardiac death and nonfatal myocardial infarction within 30 postsurgical days (Table 2-6)

D. **Estimating perioperative risk of major adverse cardiac event (MACE)**
   1. ACS NSQIP risk calculator: http://riskcalculator.facs.org/PatientInfo/PatientInfo
   2. Gupta: https://qxmd.com/calculate/calculator_245/gupta-perioperative-cardiac-risk
   3. Revised Cardiac Risk Index (RCRI) (Table 2-7)
   4. Low risk if <1%, high risk if >1%

E. **Estimate functional capacity:** Metabolic equivalents (METs) are used to measure functional capacity (Table 2-8).

F. **American College of Cardiology/American Heart Association (ACC/AHA) Guideline**
   1. Perioperative cardiovascular evaluation and management in noncardiac surgery
   2. Follow algorithm in Figure 2-1.

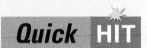

Quick HIT

Activities ≥ 4 METs include climbing a flight of stairs, walking up a hill, walking >4 mph, and performing heavy work around the house.

Preventive Care

TABLE 2-6 Surgical Risk Estimate for Noncardiac Surgery		
Low Risk (<1%)	**Intermediate Risk (1%–5%)**	**High Risk (>5%)**
• Breast • Dental • Endocrine • Eye (eg, cataract surgery) • Gynecologic • Orthopedic (minor) • Urologic (minor)	• Abdominal • Carotid • Peripheral arterial angioplasty • Endovascular aneurysm repair • Head and neck surgery • Major orthopedic surgery (eg, hip and spine) • Urologic (major)	• Aortic and major vascular surgery • Peripheral vascular surgery

Adapted from Task Force for Preoperative Cardiac Risk Assessment and Perioperative (TRUNC), European Society of Anaesthesiology, Poldermans D, Baxx JJ, et al. Guidelines for pre-operative cardiac risk assessment and perioperative cardiac management in non-cardiac surgery: The Task Force for Preoperative Cardiac Risk Assessment and Perioperative Cardiac Management in Non-cardiac Surgery of the European Society of Cardiology (ESC) and endorsed by the European Society of Anaesthesiology (ESA). *Eur Heart J.* 2009;30(22):2769–2812; Feely MA, Collins S, Daniels PR, et al. Preoperative testing before noncardiac surgery: guidelines and recommendations. *Am Fam Physician.* 2013;87(6):414–418.

TABLE 2-7 Revised Cardiac Risk Index
One point for each of the following: • History of ischemic heart disease • History of congestive heart failure (CHF) • History of cerebrovascular disease • History of diabetes mellitus (DM) requiring perioperative insulin use • Creatinine >2 mg/dL • Undergoing suprainguinal vascular, intraperitoneal, or intrathoracic surgery

Risk for major adverse cardiac event: 0 = 0.4%; 1 = 0.9%; 2 = 6.6%; ≥3 = >11%.

TABLE **2-8**	Metabolic Equivalents Table	
Light (<3 METs)	**Moderate (3–6 METs)**	**Vigorous (>6 METs)**
Walking at slow pace (2 METs)	Brisk walking (5 METs)	Jogging at 6 mph (10 METs)
Computer work—Sitting (1.5 METs)	Heavy cleaning (eg, vacu-uming) (3–3.5 METs)	Shoveling (7–8.5 METs)
Cooking and washing dishes (2–2.5 METs)	Mowing lawn (5.5 METs)	Fast bicycling (10 METs)
Playing most instruments (2–2.5 METs)	Tennis (doubles) (5 METs)	Tennis (singles) (8 METs)

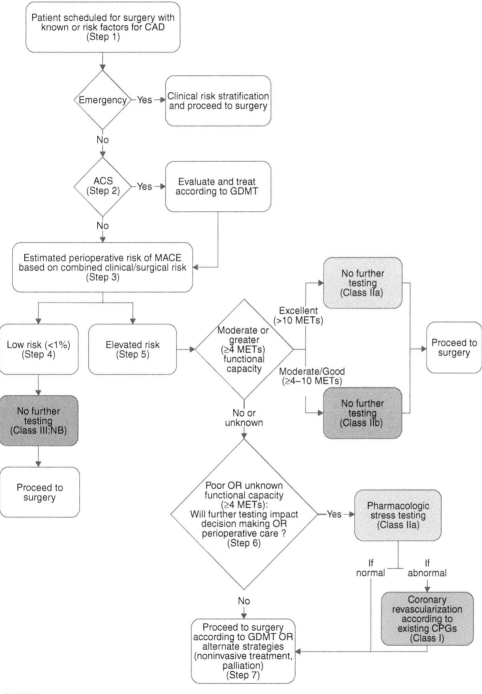

FIGURE

2-1 **ACC/AHA Stepwise approach to perioperative cardiac assessment.**

ACS, acute coronary syndrome; CAD, coronary artery disease; CPGs, clinical practice guidelines; GDMT, guideline-directed medical therapy; MACE, major adverse cardiac event; METs, metabolic equivalents; NB, no benefit.

(Reprinted with permission, *Circulation.* 2014;130:2215–2245. © 2014 American Heart Association, Inc.)

3. Figure 2-2 is the algorithm for patients with a previous percutaneous coronary intervention.
4. Electrocardiogram (ECG) is not needed in asymptomatic patients undergoing a low-risk surgery.

G. **Other chronic medical conditions:**
   1. Evaluate the stability/control of all chronic medical conditions of the patient.
   2. Optimize all therapies.
   3. Consider canceling/delaying surgery if the patient is having an exacerbation of a comorbid condition or if more time is needed to stabilize a condition.

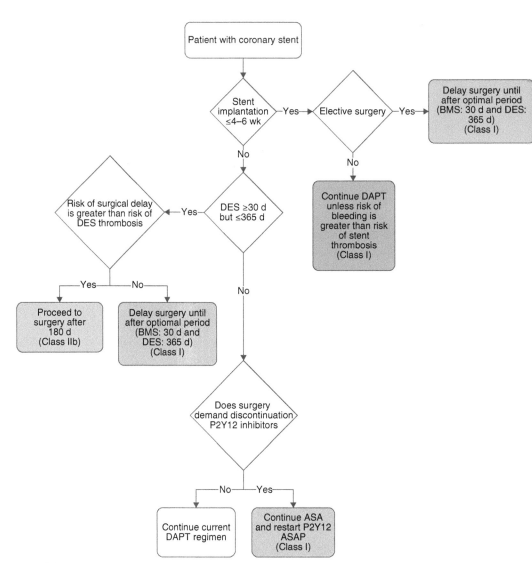

FIGURE 2-2 ACC/AHA algorithm for antiplatelet management in patients with percutaneous coronary intervention (PCI).

ASA, aspirin; BMS, bare metal stent; DAPT, dual antiplatelet therapy; DES, drug eluding stent; P2Y12, antiplatelet medicine such as clopidogrel.

(From Fleisher LA, Fleischmann KE, Auerbach AD, et al. 2014 ACC/AHA Guideline on perioperative cardiovascular evaluation and management of patients undergoing noncardiac surgery: executive summary. *J Am Coll Cardiol.* 2014;64(22):2373–2405.)

QUESTIONS

1. Which of the following screening recommendations is true during infancy and childhood?
   A. Blood pressure screening should start at the age of 4.
   B. Tuberculosis screening is universally recommended for all children at age 12 months.
   C. Autism screening should be conducted in all children.
   D. Fluoride varnishes should be considered for use in high-risk children to prevent dental caries.

2. Which of the following is correct regarding immunizations in infancy and childhood?
   A. The first dose of the Mumps, Measles, and Rubella (MMR) vaccine should be administered at 12 to 15 months of age.
   B. The first dose of the Varicella vaccine is recommended at age 9 months.
   C. The Pneumococcal 23-valent vaccine is routinely administered during the first 15 months of life.
   D. The Human papilloma virus vaccine is approved for use only in female children.

3. By the age of 6, a child should have received which of the following series of vaccinations?
   A. 3 Hepatitis B doses, 4 DTaP doses, and 2 Polio doses.
   B. 3 Hepatitis B doses, 5 Dtap doses, and 4 Polio doses.
   C. 2 Hepatitis B doses, 3 Dtap doses, and 5 Polio doses.
   D. 2 Hepatitis B doses, 4 Dtap doses, and 5 Polio doses.

4. Which of the following is true regarding screening recommendations for adolescents or young adults?
   A. HIV testing is recommended in teenagers once parents give permission.
   B. Lipid screening should not occur prior to the age of 21.
   C. Depression screening for all adolescents and young adults.
   D. Hearing screening should be regularly performed during the adolescent years.

5. A 55-year-old female lawyer comes to see you for a complete physical exam. Aside from a 30-pack year history of cigarette smoking, her Past Medical History is unremarkable. Her physical exam is completely normal. You tell her that you will be making recommendations based on guidelines issued by the U.S. Preventive Services Task Force. Which of the following do you definitely recommend?
   A. Abdominal aortic aneurysm screening because of her smoking history.
   B. Annual mammogram.
   C. Referral for colonoscopy.
   D. Screening for osteoporosis.
   E. All of the above are true.

6. Which of the following is true regarding screening for Sexually Transmitted Infections and HIV in adults?
   A. All adults should be screened for HIV before age 65.
   B. Sexually active men should be screened for Chlamydia.
   C. Chlamydia screening in sexually active young adult women is not recommended before the age of 24.
   D. Syphilis screening is only recommended in areas of high geographic prevalence.

7. Which of the following is true regarding the preparticipation evaluation?
   A. The physical exam is the most important part of the preparticipation evaluation.
   B. The history is the most important part of the preparticipation evaluation.
   C. The history and physical examinations are equally important parts of the preparticipation evaluation.
   D. None of the above are true.

ANSWERS

1. **Answer:** D. The AAP recommends BP screening starting at 3 years old. TB screening is not recommended for average risk patients in the United States. While some experts recommend screening all children for autism, the USPSTF gives it an I rating.

2. **Answer:** A. The first dose of varicella is recommended at 12 months. Pneumococcal 13 valent is given during the first 15 months. HPV vaccine is approved and recommended by the CDC for both females and males.

3. **Answer:** B. Choice B is the correct number for children with standard recommendations. If using some combination vaccines, a child may receive a 4th dose of hep B.

4. **Answer:** C. The CDC recommends screening everyone aged 15 to 65 years for HIV. Lipid screening is recommended for adolescents by the AAP but not by the USPSTF. Universal hearing screen is not recommended for adolescents or young adults. Depression screening is recommended for all 12 years or older.

5. **Answer:** C. AAA screening is not recommended in women. Mammogram screening is recommended biannually. Osteoporosis screening is not recommended in women until 65 years old unless she is at high risk.

6. **Answer:** A. HIV screening is recommended in all adults younger than 65. Chlamydia screening is not recommended in asymptomatic men per the USPSTF guidelines. All sexually active women should be screened for chlamydia. Syphilis screening is recommended for high-risk patients regardless of geographic location.

7. **Answer:** B. The history is the most important part of the preparticipation physical. The history should include any symptoms during exercise, syncope, chest pains, history of injuries, previous concussions, family history of early deaths or cardiac conditions, past medical problems, etc.

COMMON SYMPTOMS

Zachary Thurman • Robert V. Ellis • Michael B. Holliday

I. Approach to Abdominal Pain

A. **General characteristics**

1. One of the most frequent chief complaints in primary care accounting for approximately 10 million office visits a year in the United States
2. Accounts for approximately 2% of ambulatory visits
3. An "acute abdomen" is abdominal pain that has only been present for less than a few days and is progressively worsening. Patients with an "acute abdomen" need to be evaluated for urgent causes that require surgery (Table 3-1).

B. **Clinical features**

1. Historical findings:
   a. Timing and duration: gradual versus sudden onset
   b. Location and radiation (see Table 3-1)
   c. Quality of pain and severity: burning pain can be gastroesophageal reflux disease (GERD) or peptic ulcer disease (PUD) versus colicky for gall/kidney stone, gastroenteritis, or intestinal obstruction
   d. Aggravating/alleviating factors: Food can help PUD and worsen gall bladder problems and mesenteric ischemia. Movement makes peritonitis worse. It is affected by diet changes (celiac, lactose intolerance)
   e. Associated symptoms: nausea, vomiting, diarrhea, constipation, blood in stool/melena, bowel changes, rash, jaundice, change in urine/stool color, urinary tract symptoms, fatigue, weight loss

TABLE 3-1 Differential Diagnosis of Abdominal Pain Based on Location	
Location of Pain	**Differential**
Diffuse	Pancreatitis, early appendicitis, gastroenteritis, intestinal obstruction, mesenteric ischemia, peritonitis, IBD/IBS, malignancy, celiac disease, constipation
RUQ	Biliary colic, cholecystitis, hepatitis, congestive hepatomegaly (CHF), cholangitis, pancreatitis, duodenal ulcer with perforation
Epigastric	Pancreatitis, myocardial infarction (MI), gastritis, PUD, GERD, gastroparesis, dyspepsia
LUQ	Gastritis, gastric ulcer, splenic injury/infarction/megaly/abscess, pancreatitis
Umbilical	Hernia, early appendicitis
RLQ	Appendicitis, cecal diverticulitis, hernia with incarceration/strangulation, tubo-ovarian abscess/ovarian torsion, testicular torsion, endometriosis, nephrolithiasis, PID, Mittelschmerz, ectopic pregnancy
LLQ	constipation, hernia with incarceration/strangulation, sigmoid diverticulitis, tubo-ovarian abscess, testicular torsion, endometriosis, nephrolithiasis, PID, Mittelschmerz, ectopic pregnancy
Suprapubic	Cystitis

f. Medical history: diabetes mellitus (DM), coronary artery disease (CAD), congestive heart failure (CHF), liver problems, pregnancy, etc

g. Social history: sexual history for sexually transmitted infection (STI) risk, alcohol intake, travel history, sick contacts

h. Family history: inflammatory bowel disease/irritable bowel syndrome (IBD/IBS), malignancy

2. Physical exam findings:

a. Vital signs: Unstable signs are an indication for emergency department evaluation. Evaluate for weight changes.

b. Abdominal exam:

i. High-pitched hyperactive sounds could indicate an obstruction or gastroenteritis. Hypoactive sounds are heard in ileus.

ii. Percussion: Dullness could signify a mass or organomegaly while tympany is found in bowel distention.

iii. Note any tenderness to palpation. Rebound tenderness and guarding could signify peritonitis.

c. Pelvic exam: Cervical motion tenderness could signify pelvic inflammatory disorder (PID). Adnexal pain or mass could signify etopic pregnancy, PID, endometriosis, or ovarian mass, cyst or torsion.

d. Rectal exam: for mass, fecal impaction, and occult blood

3. Diagnostic findings should be based on history and physical exam.

a. Labs: may include pregnancy test, comprehensive metabolic panel (CMP), complete blood count (CBC) with differential, amylase, lipase, U/A

b. Imaging:

i. Ultrasound for those with suspected gall bladder or liver pathology

ii. Computed tomography (CT) often used for the workup of non-RUQ abdominal pain

c. Endoscopy: upper and/or lower endoscopy for certain conditions such as GERD, dyspepsia, gastric ulcer, gastrointestinal (GI) bleed, and IBD

C. Treatment

1. Treat the underlying condition.

2. Chronic abdominal pain:

a. Requires careful evaluation for other causes

b. Commonly caused by IBS; treatment based on predominant symptoms.

II. Approach to Back Pain

A. General characteristics

1. Extremely common: About 84% of adults will have back pain at some time in their lives. It is in the top five most common diagnoses in primary care.

2. Most episodes are self-limited.

3. Definitions:

a. Cauda equina syndrome: loss of bowel/bladder control, saddle anesthesia, weakness in the legs owing to compression of the lower spine/nerve roots

b. Lordosis: inward curve of the lumbar spine

c. Kyphosis: outward curve of the thoracic spine

d. Radiculopathy: compression of a nerve root that may cause pain, weakness, and numbness in a specific nerve distribution

e. Sciatica: pain or numbness in the sciatic nerve distribution

f. Spinal stenosis: degeneration of the spine causing narrowing of the spinal canal and neural outlets often resulting in compression of nerve roots

g. Scoliosis: sideways curvature of the spine

h. Spondylosis: arthritis of the spine

i. Spondylolisthesis: anterior displacement of a vertebra compared to the one beneath it

j. Spondylolysis: fracture of the pars interarticularis (Scottie dog fracture)

4. Table 3-2 lists common etiologies of back pain.

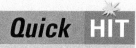

Red flags for an acute abdomen:
Distention
Rigid/firm abdomen
Rebound tenderness
Guarding
High-pitched or absent bowel sounds
History of abdominal surgery

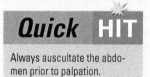

Always auscultate the abdomen prior to palpation.

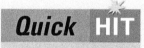

All women of childbearing age with abdominal pain should have a pregnancy test.

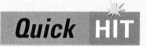

Ultrasound is the first-line imaging modality for most pediatric patients.

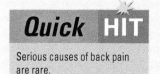

Serious causes of back pain are rare.

TABLE 3-2 Etiology of Back Pain in the Primary Care Setting	
Cause	**Frequency (%)**
Mechanical	**97**
• Strain/sprain	• 70
• Degenerative disc disease (DDD)	• 10
• Herniated disc	• 4
• Compression fracture	• 4
• Spinal stenosis	• 3
• Spondylolisthesis	• 2
Nonmechanical Spinal Conditions	**1**
• Neoplasia	• 0.7
• Inflammatory arthritis	• 0.3
• Infection	• 0.01
Visceral Disease	**2**
• Pelvic organ	
• Renal	
• Aortic aneurysm	
• GI	

TABLE 3-3 Red Flags of Back Pain
Red Flags of Back Pain That Require Further Workup Such as Imaging
Bowel or bladder incontinence
Fever
Sudden pain with spinal tenderness
Trauma
Unintentional weight loss
History of cancer
IV drug use
Immunocompromised/immunosuppressed
Major motor weakness of lower extremities

B. **Clinical features**
  1. Historical findings:
     a. Timing:
        i. Acute: <4 weeks
        ii. Subacute: 4 to 12 weeks
        iii. Chronic: >12 weeks
     b. History of present illness (HPI): Ask about trauma or inciting injury, weight loss, fevers, night sweats, falls, weakness, numbness, radiation of pain, bowel or bladder changes, progression of symptoms, gait difficulties, recent infections, and immunosuppressant use (Table 3-3).
     c. Past medical history: immunocompromising conditions, osteoporosis, previous back pain or surgeries, cancer
     d. Social history: current or past IV drug use, smoker
  2. Physical exam findings:
     a. Inspection of the back for abnormal curvature
     b. Spinous process tenderness could indicate a spinal infection or fracture.
     c. Paraspinal pain is common in muscle strains.
     d. Stork test for pars defects

TABLE 3-4 Finding of Nerve Root Compromise			
Nerve Root	**L4**	**L5**	**S1**
Pain	Lateral hip to anterior thigh and shin	Low back to lateral buttock to lateral thigh and lateral lower leg	Posterior buttock to posterior thigh and lower leg
Numbness	Anterior low thigh and knee	Lateral lower leg	Posterior lower leg and lateral foot
Motor weakness	Quadriceps extension	Dorsiflex great toe and foot	Plantar flex great toe and foot
Screening exam	Squat and rise	Heel walk	Walk on toes
Reflex	Patellar diminished	None	Achilles diminished

TABLE 3-5 Indications for Imaging in Acute Low Back Pain	
Indications for X-ray	**Indications for CT/MRI**
Age > 50 History of malignancy Fever/weight loss/elevated ESR Trauma Motor deficit Steroid use IV drug abuse	Symptoms of cauda equina syndrome Concern for tumor, infection, or fracture Symptoms for >6 wk Prior back surgery

    e. Lower extremity strength and reflexes (Table 3-4)

    f. Straight leg raise for radiculopathy

C. **Diagnostic workup**

    1. Most patients with acute low back pain do not need labs or imaging.

    2. Labs: erythrocyte sedimentation rate (ESR) or C-reactive protein (CRP) for patients suspected of having an infection or malignancy

    3. Imaging: Table 3-5 lists indications for imaging modalities.

D. **Treatment**

    1. Most cases of back pain are self-limited. About half are better in 1-week, 65% are better in 6 weeks, and 95% are better in 12 weeks.

    2. Treat underlying causes.

    3. Avoid opioid medication in most cases of acute and chronic back pain.

    4. Nonsteroidal anti-inflammatory drugs (NSAIDs) and acetaminophen are likely to be effective in treating acute low back pain.

    5. Muscle relaxers have mixed data on its efficacy.

    6. Patients should remain active.

III. Approach to Chest Pain

A. **General characteristics**

    1. Chest pain has a wide range of causes ranging from benign to life threatening. The vast majority of causes are musculoskeletal or gastrointestinal (Table 3-6).

    2. The patient should be rapidly evaluated for possible life-threatening conditions and if needed begin workup prior to taking an extensive history and physical examination.

    3. A complete evaluation should be performed after life-threatening conditions have been ruled out or properly triaged.

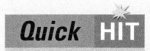

A positive straight leg raise is pain, tingling, or numbness that goes past the knee. Pain in the back, buttock, or hamstring is not considered positive.

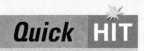

Acute cardiac ischemia only accounts for about 2% of patients presenting with chest pain in the primary care setting.

Common Symptoms

TABLE 3-6	Etiology of Chest Pain in the Primary Care Setting	
Organ System	**Prevalence**	**Common Findings**
Musculoskeletal • Chest wall pain (costochondritis) • Rib pain • Trauma	36%–49%	Tenderness to palpation of the chest wall, history of trauma
Cardiac • ACS/MI and stable angina • Aortic dissection • Heart failure • Pericarditis/myocarditis • Stress cardiomyopathy • Mitral valve disease	15%–18%	Dull squeezing pain worse with activity and relieved with rest Sharp ripping or tearing pain that radiates to the back With dyspnea, cough, fatigue, and peripheral edema Pleuritic pain Setting of physical or emotional stress Usually mild and not anginal
Gastrointestinal • GERD • Esophageal rupture/perforation • Esophagitis • Hiatal hernia	8%–19%	Squeezing or burning pain often following meals, can be improved with antacids Severe retrosternal pain that has a quick onset Retrosternal pain and odynophagia Similar to GERD symptoms
Pulmonary • Pulmonary embolism • Pneumothorax • Pneumonia • Malignancy • Asthma/COPD • Sarcoidosis • Acute chest syndrome in sickle cell	5%–10%	Dyspnea, pleuritic pain, cough, symptoms of a deep vein thrombosis (DVT) Sudden onset, pleuritic pain, and dyspnea Pleuritic pain, productive cough, fever Usually unilateral, can have hemoptysis and dyspnea Chest tightness, shortness of breath (SOB), cough, wheezing Often associated with cough and dyspnea History of sickle cell disease, associated with fever, tachypnea, cough, decrease O_2 sat
Psychiatric • Panic attack • Anxiety and depression • Somatization	8%–11%	Anxious and panic symptoms including tachycardia and hyperventilation
Other • Substance abuse • Referred pain • Herpes zoster		History of cocaine or methamphetamines use Such as cervical disc disease or biliary colic Dermatomal rash

B. **Clinical features**
  1. Historical findings:
     a. Table 3-7 shows likelihood ratios for common symptoms for acute coronary syndrome (ACS).
     b. After a rapid evaluation and appropriate workup and triage has taken place, a complete history should be taken including timing, context, quality, location, radiation, severity, and aggravating and alleviating factors.
  2. Physical exam findings:
     a. Patients with unstable vital signs (hypotension, severe tachycardia, tachypnea, hypoxia) should be transferred to the emergency department.
     b. Cardiac exam for arrhythmias, murmurs, gallops, rubs, displaced point of maximal impulse (PMI)

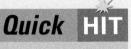

Quick HIT

Aortic dissection should be ruled out in a patient with severe chest pain that radiates to the back and is a sharp tearing/ripping pain.

TABLE 3-7 Likelihood Ratios of Common Symptoms for Acute MI	
Symptom	**Likelihood Ratio (95% CI)**
Radiation to right arm or shoulder	4.7 (1.9–12)
Radiation to both arms or shoulder	4.1 (2.5–6.5)
Associated with exertion	2.4 (1.5–3.8)
Radiation to left arm	2.3 (1.7–3.1)
Associated with diaphoresis	2.0 (1.9–2.2)
Associated with nausea or vomiting	1.9 (1.7–2.3)
Described as pressure	1.3 (1.2–1.5)
Described as pleuritic	*0.2 (0.1–0.3)*
Described as positional	*0.3 (0.2–0.5)*
Described as sharp	*0.3 (0.2–0.5)*
Reproducible with palpation	*0.3 (0.2–0.4)*
Inframammary location	*0.8 (0.7–0.9)*
Not associated with exertion	*0.8 (0.6–0.9)*

Data from Swap C, Nagurney J. Value and limitations of chest pain history in the evaluation of patients with suspected acute coronary syndrome. *JAMA.* 2005;294:2623.

     c. Pulmonary exam for air movement, wheezes, rales, and rhonchi. Check for any consolidations (egophony).

     d. Skin for rashes or signs of trauma

     e. Musculoskeletal: palpation of the chest wall. Subcutaneous emphysema could indication pneumothorax or ruptured esophagus.

     f. Abdominal exam for signs of GI or aortic etiology

C. **Diagnostic workup**

  1. Electrocardiogram (ECG): should be obtained in most patients with chest pain unless there is an obvious cause

  2. Chest X-ray (CXR): for suspected pneumonia, pneumothorax, trauma, or aortic dissection. A widened mediastinum could indicate aortic dissection

  3. Labs:

     a. Cardiac enzymes for possible ACS

     b. D-dimer can be helpful in the workup of pulmonary embolus.

  4. Chest CT: can be helpful in patients with suspected malignancy, aortic dissection, pulmonary embolism

  5. Echocardiogram: for possible CHF, valvular disease, pericarditis/myocarditis

  6. Upper endoscopy (EGD): could be useful in suspected GI disease

D. **Treatment:** Treat the underlying disorder.

IV. Approach to Cough

A. **General characteristics**

  1. Cough is the most common new symptom for which patients seek medical attention.

  2. Cough is a protective mechanism mediated by the vagus nerve; it is stimulated by mechanical irritation and inflammation.

  3. Differential diagnosis:

     a. Acute cough (<3 weeks)

       i. Viral upper respiratory infection (URI), the common cold

      ii. Bronchitis, viral or bacterial

     iii. Pneumonia, viral or bacterial

     iv. Exacerbation of underlying lung disorder:

         (a) Chronic obstructive pulmonary disease (COPD)

         (b) Asthma or reactive airway disease (children <5)

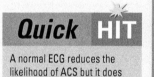

***Quick* HIT**

A normal ECG reduces the likelihood of ACS but it does not rule it out.

Common Symptoms

v. Rhinitis and upper airway cough syndrome (postnasal drip)

vi. Acute viral or bacterial sinusitis

vii. Aspiration

viii. Uncommon causes: congestive heart failure, pulmonary embolism, neoplasm, vocal cord dysfunction

b. Subacute cough (3 to 8 weeks)

i. Postinfectious cough—continues after other symptoms resolve

ii. Underlying lung disease: COPD, asthma

iii. Upper airway cough syndrome (postnasal drip)

iv. GERD or laryngopharyngeal reflux

c. Chronic cough (>8 weeks)

i. Smoking

ii. Angiotensin-converting-enzyme (ACE) inhibitor use (bradykinin accumulation)—dry, hacking cough

iii. Upper airway cough syndrome (postnasal drip)

iv. Underlying lung disease: COPD, asthma

v. GERD

vi. Interstitial lung disease

vii. In children: cystic fibrosis, recurrent aspiration—anatomic or functional causes

B. **Clinical features**

1. Historical findings:

a. Onset and duration (see differential diagnosis above)

b. Associated symptoms:

i. Rhinorrhea, nasal congestion, sneezing—consider viral cold

ii. Fever, malaise, sputum production, dyspnea—acute lung infection

iii. Postnasal drip—upper airway cough syndrome

iv. Dyspnea—consider pneumonia, bronchitis, COPD, asthma

v. Voice change—can be seen with vocal cord dysfunction, reflux

c. Circumstance of onset: sudden, especially in young children, may suggest foreign body aspiration

d. Medication history: ACE inhibitor use, previous inhaler use

e. Past medical history: lung disease, recent illnesses

f. Social history: smoking, pets or occupation exposures, TB risk

2. Physical exam findings:

a. Vitals: Evaluate for fever, tachypnea, tachycardia, or hypoxia.

b. General:

i. Assess for respiratory distress—work of breathing, mental status

ii. Children—assess for listlessness, irritability, and ability to be consoled

c. HEENT (head, eyes, ears, nose and throat):

i. Rhinorrhea, lacrimation, conjunctivitis seen in acute viral URI

ii. Cobblestone appearance of posterior pharynx suggests upper airway cough syndrome from postnasal drip.

iii. Nasal mucosal edema associated with acute URI, bacterial or viral

d. Pulmonary:

i. Normal lung sounds in upper airway infection

ii. Dullness to percussion, egophany, crackles—pneumonia

iii. Coarse crackles—bronchiectasis

iv. Wheezing—asthma, COPD, bronchitis, reactive airway disease

v. Diffuse, fine crackles—parenchymal lung disease, CHF

C. **Diagnostic evaluation**

1. Chest X-ray:

a. Not typically needed in acute cough unless worrisome signs/symptoms such as hemoptysis, weight loss, or other concern for malignancy, dyspnea

b. Consider in children if hypoxemia or concern for foreign body aspiration.

c. All patients with subacute cough if not deemed postinfectious

d. All patients with chronic cough (>8 weeks)

Quick HIT

No diagnostic testing is typically needed for the majority of patients with acute cough.

2. Laboratory studies: usually not needed for acute cough
   a. Concern for severe illness: CBC, ESR, CRP, electrolytes
   b. Rapid influenza testing if fevers, myalgia, fatigue
   c. *Bordetella pertussis* testing if cough >2 weeks and ≥1 of the below:
      i. Paroxysms of coughing
      ii. Inspiratory "whoop"
      iii. Posttussive emesis
      iv. Apnea in children <1
3. Pulmonary function testing (PFT):
   a. Consider in cases of chronic cough, dyspnea, wheezing
   b. Can distinguish between restrictive and obstructive lung disease

D. **Treatment**
1. Antitussive:
   a. Increase hydration, warm fluids.
   b. Honey—avoid in children under age 1 year
   c. Over-the-Counter (OTC): guaifenesin, dextromethorphan, pseudoephedrine (nasal decongestant)
   d. Prescription: codeine (avoid in children and adolescents)
2. Antibiotics:
   a. Indicated for pneumonia, acute sinusitis, or *B. pertussis*.
   b. Selection of agent depends on patient age and risk factors.
3. Treatments for other causes of cough:
   a. Asthma or COPD:
      i. Inhaled beta agonist, steroids, or anticholinergic
      ii. Oral corticosteroids
   b. GERD: H_2 blocker or proton pump inhibitors
   c. Upper airway cough syndrome: nasal steroids

V. Approach to Dizziness

A. **General characteristics**
1. Commonly divided into four groups based on history (Table 3-8):
   a. Vertigo
   b. Disequilibrium
   c. Presyncope
   d. Nonspecific
2. High prevalence in older adults (up to 38%) and is more frequently multicausal.

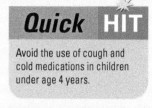

Quick HIT

Avoid the use of cough and cold medications in children under age 4 years.

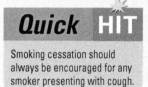

Quick HIT

Smoking cessation should always be encouraged for any smoker presenting with cough.

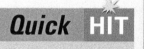

Quick HIT

History is the most important factor in determining the etiology of dizziness.

Common Symptoms

TABLE **3-8** Etiology of Dizziness in the Primary Care Setting	
Cause	**%**
Vertigo	54
• BPPV[a]	16
• Central	10
• Vestibular neuronitis	4
• Migraine	1
• Other/nonspecific	20
Psychiatric disorder	16
Multifactorial	13
Presyncope	6
Disequilibrium	2
Idiopathic	8

[a]BPPV, benign paroxysmal positional vertigo.

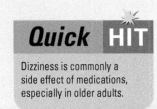

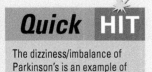

B. **Clinical features and testing**
1. Vertigo:
   a. Definition: an illusion or feeling of motion (often described as room spinning; can be tilting)
   b. History:
      i. Lack of spinning sensation does not rule out vertigo.
      ii. Time course: never continues for more than a few weeks, but it can be episodic for much longer
      iii. Detailed time course can help with diagnosis (Table 3-9).
      iv. Inquire about hearing loss or tinnitus.
      v. Presence of nystagmus (Dix-Hallpike maneuver)
   c. Evaluation:
      i. MRI/A if neurologic symptoms present consistent with stroke or mass
      ii. CT if suspect an intracranial hemorrhage
      iii. Audiology referral if having hearing loss
2. Disequilibrium:
   a. Definition: a sense of imbalance that may result from peripheral neuropathy, musculoskeletal disorder, cerebellar disorder, visual impairment, cervical spondylosis, or vestibular disorder
   b. Evaluation of muscle strength, gait, cerebellar coordination
   c. Examine for visual impairment.
   d. Examine for peripheral neuropathy. If positive, screen for DM and B_{12} deficiency.
   e. MRI of the head if cerebellar or cranial nerve function is abnormal
3. Presyncope:
   a. Definition: prodromal feeling of fainting or nearly fainting, lightheadedness that usually lasts for seconds or minutes at a time that may result from orthostatic hypotension, arrhythmias, and vasovagal attacks
   b. History:
      i. Usually occurs with standing
      ii. Patients typically describe a feeling of warmth, diaphoresis, nausea, vision blurring/tunnel vision.
      iii. Ask about palpitations, racing heart, shortness of breath, chest pain, history of a heart condition.

TABLE **3-9**	Features and Treatment for Causes of Vertigo	
Type	**Features**	**Treatment**
Vestibular neuritis (labyrinthitis)	Prolonged, severe, often associated with a viral syndrome, hearing usually normal	Antihistamines, antiemetics, oral corticosteroid
Cerebellar stroke	Prolonged, severe, sudden onset, older patient, vascular risk factors, gait impairment is prominent, headache	Follow stroke protocols
Meniere disease	Recurrent spontaneous attacks last minutes to hours, unilateral hearing loss, tinnitus	antihistamines, diuretics, antiemetics; limit salt, caffeine, nicotine, alcohol; vestibular rehab
Vestibular migraine	Recurrent spontaneous attacks last minutes to hours, usually history of migraines, headache with or following vertigo	Treat with typical migraine medicines
BPPV	Recurrent positionally triggered, brief episodes (<1 min), hearing normal	Repositioning maneuvers (Epley), home exercises
Psychogenic	Chronic persistent	SSRI and SNRI have been helpful

  c. Exam:
    i. Look for pallor.
    ii. Listen for murmurs, rubs, gallops.
    iii. Check orthostatic vital signs.
    iv. Testing: ECG, CBC, thyroid-stimulating hormone (TSH), electrolytes in most patients; Holter monitor and/or echocardiogram based on history and exam
4. Nonspecific: vague symptoms that do not fit well in the other categories; a psychiatric disorder may be the cause in many patients
    a. Most patients are younger and healthy.
    b. No specific test or physical signs

VI. Approach to Dyspnea

A. **General characteristics**
1. The American Thoracic Society defines dyspnea as a subjective experience of breathing discomfort derived from multiple physiologic, psychological, social, and environmental factors.
2. Acute dyspnea lasts hours to days, while chronic is considered lasting more than 4 to 8 weeks.
3. Usually respiratory or cardiovascular cause, but can be both (Table 3-10)

B. **Clinical features**
1. Historical findings:
    a. Past medical history: heart or lung disease, seasonal allergies, occupational/environmental exposure
    b. Smoking history
    c. Duration, exacerbating/ameliorating factors, how has it changed, associated symptoms, exertional, nocturnal, severity, fevers, ill contacts, travel history
2. Physical exam findings:
    a. Urgent workup needed for those with HR >120, RR >30, SpO_2 <90%, accessory muscle use, stridor, cyanosis, or difficulty speaking in complete sentences
    b. Heart exam: Tachy/bradycardia; murmur; gallop; decreased heart sounds in pericardial effusion or emphysema
    c. Lung exam:
        i. Stridor: upper airway obstruction
        ii. Wheeze: may indicate asthma or COPD

TABLE **3-10** Causes of Dyspnea		
	Acute Dyspnea	**Chronic Dyspnea**
Cardiovascular	MI/ACS CHF exacerbation Pericarditis Myocarditis	CHF/CAD Arrhythmia Valvular disease Anemia Deconditioning Cardiomyopathy
Respiratory	Asthma exacerbation COPD exacerbation Pulmonary infection Pulmonary embolism Pneumothorax Airway obstruction Anaphylaxis	Asthma COPD Interstitial lung disease Bronchiectasis Lung mass
Other	Guillain–Barré Myasthenia gravis Panic attack	Chronic diseases Thyroid disease Anxiety

Common Symptoms

   iii. Rhonchi: low pitched, obstruction or secretions in larger airways (can be cleared with a cough), can be heard in COPD exacerbation and bronchitis

   iv. Rales (crackles): crinkled cellophane sound, heard on inspiration, happens when closed airspaces open, heard in pneumonia and atelectasis

  d. Clubbing of the fingers: associated with bronchiectasis, pulmonary fibrosis, lung cancer, and cyanotic heart disease

  e. Jugular vein distention (JVD): heart failure

  f. Leg edema: bilateral seen on heart failure; unilateral swelling and dyspnea requires workup for pulmonary embolism (PE)

C. **Diagnostic workup**

 1. Based on history and physical exam

 2. Labs: Frequent tests include CMP, CBC, TSH, ± brain natriuretic peptide (BNP).

 3. Imaging:

  a. CXR: indicated for most patients

  b. CT chest: not a first-line test, may be helpful in subsequent workup or if there is a high level of suspicion for lung mass or pulmonary fibrosis

  c. CT pulmonary angiography (CTPA): when PE is suspected

 4. Spirometry/PFT: helpful in diagnosis of asthma, COPD. Full PFT with diffusion capacity needed for restrictive lung disease

 5. ECG: indicated in most adults with dyspnea

 6. Echo: for those suspected of heart failure, valvular disease, pericardial disease, and pulmonary hypertension (HTN)

 7. Cardiac stress test: for those suspected of CHD

D. **Treatment**

 1. Treat the underlying cause.

 2. For patients without a cause of the dyspnea following extensive workup, a conditioning program and weight loss for obese patients may be helpful. Frequent reassessment is needed to make sure a definitive cause does not reveal itself.

VII. Approach to Fever in Children

A. **General characteristics**

 1. Defined as an abnormal elevation in body temperature owing to a biologic response controlled by the central nervous system

 2. Infectious versus noninfectious causes should be considered

 3. Hospital admission for children less than 1 month old

 4. Additional outpatient workup for children less than 36 months old

B. **Clinical features**

 1. Body temperature:

  a. <36 months: Usually rectal temp: ≥100.4°F (38°C)

  b. >36 months: usually oral: ≥100°F (37.8°C)

 2. Symptoms range from asymptomatic to toxic.

 3. Usually there are other symptoms to help determine a cause.

C. **Causes**

 1. Infectious: bacterial, viral, fungal, parasite

 2. Noninfectious: recent immunizations, malignancy, medications, immunologic

D. **Physical exam findings**—variable by cause

 1. Listlessness or fatigue

 2. Dry mucous membranes, decreased skin turgor, sunken fontanelles

 3. Cervical lymphadenopathy (LAD)

 4. Tachycardia

 5. Tachypnea

 6. Abdominal distention or tenderness to palpation

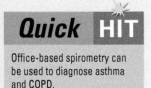

Quick HIT

Office-based spirometry can be used to diagnose asthma and COPD.

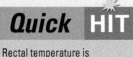

Quick HIT

Rectal temperature is considered the reference standard.

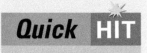

Quick HIT

The height of a fever is not associated with severity/prognosis of the cause and is less important than other signs such as a toxic appearance.

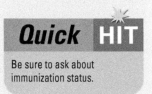

Quick HIT

Be sure to ask about immunization status.

E. **Differential diagnosis**
1. Infectious: such as urinary tract infection (UTI), pneumonia and bronchiolitis, gastroenteritis, meningitis, bacteremia
2. Noninfectious causes: recent immunizations, neoplasms (leukemia or lymphoma most common), medications, immunologic (Kawasaki disease, hereditary auto-inflammatory syndromes of periodic fever, immunodeficiency)
F. **Treatment**
1. Find and treat underlying cause.
2. Reassurance to parents that fevers do not make the illness worse and they do not cause brain damage
3. Increase fluids and rest.
4. Antipyretics if the child appears uncomfortable
   a. Acetaminophen should not be used in children <3 months.
   b. Ibuprofen should not be used in children <6 months.
   c. Aspirin is generally avoided for most pediatric patients owing to the risk of Reye's syndrome.
5. External cooling is not usually recommended with the exception of heat-related temperature elevation.

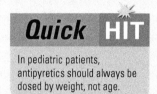

Quick **HIT**

In pediatric patients, antipyretics should always be dosed by weight, not age.

VIII. Approach to Fatigue
A. **General characteristics**
1. Definition: physical and/or mental exhaustion (lack of energy or motivation). It is distinct from somnolence, dyspnea, and muscle weakness.
2. Epidemiology:
   a. Very common: reported in 21% to 33% of primary care visits
   b. Prevalence in the United States: 6% to 7.5%; slight female predominance
B. **Clinical features**
1. Historical findings:
   a. Review medical history for causes.
   b. Ask specifically about inadequate sleep, sleep disorder, dyspnea, or muscle weakness.
   c. Determine onset, activity change, pattern, and alleviating/exacerbating factors.
   d. How much does it impact the patient's quality of life?
   e. Review prescription and OTC medications.
   f. Review drug and alcohol use.
2. Physical exam findings:
   a. General appearance: alertness, grooming
   b. Ear-Nose-Throat (ENT): Thyroid
   c. Lymphadenopathy: If positive, consider infectious illness (such as mono, HIV) or malignancy.
   d. Pulmonary: abnormal lung sounds consistent with chronic lung disease
   e. Cardiovascular: murmurs, arrhythmia, edema
   f. Neuro: muscle tone, reflexes, weakness
   g. Psych: mood and affect
C. **Diagnostic workup** (Table 3-11)
1. Screen for depression (PHQ-9).
2. Initial labs: CMP, TSH, CBC, U/A, possible ESR, and pregnancy test if indicated
3. Other tests if indicated: HIV, Lyme, B_{12}, iron studies, drug screen, TB test, ECG, echocardiogram, Hepatitis C
4. Criteria for chronic fatigue syndrome:
   a. Substantial level of impairment in preillness activities lasting >6 months, accompanied by fatigue, not related to extensive exertion, and not relieved by rest
   b. Cognitive impairment or orthostatic intolerance

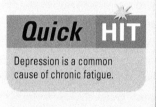

Quick **HIT**

Depression is a common cause of chronic fatigue.

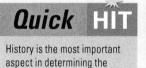

Quick **HIT**

History is the most important aspect in determining the cause of fatigue.

Common Symptoms

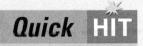

Quick HIT

No medical or psychiatric problem (idiopathic chronic fatigue) is found in 8% to 35% of patients with chronic fatigue.

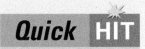

Quick HIT

Lab workup in fatigue leads to a diagnosis in only 5% of cases.

Quick HIT

Many patients presenting with sinus headaches are actually having a migraine.

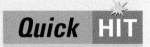

Quick HIT

Imaging is not needed in most patients presenting with headaches.

Quick HIT

SNOOP mnemonic for headache red flags:
S – systemic symptoms or illness
N – neurologic symptoms or signs
O – onset recently or suddenly
O – onset after age 40
P – prior headache history that is different or progressive headache

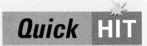

Quick HIT

Insomnia can be primary, not caused by other disorders, or secondary, caused by other disorders (eg, depression, substance abuse, chronic pain).

TABLE 3-11	Causes of Fatigue
Psychologic	Depression, anxiety, alcohol/drug abuse, somatization, adjustment disorder
Medications	Antihistamines, benzodiazepines, antidepressants, antipsychotics
Infectious	Mononucleosis, HIV, HCV, CMV, TB, Lyme, other infections
Sleep disorders	Sleep apnea, restless leg, inconsistent sleep cycle
Neoplastic	Any malignancy
Hematologic	Anemia
Cardiopulmonary	CHF, COPD
Endocrine/metabolic	Hypothyroidism, DM, adrenal insufficiency, B_{12} deficiency, renal failure, liver failure
Neurologic	Multiple sclerosis, Parkinson's, myasthenia gravis

D. **Treatment**
  1. Treat the underlying problem if found.
  2. For patients with chronic fatigue syndrome or idiopathic fatigue, antidepressants, cognitive behavioral therapy (CBT), and graded exercise therapy have been shown to be helpful.

IX. Approach to Headaches

A. **General characteristics**
  1. Very common complaint: 1-year prevalence in the general population is 65% (Table 3-12)
  2. Tension type and migraine account for the majority of headaches.

B. **Clinical features**
  1. Historical findings: A detailed history should be performed including duration, onset, age of onset, location, triggers, frequency, intensity, quality of pain, food/drug/alcohol history, medications, vision changes, neurologic symptoms, trauma, sleep, weight changes, work and lifestyle, relation to menstrual cycle, fevers, and response to medications.
  2. Exam findings: Check blood pressure, pulse, temperature, HEENT, and nuchal rigidity, and perform a comprehensive neurologic exam.

C. **Diagnostic workup**
  1. Often not needed if there are no red flags
  2. Reserve imaging for those with red flags based on the SNOOP mnemonic.
  3. MRI is the preferred test, but CT can be done in urgent situations or when there is a contraindication to MRI.
  4. Lumbar puncture for those with clinical suspicion for infection, subarachnoid hemorrhage, or idiopathic intracranial hypertension and a normal CT

D. **Treatment** (Table 3-12)
  1. Treat underlying cause.
  2. Headache hygiene: good sleep hygiene, stay well hydrated, regular meals, regular exercise, avoid triggers, biofeedback, meditation, stress reduction

X. Approach to Insomnia

A. **General characteristics**
  1. Definition: difficulty initiating or maintaining sleep or waking up too early despite adequate opportunity for sleep and it impairs daytime functioning
  2. Types:
     a. Short term: lasting <3 months and often caused by an inciting factor such as stress, acute pain, or a major adjustment
     b. Chronic: Symptoms occur greater than three times a week for >3 months.
     c. Other: for those not fitting in the above categories

TABLE **3-12** Causes, Features, and Treatment of Headaches			
Type	**Primary Care Frequency**	**Features**	**Treatments**
Migraines	45	Photo/phonophobia, often unilateral, throbbing, nausea/vomiting, may have an aura	Acute: NSAIDs, triptans, acetyl-para-aminophenol (APAP)/acetylsalicylic acid (ASA)/caffeine, antiemetics Proph: beta blocker, amitriptyline, venlafaxine, valproate, topiramate, verapamil
Tension	25	Most common but most do not go to the doctor, mild to moderate, usually bilateral, nonthrobbing	NSAIDs, ASA, APAP, NSAID/caffeine; avoid overuse of acute medicines; amitriptyline for prophylactic use
Chronic daily	5	Not truly a separate category but encompasses the other categories. 15 or more days a month for >3 mo. Often associated with daily overuse of headache medications.	Do not use acute headaches meds more than twice a week
Cluster	5	Severe, unilateral, autonomic symptoms such as ptosis, miosis, lacrimation, conjunctival injection, rhinorrhea, nasal congestion	1st line: oxygen or triptans 2nd line: intranasal lidocaine, ergotamine, prednisone Proph: verapamil
Viral/sinusitis	8	Other signs of infection	Symptomatic treatment
Withdraw syndromes	7	Sudden cessation of a substance such as drugs, pain meds, alcohol, caffeine	Slowly weaning of substances if possible
Posttraumatic head injury	3	History of trauma	Amitriptyline and propranolol; analgesia overuse headache is common and responds to analgesia withdrawal
Meningitis/ Encephalitis	<1	Fever, neck stiffness, mental status changes	Immediate antibiotics following LP
Hemorrhagic stroke	<1	Sudden severe headache, older age is a risk factor, may have neurologic deficit	Treat cause
Tumor	<1	Insidious onset, usually other neurologic symptoms	Treat cause
Temporal arteritis	<1	Temporal pain, always >50-year-old	Treat cause

Common Symptoms

3. Epidemiology:
    a. One of the most common disorders. About 35% to 69% of adults report insomnia in the previous year.
    b. More common in women and incidence increases with age
    c. Risk factors include previous history of insomnia, family history, pain, being easily aroused from sleep, and poorer self-report of health.
B. **Clinical features**
    1. Historical findings: The diagnosis of insomnia is a clinical diagnosis, so the history is the most important part of the workup.
       a. How long does it take to go to sleep (sleep latency)?
       b. How often do they wake up and for how long?

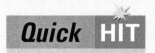

Quick HIT

Other sleep disorders such as obstructive sleep apnea and restless leg syndrome need to be ruled out in the workup of insomnia.

    c. Do they wake up earlier than they intend to?

    d. What keeps them from going to sleep?

    e. What are their sleep practices? When do they go to bed/get up? Does it vary? Do they watch TV in bed? Do they read in bed? Etc.

    f. Drug and alcohol use?

    g. Do they take daytime naps?

    h. How does this affect daytime activities?

    i. Weight loss?

  2. Physical exam findings:

    a. Possible signs of obstructive sleep apnea (OSA): body habitus, neck size, OP exam

    b. Look for/examine any painful areas.

    c. Possible signs of CHF: lower-extremity swelling, lung exam

    d. Mental status

C. **Diagnostic workup**

  1. No tests are required to diagnose insomnia. Some tests may help to rule out other sleep disorders if there is a question.

  2. Sleep study (polysomnography) can help rule out sleep disorders such as OSA and restless legs syndrome (RLS).

  3. Epworth Sleepiness Scale can help with quantifying daytime symptoms.

  4. Standardized depression and anxiety inventories

  5. Other labs or studies based on history: echo, TSH, A_{1c}, BUN/Cr, iron studies

D. **Treatment**

  1. Sleep hygiene: regular sleep cycle, avoid caffeine/alcohol/nicotine, decrease bedroom stimuli, regular exercise, avoid light emitting screen prior to bedtime, avoid napping, relaxation techniques

  2. Cognitive behavioral therapy

  3. Medications:

    a. Sedating antihistamines: do not use in older adults

    b. Benzodiazepines: very effective but problems with dependence and abuse potential

    c. Melatonin agonists (melatonin and ramelteon) can help with sleep latency

    d. Zaleplon, zolpidem, and eszopiclone: can have hangover effect and sleep walking

    e. Orexin receptor antagonist: suvorexant

    f. Antidepressants: doxepin, amitriptyline, trazodone, mirtazapine

XI. Approach to the Red Eye [Table 3-13]

A. **Chalazion and hordeolum**

  1. General characteristics:

    a. Chalazion: a blockage of the meibomian gland, a granulomatous process

    b. Hordeolum: a blockage of an oil gland or eyelash follicle, an inflammatory process

  2. Clinical features (Figure 3-1):

    a. Painful bump on the upper or lower eye lid

    b. Visual acuity is normal

TABLE 3-13 Differentiating Between Serious Eye Conditions

More Serious	Less Serious
Focal	Diffuse
Itching or irritated	Severe pain
Normal vision	Vision loss
Chronic or recurrent	Acute and progressive
Normal pupils	Abnormal pupils

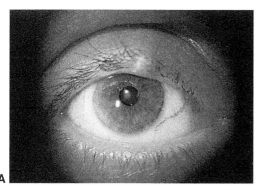 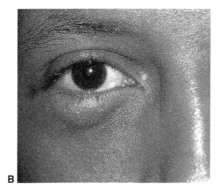

FIGURE
3-1 A: Stye (acute hordeolum). B: Chalazion.

(From Bickley LS. *Bates' Guide to Physical Examination and History Taking.* 12th ed. Philadelphia, PA: Lippincott Williams & Wilkins; 2016.)

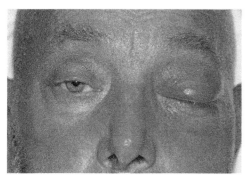

FIGURE
3-2 Left orbital cellulitis with marked periorbital edema, erythema, and proptosis.

(From Chern KC, Saidel MA. *Ophthalmology Review Manual.* 2nd ed. Philadelphia, PA: Lippincott Williams & Wilkins; 2012.)

  3. Treatment:
   a. Warm moist compresses at least four times a day for 15 minutes
   b. Topical antibiotics are rarely needed but can be used for persistent symptoms: erythromycin ophthalmic gel four times a day.
   c. Refer to ophthalmology if lasts for >2 weeks or for recurrent lesions.
   d. Most resolve in 1 to 2 weeks.
 B. **Periorbital cellulitis**
  1. General characteristics:
   a. Periorbital cellulitis is a deep-tissue infection around the eye.
   b. Risk factors include sinusitis, URI, and trauma to the face or eye.
   c. Most commonly caused by *Streptococcus pneumoniae*, *Staphylococcus aureus*, and other streptococcal species
  2. Clinical features (Figure 3-2):
   a. Presents with pain, tenderness, swelling, erythema of the eyelids and surrounding tissue, and fever
   b. Decreased vision or proptosis may indicate orbital cellulitis which requires hospitalization.
  3. Treatment:
   a. Nontoxic adults and children >1 year with mild symptoms, treat as outpatient
   b. Children <1 year and patients with systemic symptoms, admit for IV antibiotics
   c. Amoxicillin-clavulanate, cefpodoxime, or cefdinir for 7 to 10 days
 C. **Blepharitis**
  1. General characteristics: characterized by inflammation of the eyelids owing to one of the following
   a. Staphylococcal colonization
   b. Seborrheic or dandruff like
   c. Meibomian gland dysfunction

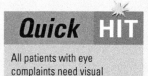

Quick HIT

All patients with eye complaints need visual acuity tested.

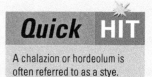

Quick HIT

A chalazion or hordeolum is often referred to as a stye.

Common Symptoms

2. Clinical features (Figure 3-3):
   a. Red eyes or eyelids, itchy eyes, crusting worse in the morning, flaking or scaling of eyelids
   b. Examine for signs of seborrheic dermatitis.
   c. Eyelids often pink and scaly
3. Treatment
   a. Warm, moist compresses four times a day for 15 minutes
   b. Eyelid massage
   c. Eyelid washing with mild soap such as baby shampoo
   d. Topical antibiotics such as tetracycline and erythromycin
   e. Topical glucocorticoids for short-term acute exacerbations

D. **Subconjunctival hemorrhage**
1. General characteristics:
   a. Very common
   b. Caused by trauma, anticoagulant (ASA, warfarin, etc.), cough or sneeze, idiopathic
2. Clinical features (Figure 3-4):
   a. Minimal symptoms except as a result of trauma
   b. Does not involve cornea or anterior chamber
   c. Focal, flat, red area on surface of sclera
   d. Visual acuity normal
   e. Need to rule out ulcer, foreign body, or hyphema
3. Treatment: self-limited, patient reassurance

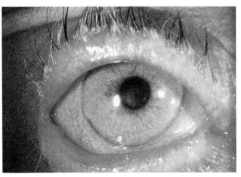

FIGURE
3-3 Blepharitis is associated with crusting of the eyelashes, thickening of the eyelids, telangiectatic vessels along the lid margins, and plugging of the meibomian glands.

(From Tasman W, Jaeger E. *The Wills Eye Hospital Atlas of Clinical Ophthalmology.* 2nd ed. Philadelphia, PA: Lippincott Williams & Wilkins; 2001.)

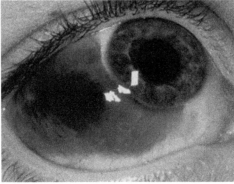

FIGURE
3-4 Subconjunctival hemorrhage.

(From Onofrey BE, Skorin L, Jr, Holdeman NR. *Ocular Therapeutics Handbook: A Clinical Manual.* Philadelphia, PA: Lippincott-Raven Publishers; 1998.)

E. Conjunctivitis
1. General characteristics:
   a. Characterized by inflammation of the conjunctiva
   b. Infectious versus noninfectious
   c. Differential diagnosis includes foreign body, ulcer, iritis, and glaucoma.
2. Clinical features:
   a. Normal visual acuity (although may have slight blurriness for the discharge)
   b. Viral: watery discharge, crusty in the AM, minimal swelling, gritty eye feeling
   c. Bacterial: thick purulent discharge, discharge returns within minutes of wiping away, significant conjunctival swelling (Figure 3-5)
   d. Allergic: history of allergies, often seasonal, itchy watery eyes, going on for weeks, cobble stones on conjunctival exam
3. Treatment:
   a. Discontinue use of contact lenses until symptoms resolve.
   b. Viral:
      i. Self-limited, no treatment needed, lubricating drops may be beneficial
      ii. Usually 5 to 7 days but can last up to 3 weeks
   c. Bacterial: (Table 3-14)
      i. Common pathogens include *S. aureus*, *S. pneumoniae*, *Haemophilus influenzae*, and *Moraxella catarrhalis*.
      ii. First line: erythromycin ophthalmic ointment or polymyxin/trimethoprim drops
      iii. Alternatives: bacitracin ointment, polymyxin-bacitracin ointment, fluoroquinolone drops, azithromycin drops, sulfa ophthalmic drops
   d. Allergic:
      i. Avoid triggers.
      ii. Acute exacerbation: over-the-counter topical antihistamine/vasoconstrictors such as naphazoline HCl/pheniramine maleate eye drops
      iii. Frequent episodes

Quick HIT

A hyphema is blood in the anterior chamber of the eye.

Quick HIT

The conjunctiva is the surface of the inner lid and eye to the limbus.

Quick HIT

Erythromycin eye ointment is recommended for all newborns to prevent infectious congenital conjunctivitis.

Quick HIT

Adults usually do not like erythromycin eye ointment owing to a film left over the eyes making it hard to see.

Common Symptoms

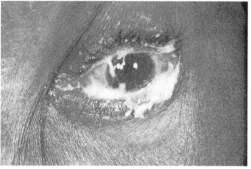

FIGURE
3-5 **Acute bacterial conjunctivitis with mild lid swelling, conjunctival injection, and discharge along the lid margin.**

(From Fiebach NH, Kern DE, Thomas PA, et al. *Barker, Burton, and Zieve's Principles of Ambulatory Medicine.* 7th ed. Philadelphia, PA: Lippincott Williams & Wilkins; 2007.)

TABLE **3-14** Causes of Neonatal Conjunctivitis	
Timing After Birth	**Most Likely Cause of Conjunctivitis**
<24 h	Chemical
24–48 h	Gonorrhea
>48 h	Other bacteria
1–5 d	Herpes simplex virus
5–10 d	Chlamydia

(a) Topical H$_1$-selective antihistamine/mast cell stabilizers such as olopatadine

(b) Oral nonsedating antihistamine such as loratadine

(c) Concomitant rhinitis: intranasal glucocorticoid or antihistamine

F. **Corneal abrasion/ulcer**

1. General characteristics:

   a. Most common eye injury

   b. Usually from trauma, foreign body, or contact lens

2. Clinical features:

   a. Intense eye pain, watery eye, difficulty keeping eye open

   b. Use of numbing drop (eg, proparacaine) relieves the pain and makes the patient more comfortable.

   c. Can be differentiated from acute glaucoma as topical analgesics will not relieve the pain in glaucoma

   d. Look for foreign bodies.

   e. Evert eyelid to check inner surface of lid.

   f. Fluorescein eye staining: pooling of the green stain under a Wood's lamp indicates an ulcer or abrasion (Figure 3-6, Table 3-15)

   g. Dendritic lesion is suggestive of a herpetic lesion (see herpetic keratitis).

3. Treatment:

   a. Removal of foreign body if needed

      i. Irrigation with water or saline

      ii. Cotton swab: dab at or gently brush away foreign body

      iii. Magnetic foreign body remover for metallic objects

   b. Topical antibiotic: erythromycin ointment, sulfacetamide, polymyxin/trimethoprim, ciprofloxacin, or ofloxacin four times daily for 3 to 5 days

   c. Patching is not recommended

   d. Analgesics

      i. Oral: acetaminophen, NSAIDs, narcotics if needed

      ii. Topical: cycloplegics (cyclopentolate): parasympatholytic drops that inhibit miosis (pupil-constriction)

   e. Minor abrasions improve in 24 to 48 hours.

   f. Large ulcers require follow-up and possible ophthalmology referral

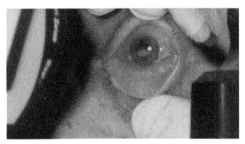

FIGURE

3-6 Corneal abrasion. Note patch of fluorescein uptake.

(From Berg D, Worzala K. *Atlas of Adult Physical Diagnosis*. Philadelphia, PA: Lippincott Williams & Wilkins; 2006.)

TABLE 3-15 Technique for Fluorescein Eye Staining

1. Remove contact lenses (will stain).
2. Place 1–2 drops of saline on the fluorescein strip.
3. Gently pull down on the lower lid with a finger.
4. Touch the strip to the inner surface of the lower lid.
5. Have the patient blink a few times.
6. With a Wood's lamp, look for pooling of fluorescein stain on the corneal surface.

Common Symptoms

G. **Herpetic keratitis**
   1. General characteristics:
      a. Corneal infection and inflammation
      b. Reactivation of varicella zoster virus or HSV
      c. Major cause of blindness worldwide
   2. Clinical features:
      a. Pain, burning, itching, and watery discharge of the eye
      b. Dendritic lesions on cornea with fluorescein staining (Figure 3-7)
      c. Suspect if shingles in the first branch of the trigeminal nerve dermatome or on the tip of the nose
         i. 65% of cases affecting the first branch of the trigeminal nerve will have ocular lesions
         ii. 40% of those with ocular lesions have iritis
   3. Treatment:
      a. All cases should be urgently referred to ophthalmology.
      b. Oral antiviral such as acyclovir
      c. Analgesics: same as for corneal abrasion
      d. Avoid topical glucocorticoids.
H. **Iritis (anterior uveitis)**
   1. General characteristics:
      a. Characterized by intraocular inflammation of the anterior chamber of the eye
      b. Causes:
         i. Infectious: toxoplasmosis, herpes zoster, CMV, syphilis, cat scratch disease
         ii. Autoimmune: sarcoidosis, juvenile idiopathic arthritis, Behcet's, systemic lupus erythematosus (SLE), others
         iii. Idiopathic
   2. Clinical features (Figure 3-8):

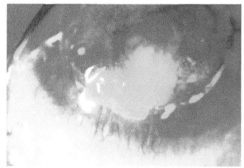

FIGURE
3-7 **Herpetic dendritic lesion.**

(From Rapuano CJ. *Wills Eye Institute Color Atlas & Synopsis of Clinical Ophthalmology: Cornea.* 2nd ed. Philadelphia, PA: Lippincott Williams & Wilkins; 2012.)

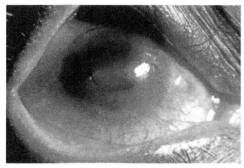

FIGURE
3-8 **Acute iritis.**

(From McDonagh D. *FMS Sports Medicine Manual: Event Planning and Emergency Care.* Philadelphia, PA: Lippincott Williams & Wilkins, 2012.)

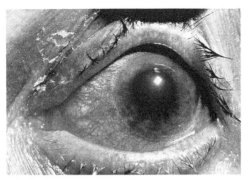

3-9 **Acute-angle glaucoma.**

(From Azuara-Blanco A, Henderer JD, Katz LJ, et al. Glaucoma. In: Tasman W, Jaeger EA, eds. *The Wills Eye Hospital Atlas of Clinical Ophthalmology.* 2nd ed. Philadelphia, PA: Lippincott Williams & Wilkins; 2001:120.)

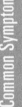

    a. Acute onset of eye pain
    b. Small, poorly reactive pupil
    c. Ciliary flush
    d. Decreased visual acuity
    e. Diagnosis requires slit lamp exam.
  3. Treatment:
    a. Referral to ophthalmology
    b. Treat underlying cause.
I. **Acute glaucoma**
  1. General characteristics:
    a. Caused by closed- or narrow-angle glaucoma
    b. About 10% of glaucoma cases in the United States
    c. Risk factors include family history, age >50, female, hyperopia (farsightedness), and Inuit and Asian populations.
  2. Clinical features (Figure 3-9):
    a. Acute onset of eye pain
    b. Headache
    c. Nausea and vomiting
    d. Dilated poorly reactive pupil
    e. Conjunctival redness
    f. Decreased visual acuity
    g. Increased intraocular pressure (eye feels hard)
  3. Treatment:
    a. Emergent ophthalmology referral
    b. Avoid anticholinergic medications.
    c. Iridotomy
    d. IV acetazolamide or mannitol

Patients with acute narrow-angle glaucoma often present with headache and nausea and can be confused with other illnesses with similar presentations such as migraines.

QUESTIONS

1. A 64-year-old male with a history of HTN and metabolic syndrome presents with a 3-day history of progressively worsening epigastric pain that radiates to the back. He has a poor appetite and the pain is worse with food. He denies fever or bowel changes. His heart and lung exam are normal. He has moderate-to-severe tenderness in the epigastric area which feels very firm and he guards that area. He does not have any rebound tenderness. What is the next best treatment step?
   A. Routine right upper quadrant ultrasound
   B. Start omeprazole
   C. Urgent upper endoscopy (EGD)
   D. Urgent CT of the abdomen

2. A 44-year-old male presents with a 3-day history of low back pain that radiated to his right upper thigh. It started the evening after moving some furniture and was worse the next day. He denies any weakness or numbness and has had no bowel or bladder changes. He smokes a half pack per day and denies drug use. On exam, he is slow to get up and move and appears very stiff. He has mild paraspinal tenderness in the right lumbar area. His strength is limited by the low back pain. He has a negative straight leg raise, 2+ patellar and ankle deep tendon reflexes (DTR), and normal lower extremity sensation. Which is the next best step in the workup and treatment of this patient?
   A. Order a lumbar MRI.
   B. Naproxen with follow-up in 1 to 2 weeks
   C. Bed rest to encourage quicker healing
   D. Order a lumbar XR
   E. Tylenol with codeine with follow-up in 1 to 2 weeks

3. A 25-year-old female presents with a 5-day history of red eyes. She has watery discharge that lasts throughout the day and has slight crusting of the eyes when waking up. Her eyes are itchy but not painful and she denies any vision changes. She has not had any sick contacts. She has mild rhinorrhea and sneezing. What is the most likely diagnosis?
   A. Viral conjunctivitis
   B. Allergic conjunctivitis
   C. Dry eyes
   D. Blepharitis

4. A 38-year-old woman presents with chronic headaches that she has on most days. It is a bilateral frontal headache and is usually dull and pressing. She has slight photo/phonophobia. She denies an aura preceding the headache. She has no vision changes or weakness, denies nausea or vomiting, and weight has been stable. She takes labetalol for HTN and ibuprofen most mornings for the headache. Which of these is the best treatment to improve her headaches?
   A. Increase the ibuprofen to three times a day.
   B. Discontinue the ibuprofen.
   C. Sumatriptan as needed
   D. Change labetalol to propranolol.

ANSWERS

1. **Answer: D.** This patient has red flags for a possible serious intra-abdominal problem including moderate-to-severe pain that radiates to the back with both voluntary and involuntary guarding. This presentation is most consistent with pancreatitis although other disorders can present similarly. An urgent abdominal CT would be important in evaluating this and ruling out other possibilities. Blood work including a CMP, CBC with differential, and lipase/amylase should be done as well. An Ultrasound could be useful, but it is not the best test to evaluate the pancreas. There is also need for urgent evaluation. An EGD may be useful in subsequent workup but not in the initial workup of this patient. It is not appropriate to simply start a PPI without workup in a patient with abdominal red flags.

2. **Answer: B.** The patient has acute low back pain without any red flags. The most appropriate next step would be to have the patient take an NSAID and to follow-up if it is not improving or if new/worsening symptoms develop. Imaging is not needed at this point. The vast majority of patients with this presentation will improve within 2 to 4 weeks. Strict bed rest is contraindicated and will prolong the recovery. Opioid-containing medications are not considered first-line medications for treatment of acute low back pain without red flags.

3. **Answer: B.** This presentation is most consistent with allergic rhinitis with the lack of sick contacts, bilateral symptoms, and associated rhinorrhea and sneezing. Viral conjunctivitis is a possibility but is much less likely with this presentation. Dry eye will have less redness and will have a chronic timeframe. Blepharitis is characterized by inflammation of the eyelids rather than the conjunctiva.

4. **Answer: B.** Her symptoms are most consistent with a withdrawal-type headache owing to the use of the ibuprofen. Discontinuing the ibuprofen or limiting it to no more than two to three times a week will likely improve her symptoms once she gets past the acute withdrawal stage (usually within a few days). Increasing the ibuprofen to three times a day may initially help but the headaches will eventually come back and it does not solve the actual cause. Sumatriptan is used to treat migraine-type headaches, which is not consistent with this presentation. While propranolol is used in headache prophylaxis, changing the labetalol to propranolol is unlikely to significantly benefit this patient.

Answers

IMMUNOLOGIC
DISORDERS
Christopher Lewis • Leila J. Saxena

4

I. Food Allergies
A. **Characteristics**
1. Definitions:
    a. Food allergy: an adverse health effect arising from a specific immune response that is reproducible on exposure to a given food
    b. Food: any substance intended for human consumption
      i. Includes drinks, chewing gum, and dietary supplements
      ii. Does not include drugs, tobacco products, or cosmetics
    c. Food allergen: specific components of the food (protein, chemical hapten) that are recognized by an allergic-specific immune cell that causes characteristic symptoms
2. Prevalence:
    a. More than 170 foods have been reported to cause immunoglobulin E (IgE)-mediated reactions.
    b. The most common foods to cause allergies are hen's eggs, cow's milk, peanuts, tree nuts, soy, wheat, fish, and crustacean shellfish.
    c. True prevalence is difficult to ascertain. Up to 15% of parents believe that their children have food allergies; however, allergies can be confirmed in only 1% to 3%.
3. Other food reactions that are not true food allergies:
    a. Malabsorption syndromes: celiac sprue
    b. Metabolic conditions: lactose intolerance, phenylketonuria
    c. Hemolytic conditions: G6Pd deficiency
    d. Preexisting conditions: ulcer, gallbladder disease, irritable bowel disease, or inflammatory bowel disease
    e. Food dislikes
B. **Clinical features**
1. Cutaneous reactions:
    a. Acute urticaria (see Figure 14-20)
      i. Pruritic wheals that develop rapidly
      ii. Occurs minutes to hours after ingesting a specific food.
      iii. Can be IgE- or non-IgE mediated
    b. Angioedema
      i. IgE mediated, nonpitting, nonpruritic, swelling of the face, hands, buttocks, genitals, or larynx
      ii. Laryngeal edema is a medical emergency.
      iii. This is a manifestation of anaphylaxis.
    c. Atopic dermatitis/eczema
      i. Areas of pruritic skin, which rash owing to scratching
      ii. Avoidance of food does not alter the course of the reaction, but can reduce the severity of atopic dermatitis.
2. Food-induced anaphylaxis:
    a. IgE mediated

> **Quick HIT**
> - More than 70% of children will outgrow milk and egg allergies by early adolescence, but only 20% will outgrow peanut or tree nut allergies.
> - About 50% to 90% of self-reported food allergies are not true allergies.
> - Adverse reactions that are not immune mediated are not food allergies.

b. Rapid onset within minutes; a second reaction can occur 8 to 72 hours later
   c. Life-threatening systemic condition
3. Gastrointestinal (GI) food allergies:
   a. Dietary protein-induced proctitis/proctocolitis
      i. Non-IgE mediated, following feedings with breast, cow's, goat's, or soy milk
      ii. Occurs in healthy infants
      iii. Blood in the stool is often the only GI symptom.
   b. Eosinophilic esophagitis
      i. IgE- and non-IgE-mediated eosinophilic inflammation of the esophagus
      ii. Causes feeding disorder, vomiting, reflux symptoms, and abdominal pain
      iii. In adolescents and adults, the presentation is dysphagia and esophageal food impactions.
   c. Eosinophilic gastroenteritis
      i. IgE- and non-IgE-mediated eosinophilic infiltration of the gut
      ii. Can be localized or widespread
      iii. Food avoidance reduces severity.
   d. Food protein–induced enterocolitis syndrome
      i. IgE- and non-IgE mediated
      ii. From intake of cow's or soy milk, rice, oats, or other grains
      iii. Diarrhea and vomiting, causing severe dehydration
   e. Oral allergy syndrome
      i. Caused by cross-reactivity between aeroallergens (pollen) and certain fruits and vegetables
      ii. Symptoms of swelling or tingling limited to lips or oropharynx occur while eating.
      iii. Symptoms resolve after food is swallowed or spit out.
      iv. Cooking prevents the reaction.
4. Respiratory manifestations:
   a. IgE mediated, affects upper and lower respiratory tract
   b. Symptoms include nasal congestion, rhinorrhea, sneezing, laryngeal edema, cough, wheezing, chest tightness, and dyspnea.
C. **Diagnosis**
   1. Requires a clear and specific history
   2. Food allergy must be confirmed—50% to 90% of self-reported food allergies are not true food allergies.
   3. Methods:
      a. Skin prick test, intradermal testing, and IgE testing
         i. Only detect the presence of allergic sensitization
         ii. Not sufficient by themselves to make diagnosis of food allergy
         iii. One-half of U.S. population has detectable allergen-specific IgE against a food allergen.
         iv. Only 4% to 6% have clinical food allergy.
      b. Food elimination diets
         i. Eliminate one or a few specific foods from the diet for a week.
         ii. Gradually reintroduce food and monitor for symptoms.
         iii. Risk of nutritional deficiency if too restricted
      c. Oral food challenges
         i. Performed by a trained healthcare professional
         ii. Need immediate access to resuscitative equipment
         iii. Gold standard for diagnosis
D. **Treatment and prevention of food allergies**
   1. Elimination:
      a. Avoidance is the main treatment.
      b. Food labeling education is needed to interpret ingredient lists.
      c. Products may contain trace amounts of allergen from processing.

Quick HIT

- Suspect food allergy when patients present with anaphylaxis or a combination of symptoms occurring in a few minutes after ingestion of certain foods.
- Suspect children diagnosed with moderate-to-severe atopic dermatitis, eosinophilic dermatitis, eosinophilic esophagitis, or enterocolitis.

2. Medication:
   a. There are no recommended medications to prevent reactions.
   b. Mild reactions treated with supportive care.
   c. Anaphylactic reactions require epinephrine.
3. Immunotherapy:
   a. Allergen-specific immunotherapy is not recommended.
   b. Clinical trials are in progress.
4. Childhood prevention:
   a. No dietary restrictions are necessary during pregnancy and lactation.
   b. Exclusive breastfeeding is best until 4 to 6 months of age.
   c. If unable to breastfeed, cow's milk infant formula is used.
   d. The use of soy infant formula does not prevent food allergies.
   e. Solid-food introduction should not be delayed >6 months of age.
   f. Introduce peanut-containing foods to infants between ages 4 and 11 months.
5. Mild reactions: outpatient setting treatments
   a. Histamine H_1 antagonist
      i. Diphenhydramine
      ii. Less sedating second generation
   b. Bronchospasm: albuterol metered dose inhaler or nebulized
   c. Corticosteroids
6. Anaphylaxis:
   a. Epinephrine is the first-line treatment, all others are adjunct.
      i. Do not delay.
      ii. Autoinjector intramuscular
   b. Bronchodilator: albuterol metered dose inhaler or nebulized.
   c. Histamine H_1 antagonist
   d. Corticosteroids: oral prednisone and/or intravenous (IV) solumedrol
   e. Supplemental oxygen and IV fluids as needed for support

II. Environmental Allergies

A. **Characteristics**
   1. Definition: immune-mediated reactions of varying severity owing to exposure to allergens in the environment, such as *pollen, dust mites, pets and animals, mold and mildew, and cockroaches*
   2. Epidemiology: Environmental allergies affect 10% to 30% of children and adults in the world each year. Roughly *40 million Americans* suffer from environmental allergies.
   3. Cause: When allergens in the indoor and outdoor environments enter the nose, sinuses, and lungs, the body's immune system overreacts to these allergens in an *IgE-mediated reaction.*
   4. Genetics: Genetic factors likely contribute to the pathogenesis of environmental allergies. A family history of atopy infers an increased risk for environmental allergies.
   5. Risk factors: These include air pollution, house dust, pet ownership, history of asthma or eczema.
   6. Pathophysiology: Exposure to environmental allergens causes the production of IgE antibodies specific to the particular allergen *(sensitization)*. Subsequent exposure to the allergen leads to an allergic response with an *early and late phase*. The early response typically lasts 1 hour and includes sneezing, clear rhinorrhea, and pruritus. The late response can have similar symptoms but typically includes more nasal congestion.

B. **Clinical features**
   1. Historical findings:
      a. Nasal: sneezing, rhinorrhea (typically clear, watery), congestion, pruritus
      b. Eyes: pruritus, redness, watery, swollen lids
      c. Throat: postnasal drip, pruritus
      d. Sinus: pressure or pain, frequent sinus or ear infections

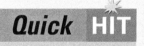

Quick HIT

All patients with a history of food allergy–induced anaphylaxis should be given an epinephrine auto-injector prescription and training.

Quick HIT

The saliva of cockroaches is more allergenic than the body and feces.

Quick HIT

Pet allergens can remain on carpets and furniture and circulate in the air for months after the pet is removed from the environment.

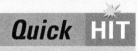

Quick HIT

Pollen counts are typically highest between 5 and 10 am and on hot, dry, windy days.

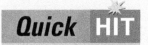

Quick HIT

The major mediator for early response is histamine.

Immunologic Disorders

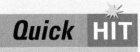

Quick HIT

The late response depends on other mediators, including chemokines, cytokines, eosinophils, basophils, and leukotrienes.

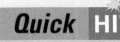

Quick HIT

Creases along the nasal bridge can result from rubbing the nose to relieve itching.

Quick HIT

Vascular congestion below the skin around the eyes can cause swelling and discoloration known as allergic shiners.

Quick HIT

Throat cobblestoning results from postnasal drip and allergens' direct effect on mucosa.

Quick HIT

Skin testing can be more accurate than blood testing owing to higher sensitivity.

Quick HIT

Second-hand smoke increases the risk of allergic complications including sinusitis and bronchitis.

Quick HIT

Air conditioning can reduce indoor humidity and mold and dust mite allergen levels.

e. Respiratory: wheezing, congestion

f. General: fatigue, snoring, irritability

2. Physical exam findings:

   a. Nasal: pale, boggy mucosa, clear rhinorrhea, nasal crease

   b. Eyes: conjunctival injection, watery, swollen lids, allergic shiners

   c. Throat: postnasal drip, cobblestoning, erythema

   d. Sinus: tenderness to percussion

   e. Respiratory: wheezing, mouth breathing

C. **Diagnosis**

1. Skin testing: bioassay in which positive results (wheal and flare) indicate the presence of allergen-specific IgE on the patient's mast cells

   a. Prick/puncture method: Drops of allergen extract are placed on the skin of the forearms or back and then pricked with a plastic device or small needle.

      i. Quick, inexpensive, no bleeding, nearly painless

      ii. Typically the most appropriate initial test and can be done in a clinical setting.

      iii. Sensitivity and specificity are dependent on type of allergen. Inhalant allergens have >85% sensitivity and specificity; for food allergens, can be <50% specificity.

   b. Intradermal method: injection of allergen extract directly into the skin

      i. Typically performed after a negative prick test

      ii. More sensitive than the prick test for inhalant allergens but has a high false-positive rate

      iii. Not used for food allergy detection owing to the possibility of systemic reactions

2. Blood (in vitro) testing: Measure patient's blood for allergen antibodies, usually via enzyme-linked immunosorbent assays (ELISA).

   a. Results are typically given as a number from 0 to 100, with a higher number denoting a higher likelihood of allergy.

   b. Number is not indicative of the severity of the response.

   c. Sensitivity and specificity vary depending on the type and quality of allergen and the type of test being used, with inhalant allergens generally producing more accurate results.

D. **Differential diagnosis**

1. Upper respiratory tract infection (URI)

2. Acute or chronic sinusitis

3. Rhinitis of other causes (vasomotor, irritant, gustatory, atrophic, drug- or disease-related)

E. **Treatment**

1. Environmental control: *avoidance* of allergens

   a. Limit outdoor activity during heavy pollen seasons.

   b. Remove pets/animals from home (although studies suggest that exposure to pets in the first year of life can decrease the risk of sensitization to allergens).

   c. Use impermeable dust-mite mattress and pillow cases.

   d. Use hard floors instead of carpet.

   e. Wash bedding weekly in hot water.

   f. Avoid smoking and second-hand smoke.

   g. Use high-efficiency particulate air (HEPA) filters.

   h. Keep doors and windows closed and use air conditioning.

2. Medications:

   a. Oral

      i. Antihistamines

         (a) First-generation H_1 blockers: more anticholinergic and central nervous system (CNS) effects

         (b) Second-generation H_1 blockers: fewer side effects, generally preferred

    ii. Decongestants reduce nasal congestion and lessen postnasal drip.

    iii. Antileukotrienes (eg, montelukast)

  b. Topical

    i. Decongestants significantly reduce nasal congestion (eg, oxymetazoline).

    ii. Intranasal corticosteroids (INS): most effective agents for allergic rhinitis

    iii. Intranasal ipratropium effective for rhinorrhea only

    iv. Intranasal cromolyn prevents inflammation rather than reversing it.

3. Allergen immunotherapy:

  a. Incremental administration (injection or oral) of allergens to affected individuals to lessen the immune response

  b. Because of **risk of anaphylaxis**, should only be given in clinical setting when capable of treating anaphylactic reactions

  c. Consider for patients with severe symptoms, concomitant asthma, medication intolerance or noncompliance, and secondary complications (sinusitis, otitis).

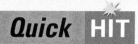

Quick HIT

HEPA filters remove 99% of dust, dander, and pollens 0.3 microns or larger.

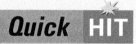

Quick HIT

Rebound congestion can occur with extended use of topical decongestants (>3 to 4 days).

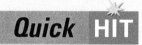

Quick HIT

INS reduces nasal symptoms and can also relieve ocular symptoms.

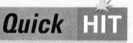

Quick HIT

Avoid antihistamines in older adults owing to anticholinergic side effects.

Immunologic Disorders

QUESTIONS

1. A 21-year-old woman presents with a history of hives that occurred soon after eating a shrimp cocktail. Which one of the following would be a correct recommendation?
   A. Serum Ig-E testing is recommended to confirm a shellfish allergy.
   B. A daily cetirizine can prevent reoccurrence.
   C. A double-blind, placebo-controlled oral food challenge is helpful to diagnose a shellfish allergy.
   D. Allergen-specific immunoglobulin G testing for shellfish would be diagnostic.

2. Which one of the following signs is NOT consistent with a food allergy?
   A. Worsening eczema after eating eggs
   B. Lip swelling after eating crab legs
   C. An infant with bloody diarrhea who takes cow's milk infant formula
   D. An adult who has developed abdominal pain and diarrhea after drinking milk

3. A 31-year-old female with a family history of a peanut allergy is considering pregnancy and asks you what she can do to prevent food allergies in her infant. Your recommendations include:
   A. Breastfeed exclusively for the first 2 years.
   B. Recommend she avoid peanuts during pregnancy and while breastfeeding.
   C. Tell her that she should hold off on starting solid foods until the infant is 9 months old.
   D. Tell her that dietary restrictions are not necessary during pregnancy and lactation.

4. A 21-year-old female patient exhibits paroxysmal sneezing, nasal pruritus, and watery rhinorrhea every morning when walking to class in the fall. What is the most likely cause of her symptoms?
   A. Vasomotor rhinitis
   B. Dust mite allergy
   C. Chronic sinusitis
   D. Ragweed allergy
   E. Mold exposure

5. A 13-year-old boy receives a pet dog for his birthday. Several weeks later, he experiences mild symptoms of rhinorrhea, postnasal drip, and nasal congestion. Which of the following measures is most appropriate to improve his symptoms?
   A. Oral loratadine
   B. Intranasal ipratropium
   C. Allergen immunotherapy
   D. Impermeable mattress and pillow covers
   E. Brushing the dog frequently

6. You determine that your 14-year-old patient is struggling to control recurrent symptoms of rhinorrhea, itchy eyes, and sneezing. She is afebrile and exam reveals pale, boggy nasal mucosa, clear rhinorrhea, and PND. You recommend which of the following as an initial step in management of her symptoms:
   A. ENT consultation
   B. Avoidance of allergens like pollen, mold, dust mites, and pet dander
   C. Oral decongestant
   D. Oral antibiotic
   E. Nasal saline irrigation

ANSWERS

1. **Answer:** C. Hives or allergic urticaria are IgE mediated and can be a cutaneous reaction to a food allergy. A careful history is needed to make a diagnosis. In this case, the urticaria occurred after eating shrimp. Ig-E testing only detects the presence of allergic sensitization and is not diagnostic for clinical food allergy. There is no medicine proven to prevent a food allergy. Allergen-specific immunoglobulin G is an unproven test for diagnosing food allergy. A double-blind, placebo-controlled food challenge is the gold standard in diagnosing a particular food allergy.

2. **Answer:** D. Eczema, angioedema, upper and lower respiratory symptoms, and upper and lower gastrointestinal symptoms are all symptoms of food-induced allergic reactions that are immune mediated. Infants who have dietary protein-induced proctitis will present with blood in the stool and no other GI symptoms. This is a non-IgE-related food allergy. Individuals with lactose intolerance are unable to digest the sugar lactose. This leads to excess fluid production in the gastrointestinal tract and diarrhea. This is not a food allergy but an intolerance.

3. **Answer:** D. Dietary restrictions are necessary during pregnancy and lactation to prevent food allergies. Family history of atopy and the presence of atopic dermatitis are risk factors for the development of food allergies. The American Academy of Pediatrics recommends breastfeeding for the first 2 years of life; however, solid foods should be started by 4 to 6 months of age.

4. **Answer:** D. The seasonal nature of the symptoms suggest an environmental allergy. The early morning timing suggests a pollen allergen, which are most prevalent between 5 and 10 am. The impact of a mold or dust mite allergy would likely impact the patient when indoors.

5. **Answer:** A. An oral antihistamine will work well to control the mild symptoms. Intranasal ipratropium can control the rhinorrhea, but not the postnasal drip and congestion. Allergen immunotherapy is indicated for more severe symptoms or patients who cannot tolerate medications. Brushing the dog frequently may actually expose the patient to more pet dander and make symptoms worse.

6. **Answer:** B. This patient's symptoms are most consistent with allergic rhinitis/environmental allergies, for which avoidance of allergens is an important initial step in management. Oral decongestants may help with her nasal symptoms, but not her eye itching. Lack of fever and clear rhinorrhea suggest allergies more than bacterial sinusitis. Nasal saline irrigation may help with congestion but is unlikely to alleviate all the patient's symptoms.

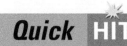

Anemia is often categorized by red blood cell size or mean corpuscular volume (MCV).

Iron deficiency without a source needs a workup for occult GI bleed.

Iron deficiency is a common cause of restless leg syndrome.

Transfusion is usually only indicated with hemoglobin less than 7 g/dL.

I. Anemia

A. Microcytic anemia

1. Iron deficiency:

   a. Characteristics

      i. Most often caused by bleeding (gross or occult)

      ii. Less commonly caused by decreased absorption owing to:

         (a) Gastric bypass

         (b) Celiac disease

         (c) Medications: proton pump inhibitors (PPIs), H_2 blockers

   b. Clinical features

      i. Weakness, fatigue, dyspnea on exertion or at rest, dizziness, pica

      ii. Commonly black or bloody stools

      iii. May have pallor, tachycardia, hypotension

   c. Diagnosis (Table 5-1)

      i. Decreased iron, ferritin, and percent saturation, increased total iron binding capacity

      ii. Consider testing for occult stool or obtaining a colonoscopy in older patients.

   d. Treatment

      i. Find and treat the source of any blood loss.

      ii. For replacement, start with oral iron. There should be a response in 2 weeks.

      iii. Consider intravenous (IV) iron in patients with continued bleeding, irritable bowel disease, or chronic kidney disease.

2. Thalassemia:

   a. Characteristics

      i. Caused by mutations in the alpha globulin or beta globulin chains of hemoglobin

      ii. Categorized as minor, intermediate, or major

TABLE 5-1	Lab Characteristics of Iron-Deficiency Anemia and Anemia of Chronic Disease	
	Iron Deficiency	**Anemia of Chronic Disease**
MCV	Low	Normal to low
Ferritin	Low	Normal to high
Serum iron	Low	Low
TIBC (transferrin)	Increased	Low
Percent saturation	Low	Normal to low

b. Clinical features
   i. Alpha and beta thalassemia minor are generally asymptomatic.
   ii. Beta thalassemia major requires lifelong transfusions.
   iii. Alpha thalassemia major is not compatible with life.
c. Diagnosis
   i. Hypochromic, microcytic anemia with normal iron stores
   ii. Red blood cell count will be disproportionately high.
d. Treatment: no specific treatment for minor thalassemias
3. Lead poisoning:
   a. Characteristics
      i. In children, it is most often from paint in older buildings
      ii. Adults may have occupational exposure.
   b. Clinical features
      i. Most children are asymptomatic.
      ii. Besides anemia, lead poisoning can also cause gastrointestinal (GI) complaints and developmental delay.
   c. Diagnosis
      i. Serum lead level equal or greater than 5 μg/dL
      ii. Basophilic stippling noted on peripheral smear
   d. Treatment
      i. It is important to find the source of exposure and remove it from the environment.
      ii. Lead levels less than 45 μg/dL should be followed closely with education of the family to ensure they are falling.
      iii. Lead levels greater than 45 μg/dL require chelation therapy.
B. **Normocytic anemia**
   1. Can be early forms of macrocytic or microcytic disease
   2. Anemia of chronic disease:
      a. Characteristics
         i. Thought to be owing to the body's response to chronic infections—classically tuberculosis
         ii. Hide iron in forms not available to bacteria, but also not available to the body
         iii. Can be caused by any disease state that causes chronic inflammation: chronic kidney disease, cancer, chronic infections
      b. Clinical features
         i. Weakness, fatigue, dyspnea on exertion or at rest
         ii. May have pallor
         iii. Less likely to have acute signs of blood loss such as hypotension or tachycardia
      c. Diagnosis
         i. Mean corpuscular volume 90 to 100 fL
         ii. Low iron and transferrin, normal percent transferrin saturation, and normal-to-high ferritin
      d. Treatment: Often treated with erythropoietin
C. **Macrocytic anemia**
   1. B_{12}/folate deficiency:
      a. Causes include:
         i. Pernicious anemia, gastritis/*H. pylori* infection, poor intake, alcohol
         ii. Gastric bypass surgery
         iii. Medications
         iv. Inherited
      b. Clinical features
         i. Folate deficiency can develop over months, whereas B_{12} stores are high enough that it may take years to show up.
         ii. B_{12} deficiency may lead to neurologic symptoms; folate deficiency will not. Neurologic symptoms include:
            (a) Numbness/tingling

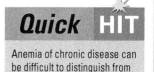

Quick HIT

Anemia of chronic disease can be difficult to distinguish from iron deficiency initially.

Disorders of the Blood

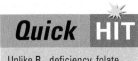

Unlike B$_{12}$ deficiency, folate deficiency does not cause confusion or delirium.

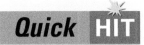

Paresthesias with B$_{12}$ deficiency are generally bilateral and in the legs more than the hands.

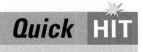

Consider checking antibodies to intrinsic factor in elderly patients with B$_{12}$ deficiency to look for pernicious anemia.

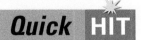

Patients with macrocytic anemia and a normal B$_{12}$/folate may need a bone marrow biopsy to further evaluate the cause.

        (b) Confusion, especially in older adults
        (c) Weakness
        (d) Impaired gait
     iii. B$_{12}$ deficiency may be associated with an increased risk for osteoporosis.
  c. Diagnosis
     i. Consider intrinsic factor antibodies in elderly patients to evaluate for pernicious anemia.
     ii. B$_{12}$ level less than 200 ng/L is always a clinically significant deficiency.
     iii. Levels between 200 and 400 ng/L may also be significant.
        (a) Methylmalonic acid (MMA) and homocysteine levels will be elevated in these cases.
        (b) MMA will be normal in folate deficiency.
  d. Treatment
     i. B$_{12}$ deficiency
        (a) Pernicious anemia must be treated with B$_{12}$ injections.
        (b) Oral replacement can be tried in other patients.
     ii. Folate deficiency: oral folate replacement
2. Other causes of macrocytic anemia to consider:
  a. Myelodysplastic disease
  b. Alcoholism, with or without B$_{12}$ deficiency
  c. Chemotherapy

II. Platelet Disorders

A. **Thrombocytopenia**
  1. Causes:
    a. Medications: heparin products, antibiotics (trimethoprim/sulfamethoxazole/penicillins), nonsteroidal anti-inflammatory drugs (NSAIDs), quinine
    b. Infection
    c. B$_{12}$/folate deficiency
    d. Pregnancy
    e. Immune thrombocytopenia (ITP)
    f. Hypersplenism
    g. Disseminated intravascular coagulation (DIC)
    h. Thrombotic thrombocytopenic purpura (TTP)/hemolytic uremic syndrome (HUS)
    i. Malignancy
  2. Clinical features:
    a. Spontaneous bleeding is unlikely with platelet counts greater than 20,000/μL.
    b. May have petechiae or purpura
    c. DIC
      i. Usually critically ill
      ii. Petechiae
      iii. Bleeding is common, although clotting is possible.
      iv. Acute kidney injury
      v. Liver dysfunction
    d. TTP/HUS
      i. Purpura
      ii. Altered mental status/seizures
      iii. Kidney failure
      iv. Fever may or may not be present
    e. Heparin-induced thrombocytopenia (HIT)
      i. Usually develops 5 to 10 days after starting heparin
      ii. Thrombosis, not bleeding
        (a) Can be venous or arterial clots
        (b) Extremity necrosis or end-organ damage possible

f. ITP
  i. Purpura and mucosal bleeding
  ii. May have infection in the preceding weeks
  iii. Evan syndrome with associated anemia
3. Diagnosis:
  a. Severe if less than 50,000/μL.
  b. Repeat complete blood count (CBC) as platelets may be falsely low owing to clumping.
  c. Rapid decreases in hospitalized patients warrant prompt workup.
    i. Peripheral smear
    ii. Coagulation studies: prothrombin time, partial thromboplastin time, and activated partial thromboplastin time
    iii. D-dimer
    iv. Fibrinogen
    v. Haptoglobin/lactate dehydrogenase (LDH)
    vi. HIT panel if appropriate
  d. ITP is a diagnosis of exclusion.
  e. May need bone marrow biopsy in elderly patient without other cause
4. Treatment:
  a. Treat the underlying disorder.
  b. Transfuse platelets only with bleeding if platelets are less than 50,000/μL.
  c. Transfuse less than 20,000/μL even without bleeding.
  d. May require splenectomy if persistent

B. **Thrombocytosis**
1. Causes:
  a. Most often reactive owing to inflammatory process: infection (acute and chronic), iron deficiency, cancer, burns, trauma, pancreatitis, surgery, asplenism, exercise
  b. Essential thrombocythemia: myeloproliferative disorder
  c. Can be falsely elevated in cryoglobulinemia
2. Clinical features: generally asymptomatic, but may see headache, vision changes, chest pain, thrombosis, bleeding
3. Diagnosis:
  a. Repeat a CBC
  b. Check ferritin and iron studies (see workup for iron-deficiency anemia)
  c. Not usually significant below 400,000 to 450,000/uL
4. Treatment:
  a. Treat the underlying disorder.
  b. Only treat if symptomatic or platelets extremely high. Use platelet-lowering drugs with a goal of 400,000/uL.

III. Disorders of Sodium

A. **Hyponatremia**
1. Causes:
  a. Hypovolemic: diuretics, dermal losses, GI losses, pancreatitis, hyperaldosteronism
  b. Euvolemic: syndrome of inappropriate ADH (SIADH) secretion, pregnancy, hypothyroidism, secondary adrenal insufficiency, primary polydipsia
  c. Hypervolemic: acute heart failure, cirrhosis
  d. Pseudohyponatremia: hyperglycemia, elevated lipids, high serum protein concentrations
2. Clinical features: nausea, headache, confusion, malaise/weakness, seizures, coma
3. Diagnosis:
  a. Serum osmolality
    i. Low in true hyponatremia
    ii. Normal indicates high lipids or protein.

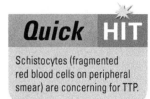

Schistocytes (fragmented red blood cells on peripheral smear) are concerning for TTP.

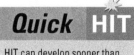

HIT can develop sooner than 5 days in patients who have been exposed to heparin in the last 30 days.

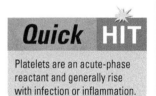

Platelets are an acute-phase reactant and generally rise with infection or inflammation.

Disorders of the Blood

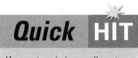

Hyponatremia is usually categorized by volume status.

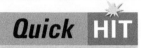

Hyponatremia is more often a problem of water regulation than a true loss of sodium.

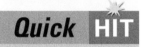

Volume-depleted patients will have similar lab studies to patients with SIADH owing to *appropriate* ADH release.

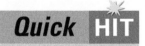

Because of thirst, hypernatremia is usually seen in people who are not able to manage their fluid intake, usually the very old and the very young.

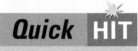

Low magnesium level is a common cause of persistent hypokalemia.

iii. High:
- (a) Hyperglycemia: Na should fall 1.6 mEq for every 100 mg/dL > 100
- (b) Alcohol ingestion
- (c) Azotemia: Corrected SOsm = SOsm − (BUN/2.8)

b. Urine osmolality: Greater than 100 mOsmol/kg indicates antidiuretic hormone (ADH) release
c. Urine Na
  i. Less than 25 mEq/L indicates hypovolemia or fluid overload.
  ii. Greater than 40 mEq/L usually indicative of SIADH
d. Thyroid-stimulating hormone
e. Cortisol

4. Treatment:
a. Avoid rapid correction, which can cause osmotic demyelination syndrome (the goal is less than 8 mEq in 24 hours).
b. Calculate the change in sodium—the expected sodium change with 1 L of fluid.
  i. The calculation is: (Fluid Na − serum Na)/(total body water + 1).
  ii. Total body water = 60% of body weight in males, 50% of body weight in females.
c. SIADH: Fluid restriction, oral salt tablets, tolvaptan

B. **Hypernatremia**
1. Causes:
a. Free water loss: sweat, GI losses, diabetes insipidus, osmotic diuresis
b. Increased salt intake: usually iatrogenic
2. Clinical features: lethargy, seizure, coma
3. Diagnosis is made by urine osmolality.
a. Should be greater than 600 mOsmol/kg
b. Less than 300 mOsmol/kg is consistent with diabetes insipidus.
4. Treatment:
a. Goal is to decrease sodium by no more than 10 mEq in a day.
b. Check Na frequently to ensure that treatment is not overcorrecting.
c. Calculate water deficit:
  i. Total body water = 60% of body weight in males, 50% of body weight in females
  ii. Water deficit = Total body water × [(Serum Na/140) − 1]
  iii. Rate of correction = Water deficit × [10 mEq/(Serum Na − 140)]

IV. Disorders of Potassium

A. Hypokalemia
1. Causes:
a. Alkalosis
b. Hypothermia
c. GI losses
d. Renal losses: low magnesium levels, diuretics, hyperaldosteronism, renal tubular acidosis
e. Iatrogenic: volume replacement with low K solutions, insulin
2. Clinical features: weakness, cramping, constipation, arrhythmias
3. Diagnosis:
a. Low potassium level
b. Electrocardiogram (ECG) changes: flattened T waves, U waves, QT prolongation
c. 24-hour urine potassium
  i. <20 mEq: nonrenal cause
  ii. >20 mEq: renal losses
4. Management:
a. Oral replacement is preferred over IV unless the K is very low (less than 2.5 mmol/L).
b. Assume a 0.1-mEq increase in serum K for every 10 mEq replaced.

Checking urine potassium is usually unnecessary unless the cause is not clear from the history.

B. **Hyperkalemia**
1. Causes:
   a. Acidosis
   b. Exercise
   c. Diabetic ketoacidosis
   d. Trauma/tissue damage
   e. Kidney failure/injury: acute and chronic
   f. Medications: potassium-sparing diuretics, angiotensin-converting-enzyme (ACE) inhibitors, NSAIDs
   g. Hypoaldosteronism
2. Clinical features: paresthesias, weakness, ascending paralysis, bradycardia/arrhythmias
3. Diagnosis:
   a. Elevated potassium level
   b. ECG changes, which progress as K increases
      i. Peaked T waves
      ii. Lengthening PR
      iii. QRS widening
      iv. Sine wave pattern
4. Management:
   a. Check the ECG.
   b. Repeat the potassium level.
   c. Stabilize the heart rhythm with calcium gluconate.
   d. Shift potassium into cells with bicarbonate, insulin, and glucose.
   e. Remove potassium from the body with kayexalate, loop diuretics, or dialysis.

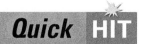

Potassium can be falsely elevated owing to hemolysis of collected blood in the tube.

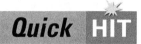

Patients in diabetic ketoacidosis (DKA) have low total body potassium, so serum potassium levels will fall rapidly with treatment of acidosis.

Disorders of the Blood

QUESTIONS

1. A 60-year-old female presents to your office with a few weeks of worsening shortness of breath with activity. She has also been feeling generally more fatigued. She denies any chest pains, abdominal pains, or melena, but has noted mildly bloody stools with increasing frequency. On exam, you note subconjunctival pallor. Lab work shows an Hb of 8.4 g/dL with an MCV of 82 fL and her stool is positive for occult blood. What would you expect her iron studies to show?

    A. High ferritin, low serum iron, low TIBC, normal percent saturation

    B. Low ferritin, high serum iron, low TIBC, low percent saturation

    C. Low ferritin, low serum iron, low TIBC, low percent saturation

    D. Low ferritin, low serum iron, high TIBC, low percent saturation

    E. High ferritin, high serum iron, low TIBC, high percent saturation

2. An 82-year-old female with a history of HTN comes to your office with complaints of bilateral hand and feet numbness as well as fatigue. She has been otherwise well. Her exam is normal with the exception of mild loss of vibration sensation in the bilateral feet. Lab work reveals fasting blood glucose of 82, an Hb of 9.9 g/dL, and MCV of 102 fL. Which of the treatments below is most likely to improve her symptoms?

    A. Metformin 500 mg PO twice daily

    B. Folic Acid 1 mg PO daily

    C. Vitamin B_{12} 1 mg IM monthly

    D. Vitamin D 50,000 U PO weekly

    E. Vitamin B_6 10 mg PO daily

3. A 41-year-old healthy female presents to the Emergency Department with rash, headache, and confusion. She has a normal cardiovascular, respiratory, and neurologic exam. Her skin exam reveals diffuse petechiae. Lab work shows hemoglobin of 9.2 g/dL, platelet count 21,000, and creatinine of 0.9 mg/dL. Peripheral smear has schisto-cytes. CT scan of the head shows no abnormalities. Which of the following lab values is likely to lead you to the correct diagnosis?

    A. Fibrinogen level

    B. ADAMTS13 activity

    C. Shiga toxin

    D. HIT antibody

    E. Anti-platelet antibody

4. An 87-year-old female with a history of HTN comes to your office with a 2-week history of worsening nausea, headache, and "feeling weak." She does not remember any inciting event. No recent illness. No vision changes or dizziness. She has had some mild weakness. She has noted some lower-extremity swelling that is worse than her baseline. She does note some shortness of breath with activity. No chest pain or palpitations. She is only tak-ing amlodipine for her blood pressure. On exam, you note dry mucous membranes. She also has mild crackles in the bases of her lungs, a 2/6 systolic murmur, and 1+ pitting edema to her knees. Lab work shows sodium of 128, potassium of 4.1, creatinine of 0.76, and hemoglobin of 11.2 g/dL. Urine osmolality is 423 and urine sodium is <20. Which of the following is the best next step to increase her sodium?

    A. Fluid restriction

    B. Lasix therapy

    C. Normal saline

    D. Hypertonic saline

    E. Salt tablets

5. A 67-year-old male with a history of HTN and ischemic cardiomyopathy presents to your office with paresthesias in his hands and feet as well as generalized weakness that has been worsening over the last few days. No other complaints and has been otherwise healthy. He was recently seen at his cardiologist's office and was started on spironolactone. His physical exam is remarkable for a 2/6 systolic murmur, but otherwise normal. Lab work reveals sodium of 142, potassium of 6.7, calcium of 8.2, creatinine of 1.47, and BNP of 102. ECG shows peaked T waves and a PR interval of 212 msec. What is the most important next step in therapy?

   A. Kayexalate

   B. Dialysis

   C. Bicarbonate

   D. Calcium

   E. Insulin

6. A 43-year-old female without past medical history comes to your office with complaints of weakness and lower extremity cramping following a 2-day GI illness involving vomiting and profuse diarrhea. The illness was self-limiting and has now resolved. Her exam is normal besides some tacky mucous membranes. Her lab work reveals a sodium of 136, potassium of 2.4, and creatinine of 0.96. ECG is normal. You prescribe potassium replacement and encourage fluids. She returns to your office 2 days later with the same symptoms. Lab work now shows sodium of 141, potassium of 2.6, and creatinine of 0.68. Which next step is most likely to help you resolve her low potassium?

   A. Repeat oral replacement

   B. Admit for IV replacement

   C. Check aldosterone level

   D. Check magnesium level

   E. Check calcium level

Questions

ANSWERS

1. **Answer: D.** You would expect the patient to have an iron-deficiency anemia likely related to a lower GI bleed. Ferritin is often the most sensitive test for iron deficiency and will be low. Ferritin is an acute-phase reactant, though, and can be elevated in situations of acute illness or inflammation. You would also expect a low iron level as well as a low percent saturation. TIBC (transferrin) is a measure of the iron transporter in the body: levels would be elevated in an attempt to make as much iron available as possible. Choice A is a typical finding for anemia of chronic disease. In this state, the body is attempting to make iron less available through the body, possibly as a way to fight chronic infections such as TB. Iron stores (ferritin) will by high, while iron and TIBC levels will be low. Choice E is a typical finding for hemochromatosis, a state of iron overload, either hereditary or secondary.

2. **Answer: C.** The patient likely has a B_{12} deficiency causing both her anemia and her neurologic complaints. She may be able to take B_{12} by mouth, but should be worked up for pernicious anemia prior to starting down that route. Diabetes Mellitus can cause a peripheral neuropathy with loss of vibration sensation; however, with a normal fasting blood sugar, this is less likely. Folic acid can cause a macrocytic anemia; however, folate deficiencies do not cause neurologic issues. Vitamin D deficiency may be associated with fatigue, but does not cause anemia or neuropathy. Vitamin B_6 deficiency is rare and is more often associated with stomatitis, cheilosis, or facial rash.

3. **Answer: B.** The patient's presentation is most consistent with TTP with petechial rash, thrombocytopenia, and neurologic symptoms. Schistocytes on peripheral smear is concerning for microangiopathic hemolytic anemia. This is when damage is caused to red blood cells as they pass through clots formed by platelets in the microvasculature. It is similar to HUS in that both will have this form of hemolysis; however, TTP generally does not result in kidney damage. Fibrinogen levels are helpful in looking for DIC. In this setting, you may have thrombocytopenia and anemia. You would expect to see elevated coagulation studies (PT & aPTT) as well as a low fibrinogen owing to consumption. The patient may also have an elevated D-dimer. Shiga toxin may be present in patients who have HUS related to Shiga toxin-producing E. coli (STEC). These patients will have microangiopathic hemolytic anemia, but will also have acute kidney injury. HIT antibody would be positive in patients who have HIT. This is most often seen in hospitalized patients 5 to 10 days after initiation of heparin, although it can be seen earlier if the patient has been exposed to heparin previously. Anti-platelet antibodies are sometimes positive in patients with ITP. These patients most often do not have anemia, though they can in Evan syndrome. They also will not have schistocytes on their peripheral smear.

4. **Answer: B.** In this case, the patient is presenting to the office with hyponatremia and signs of excess fluid on her exam. Her low sodium in this case is likely owing to fluid retention related to decreased renal perfusion from a low cardiac output. Her high urine osmolality is indicative of ADH release in this case owing to relative volume depletion. Fluid restriction is the mainstay of treatment for SIADH. These patients tend to be euvolemic as opposed to fluid overloaded as the patient above. These patients will have an elevated urine osmolality, but will also have an elevated urine sodium. Normal saline can be a good choice for treatment of hyponatremia owing to volume depletion. These patients will also have high urine osmolality and low urine sodium, but will have history and exam findings consistent with volume depletion. Hypertonic saline can be used in some cases of hyponatremia, but generally in cases of critically low sodium levels or refractory hyponatremia. Salt tablets can be helpful in some situations of hyponatremia, but in general hyponatremia is managed as a problem of water retention rather than the need for salt.

5. **Answer: D.** The patient has developed hyperkalemia likely related to the new addition of a potassium sparing diuretic. Hyperkalemia can be a life-threatening emergency owing to the likelihood of arrhythmias. The first step in treating a patient with hyperkalemia and ECG changes is to stabilize the myocardium by giving calcium gluconate. The other treatments listed are important and should be given as well to lower the potassium level and help remove excess potassium from the body, but the calcium is most important to prevent arrhythmia while the other medications take effect. Kayexalate is a medication that binds potassium in the bowels and allows it to be removed through bowel movements. It is one method of lowering potassium by removing it from the body; however, it takes time to take effect and so will not work immediately. It is also important to remember that if the patient does not have a bowel movement, then potassium will eventually be reabsorbed into the body. Dialysis is another method of reducing potassium by removing it from the body. It is generally reserved for patients whose kidneys are no longer functioning and the potassium cannot be removed by other means such as diuretics. This patient does have a mildly elevated creatinine, but likely does not meet the criteria for dialysis. Bicarbonate can be effective at lowering blood levels of potassium by shifting potassium into cells using a potassium/hydrogen transporter. It is important to remember that this method is only effective for a period of hours and that some other therapy to remove potassium from the body such as diuretics,

kayexalate, or dialysis. Like bicarbonate, insulin can lower blood levels of potassium by shifting the potassium into cells. Also like bicarbonate, it is not long acting and will need to be given with other therapy to help remove potassium from the body.

6. **Answer:** **D.** Hypomagnesemia is a common cause of low potassium levels, particularly when the potassium appears to be difficult to replace. Magnesium can be lost in similar ways to potassium such as in this case with GI losses. If her reason for potassium losses have resolved, then low potassium stores should be easy to replace, and a healthy individual may not need much in the way of replacement at all. In this case, if potassium replacement has not helped, it is best to look for another reason her potassium levels are low. The patient has not responded to PO replacement and so considering IV replacement would be reasonable. However, it is likely to have the same difficulty if her magnesium level is low. Hyperaldosteronism can cause low potassium, but in this case, GI losses are a much more likely cause. Calcium levels do not have the same impact as magnesium levels on potassium.

Answers

MENTAL DISORDERS

Jerry A. Friemoth

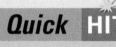

Quick HIT

Family physicians provide the majority of mental healthcare in the United States.

Quick HIT

SSRIs are the first-line medication treatment for depression and anxiety.

Quick HIT

Paroxetine is less favored in the SSRI group owing to its short half-life and increased risk of withdrawal symptoms, even with missing a few doses.

Quick HIT

Diagnosis of BAD requires a history of at least one manic episode.

I. Psychological Disorders of Adults

A. **General facts**
   1. Neuropsychiatric disorders are the leading cause of morbidity in adults.
   2. Less than one-third of adults with a diagnosable mental disorder receive treatment in a single year.
   3. Depressed patients have a largely increased risk of coronary artery disease.

B. **The major types of psychiatric disorders seen in family medicine**
   1. Affective:
      a. Major depression disorder:
         i. There is a 12-month prevalence of about 10% in women, 5% in men.
         ii. Defined as two or more weeks of persistent low mood or anhedonia causing problems in functioning, which is not a result of medical illness or substance abuse
         iii. Treatment: psychopharmacologic with selective serotonin reuptake inhibitors (SSRIs), serotonin–norepinephrine reuptake inhibitors (SNRIs), bupropion, mirtazapine; or cognitive-behavioral therapy (CBT) (Table 6-1). Ideally treatment is a combination of medication and CBT.
      b. Bipolar affective disorder (BAD):
         i. BAD I: For diagnosis, the patient needs to have a manic episode lasting *at least a week* with marked functional impairment.
         ii. BAD II: the same symptoms as BAD I, but only needs to last *at least 4 days*, and without marked functional impairment
         iii. Treatment: psychopharmacologic with lithium, lamotrigine, atypical antipsychotics; CBT and family psychoeducation
   2. Anxiety:
      a. Generalized anxiety disorder (GAD):
         i. Excessive worrying that affects functioning
         ii. Treatment: psychopharmacologic with SSRIs, SNRIs, bupropion; CBT
      b. Panic disorder:
         i. Repeated panic attacks, accompanied by fear of having another attack, or a negative change in behavior to try to avoid another attack
         ii. Treatments of choice are the same as in GAD.
      c. Social phobia:
         i. Marked distress about social situations in which the patient could be negatively evaluated by other people
         ii. These situations are avoided or endured with marked distress.
         iii. Treatment is primarily CBT, occasionally SSRIs.
      d. Agoraphobia:
         i. A marked fear of being in situations in which escape or getting help would be difficult if the patient experiences distress or embarrassing symptoms; examples include public transportation, open or enclosed spaces, being in a crowd
         ii. These situations are avoided or endured with marked distress.
         iii. Treatment is primarily CBT.

TABLE **6-1**	Cognitive-Behavioral Therapy (CBT)

CBT is a blend of two therapies: cognitive therapy (CT) and behavioral therapy. CT was developed by psychotherapist Aaron Beck, M.D., in the 1960s. CT focuses on a person's thoughts and beliefs, and how they influence a person's mood and actions, and aims to change a person's thinking to be more adaptive and healthy. Behavioral therapy focuses on a person's actions and aims to change unhealthy behavior patterns.

CBT helps a person focus on his or her current problems and how to solve them. Both patient and therapist need to be actively involved in this process. The therapist helps the patient learn how to identify distorted or unhelpful thinking patterns, recognize and change inaccurate beliefs, relate to others in more positive ways, and change behaviors accordingly.

CBT can be applied and adapted to treat many specific mental disorders.

For further information, see http://www.nimh.nih.gov/health/topics/psychotherapies/index.shtml.

3. Somatic symptom problems:
   a. Multiple distressing physical symptoms with a negative medical evaluation, causing marked worry which may become the major focus of life
   b. Illness anxiety disorder: excessive worry about having a serious medical condition
   c. Conversion disorder: problem in *voluntary muscle* or *sensory* function that is incompatible with known medical illness
   d. Treatment for all of these is primarily CBT.
4. Psychotic disorders:
   a. Schizophrenia
      i. Delusions, hallucinations, grossly abnormal speech or behavior, markedly limited emotions or motivation present for at least 6 months
      ii. Treatment: psychopharmacologic with atypical antipsychotics, family psychoeducation, CBT
   b. Brief psychotic disorder
      i. Same symptoms as above, but duration ranges from 1 day to less than 1 month
      ii. Full return to baseline functioning
      iii. Treatment as above
5. Eating disorders:
   a. Anorexia nervosa
      i. Low food intake leading to significant low weight
      ii. Fear of gaining weight/getting fat
      iii. Distorted body image
      iv. Treatment is primarily CBT and family therapy.
   b. Bulimia nervosa
      i. Excessive, binge eating in a short time interval
      ii. Loss of control of eating while binging
      iii. Harmful behaviors to prevent weight gain after binging, including fasting, excessive exercise, use of diuretics and laxatives, and forced vomiting
      iv. Treatment is primarily CBT, with SSRIs used occasionally.
   c. Binge eating disorder: binges without harmful behaviors
6. Obsessive-compulsive and related disorders:
   a. Obsessive-compulsive disorder
      i. Obsessions: recurrent distressing thoughts, images, and urges which the patient tries to alleviate by another thought or behavior
      ii. Compulsions: thoughts or behaviors like excessive hand washing, checking and rechecking, and counting, which are distressing
      iii. Treatment: psychopharmacologic with SSRIs; CBT

b. Body dysmorphic disorder
   i. Obsession with perceived flaws in appearance that others dismiss
   ii. Excessive behaviors and thoughts to address these flaws
   iii. Treatment is CBT.
c. Hoarding disorder
   i. Distress with discarding possessions of any kind
   ii. Results in such clutter that areas of the home are unusable
   iii. Treatment is CBT.
d. Trichotillomania
   i. Repeatedly pulling out hair, causing hair loss that is distressing or causes problems in functioning
   ii. Repeatedly trying to stop this behavior
   iii. Treatment is CBT.
7. Trauma and stress-related disorders:
   a. Posttraumatic stress disorder:
      i. Exposure to threatened or actual death, serious injury, or sexual violence that leads to at least 1 month of:
         (a) *Intrusive* symptoms like memories or dreams of the event, flashbacks, distress at exposure to cues of event, or
         (b) *Avoiding* any reminders of the event, or
         (c) *Negative changes* in thoughts and mood associated with the event, or
         (d) *Hyperarousal* associated with the event
      ii. Treatment: SSRIs, CBT, eye movement and desensitization reprocessing
   b. Acute stress disorder: same as above, with a duration of 3 days to 1 month after the event
8. Sexual dysfunctions:
   a. Delayed ejaculation
      i. Involuntary marked delay in or infrequency of ejaculation on nearly all occasions
      ii. Duration of at least 6 months, and causing marked distress
      iii. Treatment is primarily CBT.
   b. Erectile disorder
      i. Marked difficulty obtaining or maintaining an erection, or loss of erectile rigidity for at least 6 months
      ii. Check total testosterone.
      iii. Treatment is primarily pharmacologic: phosphodiesterase (PDE) type 5 inhibitors (sildenafil, tadalafil, vardenafil).
   c. Female orgasmic disorder
      i. Markedly delayed, infrequent, or absent orgasms
      ii. Duration of at least 6 months, and causing marked distress
      iii. Treatment is with CBT variants: sensate focus, directed masturbation.
   d. Premature ejaculation
      i. Ejaculation during sexual activity with partner within 1 minute, or before the patient wishes it
      ii. Duration of at least 6 months, occurring on almost all occasions
      iii. Treatment: SSRIs, "squeeze technique," CBT
C. **Counseling for unhealthy behaviors**
   1. Counseling can be used for smoking, alcohol and drug abuse, sedentary lifestyle, unhealthy diet, nonadherence to medical regimen, etc.
   2. Stages of change: a predictable sequence of the process of change
      a. Precontemplation: no current interest in changing behavior; give the patient a firm statement of risks and encourage thinking about the issue
      b. Contemplation: thinking about changing behavior, is ambivalent; highlight risks of behavior and benefits of change
      c. Preparation: ready to change, unsure of how to do this; help patient list options and prioritize them

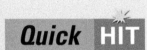

Quick HIT

Erectile dysfunction is a marker for **arteriosclerotic disease**. Check lipids and other cardiovascular risk factors.

Mental Disorders

d. Action: making positive change in behavior; applaud the change and closely monitor the patient

e. Maintenance: Change is established; review triggers of relapse and options for addressing them.

f. Relapse: common in behavior change; encourage the patient to try again. What did the patient learn in the previous attempt?

II. Substance Abuse and Addiction

A. Prevention

1. "Positive parenting":

a. Encourage parent–child interactions that work to prevent alcohol and drug initiation.

b. These include communication, encouragement, negotiation, setting limits, supervision, and knowing friends.

2. If there is a positive family history of alcohol/drug dependence, encourage abstinence.

B. Screening

1. California Society of Addiction Medicine (CAGE): One positive response requires further assessment.

a. "Have you ever felt the need to Cut down on your drinking?"

b. "Have you ever felt Annoyed by others' criticism of your drinking?"

c. "Have you ever felt Guilty about your drinking?"

d. "Have you ever needed an Eye-opener the next morning?"

2. Alcohol Use Disorders Identification Test (AUDIT): A score of 8 or higher is associated with problem use (Table 6-2).

C. **Assessment: for each class of substance, can classify as:**

1. Use disorder: problems associated with chronic use

2. Intoxication: problem symptoms of acute use

3. Withdrawal: problem symptoms of stopping prolonged or heavy use

D. **Psychopharmacology of selected substances**

1. Tobacco:

a. Nicotine replacement (gum, patches, lozenges, inhalers)

b. Varenicline (Chantix)

c. Zyban (bupropion)

2. Alcohol:

a. Disulfiram (Antabuse) interferes with the degradation of alcohol, resulting in the accumulation of acetaldehyde, which in turn produces a very unpleasant reaction including flushing, nausea, and palpitations if the patient drinks alcohol.

b. Acamprosate (Campral) acts on the gamma-aminobutyric acid (GABA) and glutamate neurotransmitter systems and is thought to reduce symptoms of protracted abstinence such as insomnia, anxiety, restlessness, and dysphoria. It is available in oral form (three-times-daily dosing).

c. Naltrexone blocks opioid receptors that are involved in the rewarding effects of drinking alcohol and the craving for alcohol. It is available in two forms: oral (Depade, ReVia), with once-daily dosing, and extended-release injectable (Vivitrol), given as once-monthly injections.

3. Opiates:

a. Methadone, a slow-acting, opioid agonist. Methadone is taken orally, so that it reaches the brain slowly, dampening the "high" that occurs with other routes of administration while preventing withdrawal symptoms. Methadone has been in use since the 1960s to treat heroin addiction and is still an excellent treatment option, particularly for patients that do not respond well to other medications; however, it is only available through approved outpatient treatment programs, where it is dispensed to patients on a daily basis.

b. Buprenorphine (Subutex, Suboxone), a partial opioid agonist. Buprenorphine relieves drug cravings without producing the "high" or dangerous side effects of other opioids. Suboxone is a novel formulation, taken

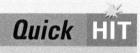

Quick HIT

Smoking is the leading preventable cause of death in the United States.

Mental Disorders

Mental Disorders

TABLE 6-2 **AUDIT**

The AUDIT

PATIENT: Because alcohol use can affect your health and can interfere with certain medications and treatments, it is important that we ask some questions about your use of alcohol. Your answers will remain confidential, so please be honest. Place an X in one box that best describes your answer to each question.

Questions	0	1	2	3	4
1. How often do you have a drink containing alcohol?	Never	Monthly or less	2 to 4 times a month	2 to 3 times a week	4 or more times a week
2. How many drinks containing alcohol do you have on a typical day when you are drinking?	1 or 2	3 or 4	5 or 6	7 to 9	10 or more
3. How often do you have 5 or more drinks on one occasion?	Never	Less than Monthly	Weekly	Daily or almost daily	
4. How often during the last year have you found that you were not able to stop drinking once you had started?	Never	Less than monthly	Monthly	Weekly	Daily or almost daily
5. How often during the last year have you failed to do what was normally expected of you because of drinking?	Never	Less than monthly	Monthly	Weekly	Daily or almost daily
6. How often during the last year have you needed a first drink in the morning to get yourself going after a heavy drinking session?	Never	Less than monthly	Monthly	Weekly	Daily or almost daily
7. How often during the last year have you had a feeling of guilt or remorse after drinking?	Never	Less than monthly	Monthly	Weekly	Daily or almost daily
8. How often during the last year have you been unable to remember what happened the night before because of your drinking?	Never	Less than monthly	Monthly	Weekly	Daily or almost daily
9. Have you or someone else been injured because of your drinking?	No		Yes, but not in the last year		Yes, during the last year
10. Has a relative, friend, doctor, or other healthcare worker been concerned about your drinking or suggested you cut down?	No		Yes, but not in the last year		Yes, during the last year
					Total

Note: This questionnaire (the AUDIT) is reprinted with permission from the World Health Organization and the Generalitat Valenciana Conselleria. De Bemestar Social. To reflect standard drink sizes in the United States, the number of drinks in question 3 was changed from 6 to 5. A free AUDIT manual with guidelines for use in primary care is available online at www.who.org.

orally, that combines buprenorphine with naloxone (an opioid antagonist) to ward off attempts to get high by injecting the medication. If an addicted patient were to inject Suboxone, the naloxone would induce withdrawal symptoms, which are averted when taken orally as prescribed. The Food and Drug Administration (FDA) approved buprenorphine in 2002, making it the first medication eligible to be prescribed by certified physicians through the Drug Addiction Treatment Act. This approval eliminates the need to visit specialized treatment clinics, expanding treatment access.

   c. Naltrexone (Depade, Revia) an opioid antagonist. Naltrexone is not addictive or sedating and does not result in physical dependence; however, poor patient compliance has limited its effectiveness. Recently, an injectable long-acting formulation of naltrexone called Vivitrol received FDA approval for treating opioid addiction. Given as a monthly injection, Vivitrol should improve compliance by eliminating the need for daily dosing. To avoid withdrawal symptoms, Vivitrol should be used only after a patient has undergone detoxification. Vivitrol provides an effective alternative for individuals who are unable to or choose not to engage in agonist-assisted treatment.

 E. **Counseling for Substance Abuse: Five A's** (Table 6-3)
 F. **Five R's** (Table 6-4)
 G. **Other drugs of abuse:** Check the web site of the National Institute of Drug Abuse www.drugabuse.gov.

III. Behavioral Problems in Children and Adolescents

 A. **Attention-deficit/hyperactivity disorder (ADHD)**
   1. A pattern of inattention and/or hyperactivity-impulsivity
   2. Duration of at least 6 months
   3. Symptoms are present before age 12.
   4. Symptoms are present in at least two settings.
   5. Symptoms cause problems with academics and relationships.
   6. Treatment:
      a. Psychopharmacologic (Table 6-5)
      b. Psychosocial
         i. Behavioral therapy: reduces problem behaviors by working with antecedents and consequences
         ii. Parent training: helps parents find ways of limiting problem behaviors by rewarding positive behaviors, doing problem-solving with the child, and setting limits on behaviors
 B. **Autism spectrum disorders**
   1. Marked deficits in social functioning and communication, as well as abnormally rigid patterns of behavior
   2. Screening with Modified Checklist for Autism in Toddlers (M-CHAT) between 16 and 30 months: http://www2.gsu.edu/~psydlr/M-CHAT/Official_M-CHAT_Website_files/M-CHAT-R_F.pdf

TABLE **6-3**	The Five A's

Successful intervention begins with identifying users and appropriate interventions based upon the patient's willingness to quit. The five major steps to intervention are the "5 A's": Ask, Advise, Assess, Assist, and Arrange.
- **Ask**: Identify and document tobacco use status for every patient at every visit.
- **Advise**: In a clear, strong, and personalized manner, urge every tobacco user to quit.
- **Assess**: Is the tobacco user willing to make a quit attempt at this time?
- **Assist**: For the patient willing to make a quit attempt, use counseling and pharmacotherapy to help him or her quit.
- **Arrange**: Schedule follow-up contact, in person or by telephone, preferably within the first week after the quit date.

Five Major Steps to Intervention (The "5 A's"). Content last reviewed December 2012. Agency for Healthcare Research and Quality, Rockville, MD. http://www.ahrq.gov/professionals/clinicians-providers/guidelines-recommendations/tobacco/5steps.html.

TABLE 6-4	The Five R's

Patients not ready to make a quit attempt may respond to a motivational intervention. The clinician can motivate patients to consider a quit attempt with the "5 R's": Relevance, Risks, Rewards, Roadblocks, and Repetition.

- **Relevance**: Encourage the patient to indicate why quitting is personally relevant.
- **Risks**: Ask the patient to identify potential negative consequences of tobacco use.
- **Rewards**: Ask the patient to identify potential benefits of stopping tobacco use.
- **Roadblocks**: Ask the patient to identify barriers or impediments to quitting.
- **Repetition**: The motivational intervention should be repeated every time an unmotivated patient has an interaction with a clinician. Tobacco users who have failed in previous quit attempts should be told that most people make repeated quit attempts before they are successful.

Patients Not Ready To Make A Quit Attempt Now (The "5 R's"). Content last reviewed December 2012. Agency for Healthcare Research and Quality, Rockville, MD. http://www.ahrq.gov/professionals/clinicians-providers/guidelines-recommendations/tobacco/5rs.html.

TABLE 6-5	ADHD Medications	
Trade Name	**Generic Name**	**Approved Age**
Adderall	Amphetamine	3 and older
Adderall XR	Amphetamine (extended release)	6 and older
Concerta	Methylphenidate (long acting)	6 and older
Daytrana	Methylphenidate patch	6 and older
Desoxyn	Methamphetamine hydrochloride	6 and older
Dexedrine	Dextroamphetamine	3 and older
Dextrostat	Dextroamphetamine	3 and older
Focalin	Dexmethylphenidate	6 and older
Focalin XR	Dexmethylphenidate (extended release)	6 and older
Metadate ER	Methylphenidate (extended release)	6 and older
Metadate CD	Methylphenidate (extended release)	6 and older
Methylin	Methylphenidate (oral solution and chewable tablets)	6 and older
Ritalin	Methylphenidate	6 and older
Ritalin SR	Methylphenidate (extended release)	6 and older
Ritalin LA	Methylphenidate (long acting)	6 and older
Strattera	Atomoxetine	6 and older
Vyvanse	Lisdexamfetamine dimesylate	6 and older

3. Early intensive behavioral therapy improves cognitive and language functioning.
4. Aripiprazole improves problem behaviors.

C. **Common behavior problems**

1. Discipline techniques: techniques work best when a *positive relationship* exists between the parent and child. Frequent brief praise or pats on the shoulder create a strong bond.

   a. Extinction: ignoring problem behavior (if not dangerous), while noticing and praising good behavior

   b. Redirecting: helping the child replace a problem behavior with good behavior (e.g., if the child is tearing leaves off house plants, pick up and show him toys)

   c. Time out: putting the child in boring location (e.g., a corner in the room) for a brief period, and making sure he has rich "time in" opportunities of engaging with parent

      d. Natural consequences: letting the child experience the consequences of misbehavior (if she breaks a toy on purpose, she doesn't have the toy anymore)

      e. Logical consequences: The parent sets the consequences (if the child throws a toy, he doesn't get to play with it any more that day).

2. Sleep issues:

      a. Very common in the first few months of age

      b. Set an established, consistent bedtime, and put the baby to bed awake.

      c. Allow a few minutes of crying when the baby awakens at night to teach the baby to "self-soothe."

3. Feeding problems:

      a. "Picky eaters"

         i. Avoid cajoling, begging, or bribing to eat nutritious foods.

         ii. Allow the child the choice of eating during the family meal; if the child doesn't eat, matter of factly take the plate away and let the child know that he can try again at the next snack/meal.

      b. Overweight/obesity

         i. Provide nutritious, balanced diet low in fat and sugar.

         ii. Limit portion size and servings.

         iii. Emphasize adequate exercise of at least 30 minutes daily and limit screen time to 2 hours a day.

4. Toilet training:

      a. Children are usually developmentally ready sometime between 18 months and 4 years of age.

      b. Avoid punitive shaming methods; use praise when the child is successful.

5. Adolescent risky behaviors: smoking, drinking, using drugs, sexual activity

      a. Make sure the teen knows your values and positions on the above behaviors.

      b. Adequate monitoring: Know where/with whom/what the teen is doing when they are out.

      c. Clear and consistent boundaries: for example, don't ride in car if the driver has been drinking

6. Exposure to adverse experiences of childhood (ACE):

      a. ACE include abuse, neglect, severe poverty, and parental absence.

      b. In these situations, with a lack of supportive caregivers, "toxic stress" results.

      c. Toxic stress has strong links to childhood and adult mental and physical diseases, and shortened lifespan.

Mental Disorders

QUESTIONS

1. You see a 35-year-old man in your office complaining of numbness in his entire right arm for last 2 days. He also states that his wife was recently in a serious motor vehicle accident and is recovering in the hospital. He has no associated neurologic symptoms and no history of neurologic disease. His neurologic exam is normal except that patient states he can't feel anything on touch and pinprick testing of his right arm. You order an electromyelogram and nerve conduction tests which are normal. What is the most likely diagnosis?

   A. Somatic symptom disorder
   B. Conversion
   C. Malingering
   D. Factitious disorder
   E. Adjustment disorder

2. A 16-year-old woman comes in with her mother who has concerns about persistent vomiting. Further history reveals that the patient has a several-month history of eating very large amounts of food and has a strong feeling of lack of control of this. Following this eating, she self-induces vomiting to help control her weight. The most likely diagnosis is:

   A. Anorexia nervosa
   B. Bulimia nervosa
   C. Binge eating disorder
   D. Body dysmorphic disorder
   E. Purging disorder

3. You see a 40-year-old man who complains of fatigue, recurrent epigastric pain, and a recent motor vehicle accident which occurred after he left a wedding reception during which he states, drank "a couple of beers." Besides asking him about the frequency and quantity of drinking alcohol, you'd like to administer a screening test for alcohol misuse. Which of these is a recognized screening test for alcohol problems?

   A. AUDIT
   B. Patient Health Questionnaire-9 (PHQ-9)
   C. Duke Health Profile
   D. Patient Health Questionnaire
   E. Life Event Checklist

4. A 28-year-old woman admits to alcohol and heroin abuse for several months. Which medication is potentially beneficial for both of these problems?

   A. Buprenorphine
   B. Remeron
   C. Naltrexone
   D. Acamprosate
   E. Disulfiram

5. A mother brings in her 24-month-old son with concerns of possible autism. You perform a thorough history which reveals some apparent problems with communication and some rigid behaviors. You wonder about administering the M-CHAT autism screen. What is the recommended age range for this?

   A. 3 to 6 months
   B. 6 to 2 months
   C. 16 to 30 months
   D. 30 to 48 months
   E. 48 to 60 months

ANSWERS

1. Answer: B. Conversion disorder is defined as a sensory or voluntary muscle symptom that is incompatible with medical explanation. Somatic symptom disorder consists of multiple distressing symptoms without a medical explanation. Malingering is a conscious feigning of symptoms for secondary gain. Factitious disorder is a conscious feigning of symptoms without secondary gain. Adjustment disorder involves emotional or behavioral symptoms related to a stressor.

2. Answer: B. Bulimia nervosa consists of recurrent food binges, which is accompanied by problematic compensatory behaviors like self-induced vomiting, misuse of laxatives or diuretics, fasting, or excessive exercise. Anorexia nervosa is avoidance of food with fear of gaining weight and distorted experience of body weight and shape; resulting in significantly low body weight. Binge eating disorder is food binging without the compensatory abnormal behavior. Body dysmorphic disorder is preoccupation with perceived flaws in appearance, but no abnormal eating patterns. Purging disorder is recurrent purging behaviors without food binges.

3. Answer: A. AUDIT is a 10-item screen which reliably identifies patients with risky drinking or alcohol abuse. PHQ-9 is a brief screen for depression. Duke Health Profile is a general health screen listing health and dysfunction measures. Patient Health Questionnaire is a general screen for behavioral health symptoms. Life event checklist screens for potentially traumatic events.

4. Answer: C. Naltrexone is an opioid antagonist with effectiveness for both opioid and alcohol dependence. Buprenorphine is a partial opioid antagonist which relieves drug craving in patients with opiate dependence. Remeron is an anti-depressant. Acamprosate acts on the GABA neurotransmitter system and reduces symptoms of protracted alcohol abstinence. Disulfiram blocks aldehyde dehydrogenase and produces noxious symptoms when alcohol is ingested.

5. Answer: C. This is the standard age range for administering the M-CHAT.

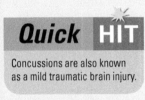

Quick HIT

Concussions are also known as a mild traumatic brain injury.

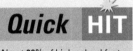

Quick HIT

About 20% of high school football players and 10% of college football players experience concussion at least once.

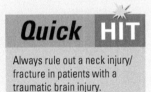

Quick HIT

Always rule out a neck injury/fracture in patients with a traumatic brain injury.

I. Concussion

A. **General characteristics**
  1. Definition:
     a. Head injury that causes a temporary loss of brain function—physical, cognitive, or emotional
     b. Felt to be a functional disruption rather than a structural disruption
     c. Imaging studies are normal.
     d. Symptoms last a very short period of time or up to 21 days (rarely longer).
  2. Causes: sports injuries, motor vehicle accidents, falls, and abuse

B. **Clinical features**
  1. May or may not have loss of consciousness
  2. Confusion or difficulty focusing (hallmark)
  3. Posttraumatic amnesia (hallmark)
  4. Headache, dizziness
  5. Nausea and vomiting
  6. Lack of coordination
  7. Photophobia
  8. Slurred speech
  9. Emotional changes—tearful, apathetic, irritable
  10. Seizure—less than 5%

C. **Diagnosis**
  1. SCAT3—Sport Concussion Assessment Tool
     a. Standardized tool used to evaluate athletes aged 13 and older who are suspected to have sustained a concussion
     b. The athlete is tested preseason to establish a baseline of the athlete's cognitive abilities, balance, and coordination abilities.
     c. After a suspected head injury, the clinician uses the assessment tool to test for symptoms and signs of concussion.
     d. This includes questions of orientation, neck exam, balance and coordination exam, and memory.
     e. The form can be found online at http://bjsm.bmj.com/content/47/5/259.full.pdf+html.
  2. Remember to check airway, breathing, and circulation status.
  3. Rule out intracranial hemorrhage.
  4. Check for immediate and delayed word recall and ability to follow commands.
  5. Check coordination, strength, speech, and recall of events of the head trauma.
  6. Check orientation such as day, week, month, and year.
  7. Check emotional status.
  8. Complete a thorough neurologic exam.

D. **Treatment**
   1. Sideline:
      a. Do not allow an athlete to return to play that day.
      b. Observe the patient for hours.
      c. Send to the emergency room if:
         i. Patient does not spontaneously open eyes on command.
         ii. Patient is not oriented.
         iii. Patient cannot follow commands.
   2. Emergency room evaluation: indications for computed tomography (CT) of the brain:
      a. Glasgow coma scale score is less than 15. This means the patient does not spontaneously open his eyes, is not oriented, or cannot follow motor commands.
      b. There has been more than one episode of vomiting.
      c. The patient is over 65.
      d. There is question of fracture.
      e. Drugs or alcohol are involved.
      f. There are any neurologic changes or seizure.
   3. Indications for hospital admission:
      a. Glasgow coma scale score is less than 15.
      b. CT is abnormal.
      c. Seizure activity occurs.
      d. Patient has increased risk of bleeds.
      e. No one is at home to observe the patient.
   4. The patient should seek immediate medical attention if:
      a. Headache increases; there is change in vision; vomiting, incontinence, stiff neck, or unexplained weakness.
      b. Seizure activity or loss of consciousness occurs.
   5. Return to play:
      a. Recovery usually takes a minimum of 7 days before an athlete can return to competition.
      b. The athlete should participate at each stage listed in Table 7-1 for at least 1 day and show no difficulty before moving to the next stage.

II. Neuropathy

A. Polyneuropathy
   1. General characteristics:
      a. Inherited or acquired diseases of the peripheral nervous system that can cause pain, decreased sensation, and disrupted motor function.
      b. Causes: See Table 7-2.

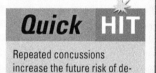

Quick HIT

Repeated concussions increase the future risk of dementia and Parkinson disease.

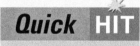

Quick HIT

Once a patient has had a concussion, he/she is more prone to get another concussion in his/her life.

TABLE 7-1	Stepwise Approach to Return to Play	
Stage	**Functional Exercise**	**Objective**
No activity	Complete rest	Recovery
Light aerobic exercise	Walking, swimming, stationary cycling	Increase heart rate
Sport-specific exercise	Skating drills for hockey, running for soccer, etc.	Add movement
Noncontact training drills	More complex drills	Exercise, coordination, and cognitive load
Full contact practice	After medical clearance	Restore confidence and skills
Normal play		

Reproduced from Consensus Statement on Concussion in Sport: the 3rd International Conference on Concussion in Sport held in Zurich. McCrory P, Meeuwisse W, Johnston K, Dvorak J, Aubry M, Mooloy M, Cantu R. 43:i76-i84. 2009, with permission from BMJ Publishing Group Ltd.

TABLE 7-2 Causes of Peripheral Neuropathy

Infectious	HIV, viral hepatitis, leprosy, Lyme disease, syphilis
Nutritional Deficiencies	B_6, B_{12}
Drugs	Amiodarone, chloroquine, heroin, hydralazine, isoniazid, metronidazole, nitrofurantoin, phenytoin, statins, vincristine
Hem/onc	Lymphoma, multiple myeloma, monoclonal gammopathy, paraneoplastic syndrome
Genetic	Charcot-Marie-Tooth
Toxins	Diphtheria, ethanol, heavy metals, organophosphates, tetanus, tic paralysis
Other	Chronic liver disease, diabetes mellitus, end-stage kidney or renal disease, hypothyroidism, amyloidosis, Guillain-Barre, porphyria

Diseases of the Nervous System

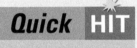

Pain and altered sensation generally precede motor symptoms.

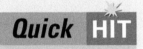

It may take 6 weeks or more of symptoms before EMG changes are detected.

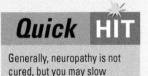

The most common cause of neuropathy is long-standing diabetes.

Quick HIT

Generally, neuropathy is not cured, but you may slow progression.

2. Clinical characteristics:
   a. Involves multiple nerves
   b. Symmetrical sensory loss, pain, or weakness in the distal lower extremities
   c. Longer nerves are usually affected first (eg, feet).
3. Diagnosis:
   a. Obtain a good history: family history of neuropathy, history of toxin exposure, past medical history (eg, diabetes or alcohol abuse), medications.
   b. May present with decreased pin prick, absent deep tendon reflex, or pain
   c. Hereditary neuropathy patients may have pes cavus or hammer toes.
   d. Electromyography (EMG) or nerve conduction studies (NCS) may help confirm the neuropathy and determine if the disease is axonal or demyelinating.
4. Treatment:
   a. Treat underlying cause if found.
   b. Duloxetine, pregabalin, gabapentin, and amitriptyline can be used to decrease pain.
   c. Physical medicine consultation may help with braces or other walking aids.
B. **Mononeuropathy**
   1. Involvement of a single nerve, usually owing to entrapment, compression, or trauma
   2. Carpal tunnel syndrome:
      a. The most common mononeuropathy seen in primary care.
      b. Risk factors: diabetes, repetitive wrist activities, rheumatoid arthritis, hypothyroidism, obesity, and family history. Some cases are idiopathic.
      c. Presents with numbness, pain, or tingling in the thumb, index, long, and half of the ring finger, often awakening the patient at night
      d. Weakness and atrophy of the thenar eminence are late findings.
      e. The diagnosis is made clinically by subjective symptoms, positive Tinel's and Phalen's signs, and EMG.
      f. Treatment: removing repetitive flexion extension action of the wrist, splints, nonsteroidal anti-inflammatories, steroid injections, and surgery if all fails
   3. Tibial tarsal syndrome:
      a. Compression of the tibial nerve
      b. Burning, pain, and numbness on the bottom of the foot, primarily the sole, but can extend to the toes and into the heel
      c. Treatment: nonsteroidal anti-inflammatory drugs (NSAIDs), orthotics, braces, cortisone shots, or surgery
   4. Sciatica:
      a. Compression of a spinal nerve as it exits the spinal canal
      b. Causes: arthritic spurs, herniation of a disc, spinal stenosis, compression fracture, or tumor

c. Symptoms: pain, burning, numbness in the posterior or lateral leg. If the pain extends to the ankle or foot, it is more likely true sciatica.

d. The most commonly compressed are lumbar spinal nerves L4-S1.

e. Treatment: physical therapy, weight loss, anti-inflammatories, epidural shots, and surgery

5. Ulnar nerve compression:

a. Presents with numbness, pain, and tingling in the fourth and fifth finger if the ulnar nerve is compromised at the elbow

b. The cause is repetitive flexion of the elbow or pressure on the ulnar nerve at the elbow.

c. Presents with pain and weakness

d. Treatment: NSAIDs, bracing arm in extension while sleeping, avoid leaning on elbow, surgery

III. Seizures

A. **General characteristics**

1. Definitions:

a. Seizure: a disorder primarily in the cerebral cortex where groups of neurons discharge in an abnormal fashion. The effect varies from jerking movements that are uncontrolled and associated with loss of consciousness (tonic-clonic) to brief episodes lasting seconds with loss of awareness but no loss of consciousness (absence seizures).

b. Epilepsy: recurrent unprovoked seizures that occur at least 24 hours apart

c. Types of seizures:

   i. Grand mal (tonic-clonic seizure): The patient quickly loses consciousness and may moan or scream followed by exaggerated muscle twitching or violent muscle jerking. The patient may bite the tongue or lose control of the bladder. This is followed by a post-ictal state, in which the patient is very somnolent, confused, may have loud snoring, and has complete amnesia for the event. The seizure can be the primary disorder or may come from generalization of a partial seizure.

   ii. Absence seizure (petit mal seizure): a brief (20 seconds or less) loss and then return to awareness. The first attack usually occurs when the patient is under age 13 years. The attack may be followed by lethargy but no post-ictal state. The patient will stop talking or slow talking, have a blank stare, and there is an abrupt stop to ongoing activity. Sometimes, the episode will end if the person is yelled at. It can be induced by hyperventilation or intermittent photic stimulation. Electroencephalogram (EEG) has classic spike and slow pattern.

   iii. Partial (focal) seizures originate in localized area of the cortex. The patient may or may not lose consciousness.

   (a) Focal seizure without impairment of consciousness (previously known as simple partial seizure)

      (i) Motor seizure: focal motor abnormality such as head or eye turning, vocalizations. Sometimes, the motor activity spreads anatomically, called Jacksonian seizure.

      (ii) Sensory seizure: feelings of vertigo, auditory or olfactory symptoms, paresthesias, or vision phenomena such as flashing lights

      (iii) Autonomic seizure: sweating, pupillary changes, and piloerection

   (b) Focal seizure with impairment of consciousness (previously known as complex-partial) does affect consciousness and is associated with actions such as aimless walking, chewing, lip smacking, or other complex motor behaviors.

2. Causes are dependent on age:

a. Neonates (less than 1 month): genetics, hypoxia at birth, intracranial bleed or trauma, infection (particularly central nervous system [CNS]),

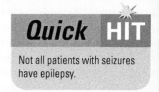

Quick **HIT**

Not all patients with seizures have epilepsy.

Diseases of the Nervous System

drug withdrawal, hypoglycemia, hypocalcemia, pyridoxine deficiency, hypomagnesemia, hyponatremia
   b. Infants and children: febrile seizures, CNS infection, genetic and developmental disorders, trauma, idiopathic, birth asphyxia
   c. Adolescents: drug or alcohol withdrawal, brain tumor, CNS infection, trauma, genetic disorder, idiopathic
   d. Adults: alcohol withdrawal and illicit drug use, brain tumor, trauma, metabolic disorder (eg, uremia, liver failure, hypoglycemia, and electrolyte abnormalities), cerebrovascular disease, degenerative CNS diseases, idiopathic (Table 7-3)
B. **Diagnosis**
   1. Differential diagnosis:
      a. Psychological conditions: hyperventilation, psychogenic seizure
      b. Basilar or confusional migraine
      c. Movement disorders: myoclonus, tics, choreoathetosis
      d. Syncope: vasovagal, arrhythmia, orthostatic hypotension, severe aortic stenosis
      e. Sleep disorders: narcolepsy, benign sleep myoclonus
      f. Drug and alcohol related: psychoactive drugs such as hallucinogens, delirium tremens, or alcoholic blackouts
      g. Transient ischemic attack (TIA)
      h. Hypoglycemia
      i. Hypoxia
      j. Pediatric situations: sleepwalking, night terrors, breath-holding spells
   2. Evaluation:
      a. Take a thorough history and physical, paying particular attention to medication and alcohol use, drug abuse, and past medical history.
      b. If the patient has a history of epilepsy and is on medication, check the serum levels of the antiepileptic therapy.
      c. Lab tests: toxicology screen and alcohol level, complete blood count (CBC), glucose, electrolytes, magnesium and calcium, liver function tests
      d. Imaging: magnetic resonance imaging (MRI) if other tests do not reveal a cause
      e. EEG may help to rule out pseudo seizures and help define the kind of seizure.
      f. If infection is suspected: lumbar puncture, blood, urine, and spinal fluid cultures
C. **Treatment**
   1. Patients with epilepsy should have a neurology consultation.
   2. Goals: controlling seizures, improved quality of life, and minimize side effects
   3. No treatment is needed for an isolated seizure with a reversible cause.
   4. Pharmacotherapy:
      a. Medication is based on the type of seizure, patient circumstances, and patient preference.

> **Quick HIT**
>
> EEG can have a high false-negative rate for detecting patients with seizures.

TABLE 7-3 Drugs and Medical Interventions That Can Cause Seizures	
Sedatives	Benzodiazepines, alcohol, barbiturates
Drugs of abuse	Cocaine, PCP, methylphenidate, amphetamines
Pain meds and anesthetics	Meperidine, tramadol, local anesthetics, class 1B agents
Psychotropics	Antidepressants, antipsychotics, lithium
Antibiotics/antiviral	B-lactam, quinolones, acyclovir, isoniazid, ganciclovir
Immunosuppressants	Cyclosporine, interferons, tacrolimus, monoclonal antibodies to T cells
Others	Flumazenil, radiographic contrast

b. Status epilepticus: The drug of choice is lorazepam IV. For children, buccal or intranasal midazolam can be used.

c. Monitor:

   i. B_{12} and folate

   ii. Drug levels: If patient is not controlled, patients has side effects, or to check for compliance

   iii. Bone density if on phenytoin, phenobarbital, primidone, or carbamazepine

d. Discontinuation: can consider stopping medication if there has been no seizure in 2 to 4 years

5. Intense education for the patient and family is mandatory. Patients should keep a diary of seizures and log triggers.

6. Patients who wish to conceive must get consultation from a neurologist as many of the drugs cause birth defects.

7. Safety:

a. Limit alcohol to two drinks per day.

b. Driving: not allowed if epilepsy is not under control

c. Work: Understanding of the patient's job requirements will help protect the patient from danger during an attack.

d. There has been an increase in suicide in epileptic patients; it is not clear if this is from the epilepsy or the treatment.

8. Impaired cognition is linked to epilepsy and to the drugs used.

IV. Febrile Seizures

A. **Characteristics**

1. Two to four percent of children under 5 will have at least one.

2. Most common at age 12 to 18 months

3. No CNS infection

4. Temperature is greater than 38°C.

5. Etiology unknown

6. May happen within 24 hours of DTaP or 8 to 14 days after MMR

7. About 10% to 20% have first-degree relatives who have had a febrile seizure.

B. **Diagnosis**

1. Benign febrile seizure lasts less than 15 minutes, there are no focal findings, and there is only one seizure in 24 hours. After the seizure, the child appears normal.

2. Complex febrile seizure lasts more than 15 minutes, there is more than one seizure in 24 hours, or there are focal features and the child may have post-ictal state.

3. Workup is recommended for complex seizure or if the child is under 12 months of age.

4. Workup includes lumbar puncture, blood cultures, glucose, and electrolytes.

C. **Treatment**

1. Prognosis is good.

2. Recurrence occurs in 30% of patients. It is more likely if the first seizure was in a younger child, there is a family history of febrile seizures, the seizure happens soon after the fever starts, and if the seizure is triggered by a relatively low fever.

3. Seizure medications are not recommended for benign seizures to prevent recurrence.

V. Stroke

A. **Characteristics**

1. Definition:

a. Stroke, or cerebrovascular accident (CVA), is a loss of brain function owing to changes of the blood circulation of the brain.

   i. Ischemic stroke is caused by a blockage of blood circulation by an arterial embolism, a thrombus, or generalized hypoperfusion.

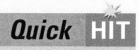

Fifty percent of patients will be adequately treated with the first drug tried. With combination treatment, 80% of patients become seizure-free.

Quick HIT

Antiseizure drugs that are enzyme-inducing, such as phenytoin, phenobarbital, and carbamazepine, have drug interactions with warfarin and some cancer drugs and antibiotics.

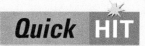

Workup is usually not necessary for febrile seizures unless they are complex.

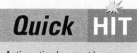

Antipyretics have not been shown to prevent febrile seizures.

Diseases of the Nervous System

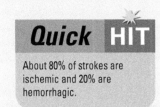

ii. Hemorrhagic stroke is bleeding into the subarachnoid space or into the brain parenchyma itself.

   b. When a patient has a stroke, the affected area of the brain cannot function, resulting in impairments of movement, vision, speech, or understanding.

2. Risk factors: hypertension, hyperlipidemia, diabetes, smoking, atrial fibrillation, advanced age, previous stroke or TIA; M:F risk 4:1

3. Causes:

   a. Thrombotic stroke: Clot forms around atherosclerotic area or around inflamed vessels (arteritis or vasculitis). Stroke happens more slowly or stepwise than a hemorrhagic stroke.

      i. May involve large vessel carotid or intracranial small vessels (lacunar); lacunar strokes are often asymptomatic and found incidentally on imaging

      ii. This is the leading cause of death in sickle cell patients.

   b. Embolic stroke: blockage of an artery by a blood clot, air emboli, bacterial clump, fat cells, or even cancer clusters that travel from a distal site

      i. Symptoms happen suddenly and are maximal at onset.

      ii. May resolve if the blockage breaks up

      iii. The most common source is the heart owing to atrial fibrillation, valvular thrombi, heart attack, valvular infection, or septal defect.

   c. Hypoperfusion: lack of adequate oxygen-carrying blood to perfuse the brain. This can be due to severe systemic bleeding, heart failure, severe hypoxia, pulmonary emboli, or myocardial infarct.

   d. Hemorrhagic stroke: subarachnoid or intracerebral bleed

      i. Often present with headache. Not true for embolic and thrombotic strokes

      ii. Most commonly from uncontrolled hypertension

      iii. Arteriovenous (AV) malformation

      iv. Secondary bleed from ischemic stroke

      v. Bleeding disorder or patient is on blood thinners

      vi. Amphetamine use (does not cause ischemic stroke) or cocaine abuse (can cause hemorrhagic or ischemic stroke)

      vii. Head trauma

      viii. Aneurysmal rupture

      ix. Tumors

B. **Clinical features**

1. Sudden onset of unilateral facial paralysis or weakness, unilateral limb weakness or paralysis, or abnormal speech

2. Cerebral stroke presents with aphasia, dysarthria, visual field defect, confusion, changes of memory, or changes in movement of face, limbs, or vision.

3. Cerebellar stroke presents with ataxia, vertigo, nystagmus, and incoordination.

4. Brainstem strokes affect the cranial nerves, impacting vision, hearing, taste, etc., depending on the location and which cranial nerve is affected.

5. Loss of consciousness can occur with increased intracranial pressure in hemorrhagic strokes but not usually in thrombotic strokes.

6. Subarachnoid hemorrhoid has an abrupt onset, usually from aneurysm rupture causing "the worse headache of my life." The patient may have loss of consciousness, seizure, stiff neck, or nausea. Usually there are no focal neurologic signs.

C. **Diagnosis**

1. Clinical neurologic findings as listed above.

2. Differential diagnosis: seizure, syncope, hypoglycemia, complex migraine, psychogenic

3. Imaging:

   a. Noncontrast CT: quick, less expensive, better at finding hemorrhagic stroke, usually done as the initial imaging study

   b. MRI with contrast: takes more time, more expensive, better for early detection of ischemic stroke

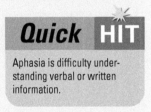

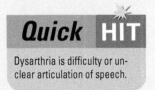

4. Labs: glucose, drug screen, prothrombin time, partial prothrombin time, complete blood count, lipids. Erythrocyte sedimentation rate (ESR) if vasculitis is suspected

5. Lumbar puncture: done if subarachnoid hemorrhage is suspected and imaging is nonrevealing

6. Carotid Doppler and echocardiogram with or without bubble study in patients with ischemic stroke

D. **Treatment**

1. General:

   a. Cautious lowering of blood pressure; aggressive blood pressure lowering can lead to worsening of the stroke

   b. Preventing aspiration; consider a swallowing study

   c. Early mobilization as clinically indicated; consult physical therapy, occupational, and speech therapy

   d. Prevent pressure sores.

2. Acute ischemic stroke:

   a. Consider thrombolysis: The risk of causing intracranial bleed is 6% and is more common in diabetics, the elderly, and in very severe strokes.

   b. Aspirin if not contraindicated

   c. Consider anti-embolus measures.

3. Hemorrhagic stroke: surgical consultation

VI. Tremors

A. **Characteristics**

1. Definition:

   a. Involuntary rhythmic muscle contractions of one or more body parts with back-and-forth movements of the hands, face, eyes, arms, trunk, legs, or voice

   b. Hand tremors are the most common.

   c. The most common of all the movement disorders

   d. Can be pathologic or physiologic owing to stress normal stimulation of adrenaline

2. Causes:

   a. Resting tremors are evident when the affected body part is completely supported against gravity and completely at rest; it disappears or lessens when the body part is voluntarily in motion.

      i. Parkinson disease:

         (a) The most common cause

         (b) Can at first be unilateral, can affect the tongue and jaw but not the head, and usually the tremor is not very obvious in the legs or feet

         (c) Other signs include bradykinesia, mask-like facies, seborrhea dermatitis, and micrographia.

      ii. Others include midbrain injury (Rubral tremor) from stroke, trauma, or demyelinating diseases, Wilson disease, and other hepatocerebral degeneration.

   b. Postural tremors are seen when the arms or head are positioned against gravity, for example, hands are held straight out in front of the patient.

      i. Physiologic tremor: seen in normal patients only when they are nervous, frightened, fatigued, have ingested caffeine, have hyperthyroidism, are on stimulants, or beta adrenergic agonists for asthma, or withdrawing from alcohol

      ii. Essential tremor:

         (a) The most common neurologic cause of postural tremor

         (b) Frequency increases with age.

         (c) Occurs in up to 5% of the population

         (d) Familial 50% of the time

         (e) Tends to be symmetrical, and can cause head tremor. It can affect the voice, chin, and trunk. It rarely affects the legs.

      (f) Worse at the end of a goal-directed activity such as finger-to-nose testing. Caffeine does not worsen but small quantities of alcohol reduce the tremor.

   iii. Cervical dystonia: head tremor but no hand tremor

 c. Kinetic tremors include action and intention tremors.

   i. Action tremors: unchanged during the voluntary movement

      (a) Essential tremors are action and postural tremors.

      (b) Primary writing tremor: exclusively while writing and not during other voluntary acts. Treatment is with anticholinergic drugs and not propranolol.

      (c) Orthostatic tremor: affects trunk and legs and occurs only while standing

      (d) Cerebellar tremors: can be action tremors and associated with ataxia and dysmetria. May have head titubation

   ii. Intention tremors: increase during the course of goal-directed movement; occur owing to upset anywhere along the cerebellar outflow pathway from the cerebellum to the thalamus

      (a) Causes include midbrain stroke or trauma, multiple sclerosis, Wilson disease, mercury poisoning, and hepatocerebral degeneration

      (b) Tremor worsens as hand moves closer to its target, large amplitude, patients often have ataxia, titubation, and dysmetria

 d. Psychogenic tremor: inconsistent findings that do not fit for known tremors, may have mixed features of resting and kinetic tremors, any part of the body can be involved and often do not respond to any treatments

B. **Diagnosis**
1. Largely based on history and clinical findings
2. Evaluate the tremor at rest, with arms extended, and with goal-directed activity.
3. Labs: may include tests for Wilson disease, thyroid disease, mercury or arsenic poisoning
4. Imaging: MRI of the brain may help if tumor or stroke is suspected.

C. **Treatment**
1. Physiologic tremors: Reduce or remove the cause.
2. If anxiety is the cause, propranolol can be used prior to activities that may increase the stress.
3. Parkinson disease:
   a. No treatment is needed for mild disease. Begin treatment when function becomes compromised.
   b. Carbidopa-levodopa is usually the first-line treatment.
   c. Dopamine agonists (ineffective in patients who do not respond to levodopa)
   d. Anticholinergic drugs: used for younger patients with tremor as the prominent problem. Do not use in older or demented patients owing to anticholinergic properties.
4. Orthostatic tremors: may respond to clonazepam or gabapentin
5. Essential tremor:
   a. First-line treatment is propranolol or primidone, as needed or continuous.
   b. Alternative medications: gabapentin, topiramate, and nimodipine
   c. Alcohol: Small amounts before meals or social events can be helpful. Tolerance to the beneficial effects can happen with regular prolonged use.
   d. Deep brain stimulation and unilateral thalamotomy are indicated for severe refractory essential tremors.
   e. Botox injections can have a modest benefit.
6. Cerebellar tremor: No good treatments are available.

QUESTIONS

1. A football player is involved in a head-to-head impact on the football field. He gets up but initially he is staring off and does not seem to know where he is and does not initially answer questions about the date or the season. However, over the next 5 minutes, he is oriented to place, date. He is able to follow commands. He has vomited three times but now states that he is fine. He is on no home medications and did not lose consciousness. Your next step is
    A. Send him to the emergency room.
    B. Allow him to return to the game in 15 minutes.
    C. Allow him to return to playing in 30 minutes.
    D. Advise him that he will not be able to play football again for a minimum of 1 year.
    E. Advise him to drink plenty of water and return to football practice tomorrow.

2. A 62-year-old overweight, hypertensive patient who smokes marijuana regularly and drinks 10 beers a day presents with an upper respiratory illness with fever, chills, cough, and congestion. He is not short of breath. He is found to have a viral infection and sent home on nonnarcotic cough medication and a decongestant. Three days later, he returns with leg weakness, leg pain, and absent knee reflexes. His exam reveals no rash, shortness of breath, and normal sensation in feet but needs help to walk. He most likely has which of the following:
    A. New onset diabetes from the sugar in the cough medication you gave him
    B. Alcoholic neuropathy brought out by the decongestant
    C. Guillain-Barre syndrome
    D. Bilateral disc herniation brought on by his excessive coughing

3. A 50-year-old iron worker presents to the emergency room after witnessed loss of consciousness and his eyes rolling back in his head. There was slight jerking that lasted 10 seconds or less. He had been off work for the last 3 days for vomiting and diarrhea and was working in a foundry that day in 110°C weather. He has no history of seizures; he did not bite his tongue nor lose bladder control. He is on no medication with the exception of anti-nausea medication and a bismuth product for diarrhea. His exam is normal in the emergency room. The most likely cause of his symptoms is:
    A. Tonic-clonic seizure triggered by his anti-nausea medication
    B. Absence seizure triggered by exposure to bismuth
    C. Partial-complex seizure from iron oxide inhalation
    D. He passed out from dehydration and did not have a seizure.

4. A 60-year-old hypertensive, diabetic, smoker presents with a sudden onset of complete paralysis of use of his left arm and leg and inability to speak.
    A. The patient most likely has a left pons infarct.
    B. The patient most likely had a right cerebellar thrombotic infarct.
    C. The patient most likely had a right subarachnoid hemorrhage.
    D. The patient most likely had a right cerebral thrombus.
    E. The patient most likely had a right cerebral embolic stroke.

5. A 69-year-old man presents with tremor of his head and hands that he has had for 5 years but is getting worse. He does not take any medications for asthma or decongestants or other stimulants. The tremor gets worse when nervous, is bilateral, and he advises you that his mother and daughter also have a tremor. On exam, he has a fine tremor of his head, some voice quivering, and fine tremor of his hands that are not worse with finger-to-nose evaluation.

A. The gentleman has classic Parkinson syndrome and treatment with carbidopa-levodopa at low dose is appropriate.

B. This man would best be evaluated with a noncontrast MRI.

C. He has a cerebellar tremor and clonazepam will help.

D. He has an essential tremor and may benefit from propranolol.

Questions

ANSWERS

1. **Answer: A.** The patient should be instructed to go to the emergency room since he had vomiting. Any loss of consciousness, prolonged disorientation, ingestion of alcohol or drugs, or if the patient was on blood thinners would warrant a trip to the emergency room.

2. **Answer: C.** He has Guillain-Barre syndrome. He has a motor neuropathy that was triggered by a viral infection. Diabetes does not present with neuropathy; it happens after years of high sugars. Alcoholic neuropathy presents with a sensory neuropathy, not a motor neuropathy. Herniated discs rarely present with bilateral symptoms.

3. **Answer: D.** He most likely passed out owing to dehydration. When a person faints, often witnesses will note that the eyes roll upward and there may be some jerking movements. To an untrained eye, this looks like a seizure. Grand mal seizures usually last longer, there is a post-ictal state and anti-nausea medication has not been known to trigger. Absence seizures do not cause loss of consciousness and there is no history of bismuth as a seizure trigger. Partial-complex seizures are not triggered by environmental exposure.

4. **Answer: E.** The patient most likely had a right cerebral embolic stroke. The presentation was on the left and that corresponds to trauma in the left brain. The sudden onset suggests embolic stroke rather than thrombotic stroke which is slower in presentation. Infarct of the pons affects cranial nerves. Infarct of the cerebellar area is most likely to cause vertigo and nystagmus. Subarachnoid hemorrhages classically present with severe headache and no focal findings.

5. **Answer: D.** Essential tremor. In Parkinson disease, there is no head tremor. There may be jaw or tongue tremor but not the head. Generally imaging does not help diagnose the cause of a tremor. Clonazepam helps orthostatic tremors and not essential tremors.

8 CARDIOVASCULAR
DISORDERS
Edward Onusko

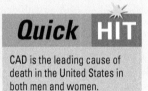

I. Coronary Artery Disease
A. General characteristics
1. Definition:
a. Coronary artery disease (CAD) is the presence of reduced blood flow through the coronary arteries owing to narrowing of the lumen.
b. Acute manifestations of CAD include unstable angina (UA), non-ST segment elevation myocardial infarction (NSTEMI), and ST segment elevation myocardial infarction (STEMI) (Table 8-1).
2. Epidemiology:
a. In the United States, about one in three adults (71 million people) have some form of cardiovascular disease (CVD).
b. Of these, about 13 million have CAD and 9 million have angina.
c. About 23% of men and 15% of women ages 60 to 79 have CAD.
d. At ages ≥ 80 years, that rises to 33% of men and 22% of women.
3. Cause:
a. The accumulation of atheromatous plaque in the coronary artery lumen causes most CAD.
b. Vasculitis, radiation exposure, cocaine, and congenital coronary anomalies may result in restricted blood flow.
c. Increased cardiac demand may also induce or worsen cardiac ischemia owing to tachycardia or sudden marked elevation of blood pressure (BP).

TABLE 8-1 Acute Coronary Events				
Acute Event	**ST Elevations on ECG**	**Cardiac Enzymes**	**% of Acute Coronary Events**	**Pathophysiology**
Unstable angina	No	Negative	60	Less severe, partial ischemia
Non-ST elevation myocardial infarction	No	Positive	27	Usually owing to a sudden narrowing of a coronary artery lumen, though it may be the result of an increased myocardial demand.
ST elevation myocardial infarction	Yes	Usually positive (unless early intervention prevents myocardial damage)	13	An acute event caused by rupture and thrombus formation in coronary artery plaque

d. Decreased coronary artery perfusion owing to hypovolemia or septic shock

e. Global hypoxia

4. Genetics: There is a significantly increased risk of CAD in patients with a first-degree relative (parent, sibling, or child) with an early clinical manifestation of CAD (<55 years of age in males, <65 years in females).

5. Risk factors:

a. Advancing age

b. Family history (as above)

c. Hyperlipidemia

d. Hypertension

e. Diabetes mellitus (DM) 1 and 2

f. Tobacco use (smoking)

g. Obesity

h. Waist circumference >40 inches for men, >35 inches for women

i. Sedentary lifestyle

j. Personal history of CVD—peripheral arterial disease, ischemic stroke, aortic aneurysm

6. Pathophysiology (Figure 8-1):

a. Coronary artery plaque may be stable ("hard") and result in slow progression of narrowing and gradual onset of symptoms.

b. The plaque material may be unstable ("soft"), and acutely rupture. This acute event causes a sudden narrowing of the vessel lumen, resulting in UA, NSTEMI, or STEMI.

B. **Clinical features**

1. Historical findings (symptoms):

a. Angina pectoris is the initial manifestation in about 50% of patients.

b. Typical angina is brought on by exertion, relieved with nitrates or rest, and is perceived as a substernal heaviness, pressure, or pain that may radiate to the jaw or shoulder.

c. CAD may present as asymptomatic "silent ischemia" or sudden cardiac death.

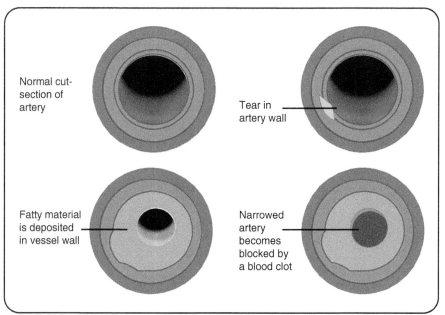

FIGURE

8-1 Coronary artery disease. Endothelial damage, followed by plaque accumulation, followed by acute hemorrhage in the plaque.

(From www.cdc.gov.)

2. Physical exam findings (signs):
   a. May be accompanied by diaphoresis or tachycardia
   b. Chest wall tenderness suggests but does not necessarily confirm a musculoskeletal etiology for the symptoms.

C. **Diagnosis**
   1. Differential diagnosis:
      a. Nonischemic cardiac causes: pericarditis, aortic stenosis, mitral valve prolapse, coronary vasospasm
      b. Gastrointestinal: gastroesophageal reflux, esophageal spasm
      c. Musculoskeletal: costochondritis, muscle strain, myositis
      d. Respiratory: pneumonia, pleuritis
      e. Vascular: pulmonary embolus, aortic dissection
      f. Neuropathic: herpes zoster
      g. Psychiatric: anxiety
   2. Laboratory (in the nonacute setting):
      a. Electrolytes, renal function, complete blood count, thyroid function (TSH), and hepatic function are usually normal.
      b. Lipid profile often shows high cholesterol levels.
   3. Imaging: Chest X-ray should be done to evaluate heart size and pulmonary status.
   4. Other findings:
      a. A 12-lead electrocardiogram (ECG) may show ischemia, previous infarction, cardiac chamber hypertrophy, or rhythm abnormality.
      b. Transthoracic echocardiogram is useful for:
         i. Estimating left ventricular ejection fraction (LVEF) to assess the functional status of the heart
         ii. Screening for valvular disease
         iii. Documenting atrial or ventricular hypertrophy
         iv. Looking for wall motion abnormalities that suggest previous myocardial infarction (MI)
      c. Cardiac stress testing (Table 8-2):
         i. Patients with a low pretest probability are likely to have an unacceptably high rate of false-positive tests. Routine screening of asymptomatic individuals is not recommended.
         ii. For patients being evaluated for chest discomfort, diagnostic stress testing is most helpful for patients with a moderate pretest probability of CAD.

TABLE 8-2 Cardiac Stress Testing		
Stressor	**Measurement of Response to Stress**	**Examples**
Exercise (usually walking on a treadmill) **Pharmacologic:** dobutamine, persantine, adenosine, regadenoson	Patient symptoms Patient appearance ECG changes: ST/T changes Bradycardia Greater than expected tachycardia arrhythmias ECG—ventricular wall motion abnormalities Nuclear perfusion studies of coronary blood flow Cardiac MRI perfusion imaging	Standard **treadmill stress test:** Patient walks on a treadmill according to a standard protocol (stressor) while symptoms, appearance, and continuous ECG monitoring are observed (measurements of response to stress) **Lexiscan:** Intravenous regadenoson is given (stressor) and coronary perfusion is measured by a nuclear perfusion test (measurement of response to stress)

     iii. In patients with a high pretest probability for CAD, for whom a negative stress result may well be a false negative, coronary angiography should be considered as an initial diagnostic test.

     iv. For patients with known CAD, stress testing can be useful in determining exercise (functional) capacity, effectiveness of treatment, and differentiation of ambiguous symptoms.

     v. When ordering a stress test, the clinician must thoughtfully consider which combination of stressor and measurement of myocardial response to that stressor will best fit the particular patient being evaluated.

     vi. Contraindications to stress testing: MI within 2 days, persistent angina, significant arrhythmias, symptomatic severe aortic stenosis, unstable congestive heart failure, acute pulmonary embolus, myocarditis, significant pericarditis, aortic dissection

D. **Treatment of stable CAD**
 1. Pharmacologic:
   a. Antiplatelet agents
     i. Aspirin, 75 to 162 mg
     ii. Clopidogrel, 75 mg daily
   b. β blockers
     i. Proven mortality benefit with metoprolol succinate, carvedilol, and bisoprolol
     ii. First choice for symptom relief
   c. Angiotensin-converting enzyme (ACE-I) or angiotensin receptor blocker (ARB)
     i. Best evidence is for patients with CAD and hypertension, diabetes mellitus (DM), LVEF < 40%, or chronic kidney disease.
     ii. Consider ARB if patient is ACE-I intolerant owing to chronic cough.
   d. Nitrates
     i. For symptom relief
     ii. Long- or short-acting preparations are available.
     iii. May be administered intravenously, orally, topically, or sublingually
   e. Calcium channel blocker: for symptom relief
   f. Ranolazine: for symptom relief
 2. Revascularization options for nonacute CAD may be used to improve *survival* and/or *symptoms*:
   a. Coronary artery bypass grafting (CABG) is recommended to improve *survival* for:
     i. >50% stenosis of left main coronary artery
     ii. ≥70% stenoses in three major coronary arteries
     iii. ≥70% stenoses in left anterior descending plus one other major coronary artery
     iv. Survivors of ischemia-mediated ventricular tachycardia and ≥70% stenosis in a major coronary artery
   b. CABG or PCI is recommended to improve *symptoms* for one or more ≥70% coronary artery stenoses amenable to revascularization and having unacceptable angina despite maximal medical management.
 3. Complications: sudden death, congestive heart failure, arrhythmias, depression
 4. Duration/prognosis: Treatment of CAD and management of alterable risk factors can be highly efficacious in preventing or delaying recurrent symptoms and CVD events.
 5. Prevention:
   a. Patient education: the focus is CVD risk reduction and promotion of wellness, to include:
     i. Medication adherence
     ii. Regular exercise (30 to 60 minutes/day, 5 to 7 days/week)
     iii. Healthy diet and weight control goal of body mass index (BMI) 18.5 to 24.9 kg/m^2
     iv. Waist circumference (<40 inches for men, <35 inches for women)

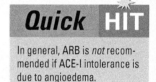

Quick HIT

In general, ARB is *not* recommended if ACE-I intolerance is due to angioedema.

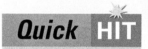

Quick HIT

Percutaneous coronary intervention (PCI) may be considered as an alternative to CABG. Intravenous thrombolysis medications may be used in the acute setting.

b. Optimal management of lipids, hypertension, DM

c. Smoking cessation (primary and second-hand exposure)

d. Screening for and managing stress or depression when present

II. Acute Coronary Syndrome

A. General characteristics

1. Definition: acute coronary events are defined by the presence or absence of

a. Objective evidence of myocardial ischemia (elevated ST segments on ECG; Figure 8-2)

b. Objective evidence of myocardial cell damage—(troponin T and troponin I are the most reliable biomarkers; Table 8-3)

2. Epidemiology: More than 1.5 million patients have an acute MI in the United States per year. Many more are hospitalized for UA or undifferentiated acute chest discomfort.

3. Pathophysiology: See Figure 8-1.

B. Clinical features

1. Historical findings: an acute coronary event, as opposed to chronic sable angina, is characterized by one or more of the following:

a. New onset of symptoms

b. Change in the pattern of previous symptoms (more intense, more frequent, more easily brought on by exertion, more persistent, accompanied by worrisome symptoms like diaphoresis or shortness of breath)

2. Physical exam findings (signs): See Section I.B.2 under CAD above.

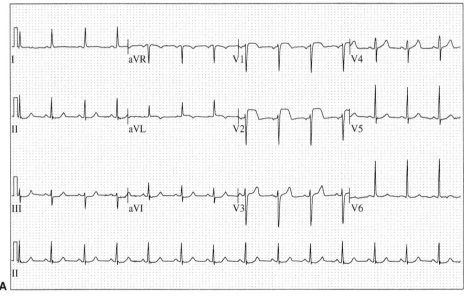

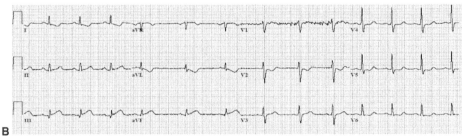

FIGURE

8-2 **ST segment elevation myocardial infarctions. A: Antero-septal ST elevations (leads V1–V3). B: Inferior ST elevations (leads II, III, and aVF).**

(**A** courtesy of Dr. Erik Powell; **B** from Baim DS. *Grossman's Cardiac Catheterization, Angiography, and Intervention.* 7th ed. Philadelphia, PA: Lippincott Williams & Wilkins; 2006.)

TABLE **8-3**	Serum Cardiac Biomarkers			
Lab Test	**Onset of Rise**	**Peak**	**Duration of Elevation**	**Comments**
Troponin	3–6 h	24–36 h	5–14 d	The "gold standard" for myocardial cell damage
Creatine phosphokinase (CPK)	2–6 h	12–18 h	24–48 h	Will rise with skeletal as well as myocardial muscle damage—MB band helps specify cardiac muscle injury
Myoglobin	1–2 h	6–8 h	12–24 h	Least frequently used of the three. Only advantage is that it rises earlier than the other biomarkers. Also not specific for cardiac muscle. Has been used to determine early discharge from the Emergency Department in low-risk patients

C. **Diagnosis**
   1. Differential diagnosis: See Section I.C under CAD above.
   2. Laboratory findings (in the acute setting):
      a. A 12-lead ECG should be done and interpreted *immediately* upon arrival for patients with chest pain.
      b. Serial ECGs in the acute care setting performed over time may be very helpful in documenting ischemia that was not evident on the initial tracing.
      c. Cardiac biomarkers: See Table 8-3.
   3. Radiology findings: Chest X-ray may demonstrate a cause for acute chest pain such as spontaneous pneumothorax, pneumonia, or rib fractures.

D. **Treatment**
   1. Therapy: The initial decision in treatment is whether to pursue an *invasive* or *conservative* management approach (Table 8-4).
      a. Initial invasive strategy—revascularize:
         i. Percutaneous coronary intervention (PCI, also known as angioplasty), usually with stent placement
         ii. Immediate intravenous thrombolytic agents (alteplase, reteplase, tenecteplase, streptokinase, or anistreplase):
            (a) With a goal of PCI or CABG within 24 to 48 hours
            (b) Thrombolysis should be *avoided* in acute coronary syndromes (ACS) unless ST segment elevation is present.
         iii. Invasive strategies are best for high-risk ACS.
      b. Initial conservative management strategy—the goal is to maximize medical therapy:
         i. Control symptoms
         ii. Then do a noninvasive stress test prior to hospital discharge.
         iii. Better reserved for lower-risk ACS
      c. CABG—See Section II.D under CAD.
   2. Complications:
      a. Rupture of ventricular wall or papillary muscle
      b. Arrhythmia
      c. Pump failure (hypotension, cardiogenic shock, congestive heart failure)
   3. Duration/Prognosis:
      a. Initial risk assessment at the time of presentation is important to determine the aggressiveness of treatment.
      b. The thrombolysis in myocardial infarction (TIMI) risk score for UA/NSTEMI estimates the risk for death, MI, or need for revascularization within 14 days.

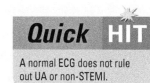

Quick HIT

A normal ECG does not rule out UA or non-STEMI.

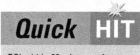

Quick HIT

PCI within 90 minutes of patient arrival has superior outcomes to fibrinolysis.

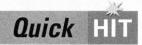

Quick HIT

Drug-eluting stents, compared to bare-metal stents, have less short-term thrombosis, but more late stent thrombosis, and so require clopidogrel for at least 1 year.

Cardiovascular Disorders

TABLE 8-4	Medical Treatment Options for Acute Coronary Syndromes		
Class	**Medication**	**Mechanism**	**Comments**
I. Antiplatelet therapy			
A. Aspirin		Blocks platelet aggregation	Rapid onset of action. Often used as a component of dual antiplatelet therapy
B. Thienopyridine P2Y12 receptor antagonists	Clopidogrel, ticlopidine, prasugrel		
C. Glycoprotein IIb/IIIa antagonists	Abciximab, eptifibatide, tirofiban	Block the interactions of fibrinogen	Available only for IV use in the acute setting
II. Anticoagulant therapy			
A. Heparin	Low molecular weight (enoxaparin) or unfractionated		
B. Direct thrombin inhibitor	Bivalirudin		
C. Selective factor Xa inhibitor	Fondaparinux		
III. Anti-anginal therapy			
A. Nitrates	IV, sublingual, topical and oral preparations available		Good symptom relief but mortality benefit is not proven
B. Narcotic	Morphine is typically used	Pain relief, sedation	Effective for relief of persistent angina in the acute setting
C. β blockers	Metoprolol, carvedilol, bisoprolol, others	Lowers the myocardial workload by downregulating the β-adrenergic system. Mortality benefit may be related to arrhythmia prevention	Should be started early in the course of treatment
D. Calcium channel blockers	Nifedipine, amlodipine, diltiazem, verapamil	Coronary vasodilation	Option for chest pain not relieved by nitrates or β blockers
IV. Other			
Statins (HMG-CoA reductase inhibitors	Atorvastatin, rosuvastatin, simvastatin, others	Appear to have benefits related to anti-inflammatory/clot stabilization as well as lipid lowering	Should be routinely administered within 24 h of an acute event

Cardiovascular Disorders

    c. A separate TIMI risk score for patients with STEMI predicts 30-day mortality following thrombolytic therapy.

    d. Calculators for both TIMI scores are available at www.mdcalc.com.

  4. Prevention: β blockers, statins, ACE-I, control alterable risk factors (eg, hypertension, hyperlipidemia, smoking)

III. Hypertension

A. General characteristics

1. Definition:

a. The level of BP at which the risk of CVD begins to increase; generally thought to be 120/80 mm Hg (may be as low as 115/75)

b. More typically, clinical hypertension is considered to be the level of BP elevation at which the benefits of treatment have been demonstrated to outweigh the risks of treatment. For the general population, this is usually ≤140/90 mm Hg.

2. Epidemiology:

a. Approximately 70 million individuals in the United States had a systolic BP ≥ 140 mm Hg and/or a diastolic BP ≥ 90 mm Hg (about 29% of the U.S. population).

b. Control rate for individuals with hypertension was about 52%.

3. Cause: Most cases of hypertension are termed *essential hypertension*—related to genetics or aging—without a clear, potentially modifiable etiology. *Secondary hypertension* implies an underlying, discoverable disease process (Table 8-5).

4. Genetics: No single gene appears to play a major role in the development of hypertension. Familial and twin studies suggest that multiple genetic as well as environmental factors have roles in the development of hypertension.

5. Risk factors: From 40 to 70 years of age, from a BP range of 115/75 to 185/115, each 20 mm Hg increase in systolic or diastolic BP doubles the risk of CVD.

B. Clinical features

1. Historical findings:

a. Often asymptomatic; about 20% of those with hypertension are not even aware that they have it.

b. Symptoms may be nonspecific (such as headache), or related to target organ damage (such as shortness of breath secondary to congestive heart failure).

TABLE 8-5	Secondary Causes of Hypertension
Renal	Renal parenchymal disease
	Renovascular disease
Endocrine	Hyperthyroidism
	Hypothyroidism
	Hyperaldosteronism
	Pheochromocytoma
	Cushing syndrome
	Acromegaly (growth hormone excess)
	Estrogens
	Testosterone
Lifestyle	Obesity
	High dietary salt intake
	Excessive alcohol intake
Medication effects	Nonsteroidal anti-inflammatory drugs (ibuprofen, naproxen, many others)
	COX-2 inhibitors (celecoxib)
	Weight loss agents/sympathomimetics (phentermine, ma huang, pseudoephedrine, amphetamines)
	Immunosuppressive agents (cyclosporine, tacrolimus, corticosteroids)
	Mineralocorticoids (fludrocortisone)
	Antidepressants (venlafaxine, phenelzine)
	Antiparkinsonian (bromocriptine)
Pulmonary	Obstructive sleep apnea
Vascular	Coarctation of the aorta

Cardiovascular Disorders

2. Physical exam findings:
   a. Look for exam findings that suggest secondary causes of hypertension (eg, truncal striae of Cushing syndrome).
   b. Look for evidence of hypertensive end organ damage (eg, peripheral edema owing to renal failure).

C. **Diagnosis**
   1. Differential diagnosis:
      a. *White-coat hypertension* implies a BP that is routinely elevated only in medical settings.
      b. See Table 8-5 for secondary causes of hypertension.
   2. Laboratory findings:
      a. Initial labs should include serum electrolytes, blood urea nitrogen, creatinine, glucose, lipid panel, and urinalysis to evaluate for end organ damage and comorbidities.
      b. Other laboratory studies may be done if there is evidence for possible secondary causes of hypertension.
   3. Radiology findings: Chest X-ray may show cardiomegaly or evidence of pulmonary edema from congestive heart failure. Not recommended as part of the initial workup.
   4. Other findings: ECG may demonstrate evidence of left ventricular strain or previous MI.

D. **Treatment:** Recommendations are based on the 2014 Evidence-Based Guideline for the Management of High Blood Pressure in Adults Report From the Panel Members Appointed to the Eighth Joint National Committee (JNC 8).
   1. Therapy:
      a. In patients aged ≥60 years, initiate pharmacologic treatment in systolic BP ≥150 mm Hg or diastolic BP ≥90 mm Hg and treat to a goal systolic BP <150 mm Hg and goal diastolic BP <90 mm Hg.
      b. In patients aged <60 years, initiate pharmacologic treatment at systolic BP ≥140 mm Hg or diastolic BP ≥90 mm Hg and treat to a goal systolic <140 mm Hg and diastolic <90 mm Hg.
      c. In patients aged ≥18 years with chronic kidney disease, initiate pharmacologic treatment at systolic BP ≥140 mm Hg or diastolic BP ≥90 mm Hg and treat to goal systolic BP <140 mm Hg and diastolic BP <90 mm Hg.
      d. In patients aged ≥18 years with diabetes, initiate pharmacologic treatment at systolic BP ≥140 mm Hg or diastolic BP ≥90 mm Hg and treat to a goal systolic BP <140 mm Hg and diastolic BP <90 mm Hg.
      e. In the general non-black population, including those with diabetes, initial antihypertensive treatment should include a thiazide-type diuretic, calcium channel blocker (CCB), ACE inhibitor, or ARB.
      f. In the general black population, including those with diabetes, initial antihypertensive treatment should include a thiazide-type diuretic or CCB.
      g. In the population aged ≥18 years with chronic kidney disease, initial (or add-on) antihypertensive treatment should include an ACE inhibitor or ARB to improve kidney outcomes.
      h. General approaches to treatment:
         i. If goal BP is not reached within a month of treatment, increase the dose of the initial drug or add a second drug.
         ii. If goal BP cannot be reached with two drugs, add or titrate a third drug.
   2. Complications: the most important health outcomes affected by the treatment of hypertension are favorable impact on the risk of:
      a. Mortality: overall, CVD-related, and chronic kidney disease (CKD)-related
      b. Cardiovascular: MI, heart failure, stroke
      c. Renal: CKD (increase in serum creatinine and decrease in glomerular filtration rate), end-stage renal disease (requirement for dialysis or transplant)

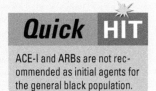

Quick HIT

ACE-I and ARBs are not recommended as initial agents for the general black population.

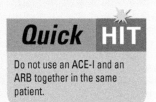

Quick HIT

Do not use an ACE-I and an ARB together in the same patient.

3. Duration/prognosis: Unless secondary factors for hypertension are identified and reversed (such as weight loss for obesity), treatment of hypertension tends to be life-long.

4. Prevention: An overall healthy diet (eg, dietary approaches to stop hypertension [DASH] diet, lowering of dietary sodium intake, and 40 minutes of aerobic physical activity three to four sessions a week have each been demonstrated to lower BP.

IV. Dyslipidemias

A. General characteristics

1. Definition:

   a. Low-density lipoprotein cholesterol (LDL-C) is the primary lipid abnormality on which risk evaluation and treatment are targeted.

   b. High-density lipoprotein cholesterol (HDL), elevated fasting triglycerides, and non-HDL cholesterol (total cholesterol minus HDL) are secondary predictors of cardiovascular risk, but are not primary targets for treatment.

2. Epidemiology:

   a. After age 40, prevalence is 49% for men and 32% for women.

   b. CVD risk seems to increase incrementally for LDL-C > 70 mg/dL.

3. Causes: diet, sedentary lifestyle, smoking, and overweight/obesity are modifiable contributing factors. Poorly controlled DM may cause elevated triglycerides.

4. Genetics: Dyslipidemias are frequently genetically determined, particularly those that are severe or appear at a young age.

5. Risk factors:

   a. Current hyperlipidemia guidelines stress that the higher the risk of CVD, the more likely the individuals to benefit from treatment of elevated or even "normal" lipids.

   b. Previous CVD and DM are the strongest risk factors for the onset of new cardiovascular events.

B. Clinical features

1. Historical findings: usually asymptomatic until it causes CVD or other sequela

2. Physical exam findings: *Xanthelasmas* are yellowish lipid deposits particularly noticeable around the eyelids that are often but not always correlated with dyslipidemia (Figure 8-3).

C. **Diagnosis**

1. Differential diagnosis: Secondary causes of hyperlipidemia are noted in Table 8-6.

2. Laboratory findings:

   a. An initial fasting lipid panel including total cholesterol, triglycerides, HDL-C, and calculated LDL-C

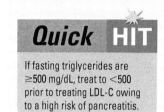

Quick HIT

If fasting triglycerides are ≥500 mg/dL, treat to <500 prior to treating LDL-C owing to a high risk of pancreatitis.

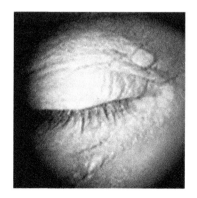

FIGURE

8-3 Xanthelasmas.

(From Ferrier D. *Lippincott Illustrated Reviews: Biochemistry.* 7th ed. Philadelphia, PA: Wolters Kluwer; 2017.)

TABLE 8-6	Secondary Causes of Dyslipidemia
Medical Conditions	**Medications**
Hypothyroidism	Oral estrogen
Diabetes mellitus	Anabolic steroids
Obesity	Oral isotretinoin
Cholestatic liver disease	Protease inhibitors
Nephrotic syndrome	Thiazide diuretics
Chronic renal failure	β blockers
Smoking	Atypical antipsychotics (clozapine, olanzapine)

    b. A second lipid panel should be done 4 to 12 weeks after starting statin therapy to assess adherence to therapy, then every 3 to 12 months as clinically indicated.

    c. Follow-up LDL-C levels and percent reduction may be used as clinically indicated to assess response to therapy and adherence, not as performance standards to reach fixed target LDL goals.

D. **Treatment**

    1. Therapy: based on the November 2013 American College of Cardiology/American Heart Association Treatment of Blood Cholesterol Guidelines

        a. The focus was to identify those most likely to benefit from statin therapy, both for secondary and primary prevention of CVD for individuals ≥21 years of age.

        b. Four major statin benefit groups were identified for whom the atherosclerotic cardiovascular disease (ASCVD) risk reduction clearly outweighs the risk of adverse events (Table 8-7).

        c. A treatment algorithm is presented in Figure 8-4 and Table 8-8.

        d. An ASCVD risk calculator is available at http://tools.acc.org/ASCVD-Risk-Estimator.

        e. United States Preventive Services Task Force (USPSTF) recommends low- to moderate-dose statin therapy for patients aged 40 to 74 years with one or more risk factors and an ASCVD risk ≥10% (B recommendation).

TABLE 8-7	Four Major Statin Benefit Groups for Atherosclerotic Cardiovascular Disease (ASCVD) Risk Reduction	
Group	**Treatment Recommendation**	**Goal**
1. Statin therapy should be initiated or continued as first-line therapy in **women and men ≤75 yr of age who have clinical ASCVD**, unless contraindicated	**≤75 yr**, unless contraindicated: **high-intensity** statin therapy **> 75 yr**: moderate-intensity statin therapy	Secondary prevention
2. Adults ≥21 yr of age with primary **LDL–C ≥190 mg/dL**	**High-intensity statin therapy** (moderate-intensity statin if high-intensity contraindicated or not tolerated)	Primary prevention
3. Statin therapy should be initiated or continued for adults 40–75 yr of age with **diabetes mellitus**	**Calculate 10-yr ASCVD risk** using the Pooled Cohort Equations: For **risk ≥7.5%**—use **high-intensity** statin therapy For **risk <7.5%**—use **moderate-dose** statin therapy	Primary prevention
4. Adults 40–75 yr of age with LDL–C 70–189 mg/dL, without clinical ASCVD or diabetes and an **estimated 10-yr ASCVD risk ≥7.5%**	**Moderate- or high-intensity statin**	Primary prevention

Cardiovascular Disorders

MAJOR RECOMMENDATIONS FOR STATIN THERAPY
(Age >21 years and no contraindications to statin therapy)

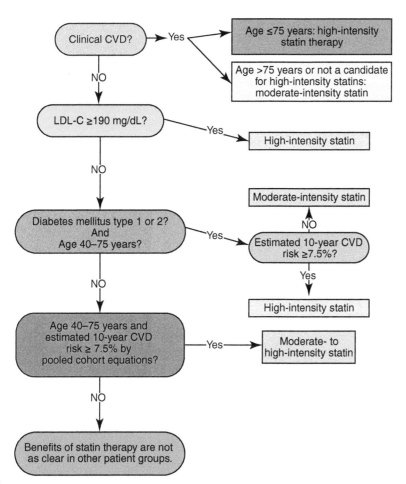

FIGURE
8-4 **Major recommendations for statin therapy (age >21 years and no contraindications to statin therapy).**

2. Complications of statin therapy:
   a. Contraindicated in pregnancy and breastfeeding
   b. Myopathy: Routine screening/monitoring of creatine kinase (CK) is not recommended.
   c. Hepatitis.
      i. Measure baseline alanine transaminase (ALT) prior to starting statin therapy.

TABLE 8-8	Intensity of LDL-C Lowering for Statins	
High-Intensity Statin Therapy	**Moderate-Intensity Statin Therapy**	**Low-Intensity Statin Therapy**
Lowers LDL–C on average ≥50%	Lowers LDL–C on average 30% to <50%	Lowers LDL–C on average <30%
Atorvastatin 40–80 mg	Atorvastatin 10 (20) mg	Simvastatin 10 mg
Rosuvastatin 20–40 mg	Rosuvastatin (5) 10 mg	Pravastatin 10–20 mg
	Simvastatin 20–40 mg	Lovastatin 20 mg
	Pravastatin 40 (80) mg	Fluvastatin 20–40 mg
	Lovastatin 40 mg	Pitavastatin 1 mg
	Fluvastatin XL 80 mg	
	Fluvastatin 40 mg bid	
	Pitavastatin 2–4 mg	

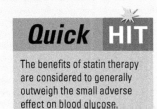

ii. Unexplained ALT elevation three times the upper limit of normal is a contraindication to statins.

iii. Routine ALT monitoring during statin therapy is not required.

d. Increased risk for new onset DM.

3. Duration/prognosis: each 39 mg/dL reduction in LDL-C by statin therapy reduces ASCVD risk by about 20%.

4. Prevention: Screen and counsel for risk factors and heart-healthy lifestyle modifications (weight loss, exercise, smoking cessation).

V. Heart Failure (HF)

A. General characteristics

1. Definition: A clinical syndrome that results from a structural or functional impairment of ventricular ejection (systolic HF) and/or filling (diastolic HF) (Table 8-9).

2. Epidemiology:

a. Approximately 5 million individuals in the United States have clinical HF.

b. Annual incidence rises with age:

i. About 2% for ages 60 to 69 years

ii. About 8% for ages ≥85 years

c. Prevalence in the Medicare-eligible population is about 12%.

d. HF places a significant burden on the healthcare system owing to frequency of hospital admission and readmissions.

3. Causes: CAD, hypertension, valvular heart disease, non-ischemic cardiomyopathy (viral causes), infiltrative disorders (amyloidosis or hemochromatosis), connective tissue disorders, IV drug abuse, idiopathic

4. Genetics: familial dilated cardiomyopathy, hemochromatosis, familial dyslipidemias resulting in CAD

5. Risk factors: Since CAD and hypertension are common causes, the risk factors for these disorders predispose to the development of HF.

6. Pathophysiology:

a. Most patients with HF have impaired ejection fraction of blood from the left ventricle (systolic HF). This may be owing to disorders of the pericardium, myocardium, endocardium, heart valves, great vessels, or metabolic abnormalities.

b. Stiffness of the ventricle results in poor filling (diastolic HF) and overall decreased cardiac output despite preserved ejection fraction.

TABLE 8-9	Classifications of Heart Failure

American College of Cardiology/American Heart Association Classifications (Based on Structural and Functional Status)

Class	Description
A	At risk for HF but no structural heart disease of symptoms of HF
B	Structural heart disease but no signs or symptoms of HF
C	Structural heart disease with current or prior symptoms of HF
D	Heart failure refractory to therapy and requiring specialized interventions

New York Heart Association Classifications (Based on Functional Status)

Class	Description
I	No limitation of physical activity (ordinary physical activity does not cause symptoms of HF)
II	Slight limitation of physical activity (comfortable at rest, but ordinary physical activity causes symptoms of HF)
III	Marked limitation of physical activity (comfortable at rest, but less than ordinary physical activity causes symptoms of HF)
IV	Unable to carry on **any** physical activity without symptoms of HF **OR** has symptoms of HF at rest

B. **Clinical features**
1. Historical findings:
   a. Related to reduced forward flow of blood from the heart: fatigue, exercise intolerance, decreased mental acuity
   b. Related to increased peripheral hydrostatic pressure owing to fluid backing up behind the impaired right ventricular: dependent edema and poor appetite (congestion of the gut)
   c. Related to increased pulmonary vascular congestion due to fluid backing up behind the impaired left ventricle: shortness of breath, orthopnea, dyspnea on exertion
2. Physical exam findings:
   a. Related to reduced forward flow of blood from the heart: hypotension, reflex tachycardia, decreased mental acuity noted on mental status exam
   b. Related to increased peripheral hydrostatic pressure owing to fluid backing up behind the impaired right ventricular: weight gain, pitting pretibial or other dependent edema, jugular venous distention, hepato-jugular reflux (manual pressure on the liver causes jugular vein distention)
   c. Related to increased pulmonary vascular congestion owing to fluid backing up behind the impaired left ventricle: rales, decreased breath sounds or dullness to percussion at base of lung owing to pleural effusion, tachypnea, S3 gallop

C. **Diagnosis**
1. Differential diagnosis:
   a. Shortness of breath/fatigue
      i. Pulmonary: chronic obstructive pulmonary disease (COPD), pneumonia, pulmonary embolus
      ii. Anemia
      iii. Muscle weakness: myopathy, hypokalemia, Guillain–Barré syndrome
      iv. Endocrine: hypo- or hyperthyroidism
      v. Other cardiac causes: aortic stenosis, cardiac tamponade
   b. Peripheral edema: venous insufficiency, low oncotic pressure, nephrotic syndrome, hepatic failure, hypothyroidism, malnutrition
2. Laboratory findings:
   a. Primarily a clinical syndrome with a variety of symptoms and physical findings
   b. Initial lab evaluation should include:
      i. Complete blood count (CBC), urinalysis, serum electrolytes including calcium and magnesium, blood urea nitrogen, serum creatinine, glucose, fasting lipid profile, liver function tests, and thyroid-stimulating hormone
      ii. A 12-lead ECG to look for left ventricular hypertrophy (LVH), arrhythmias, or evidence of ischemia
      iii. B-type natriuretic peptide (BNP) or N-terminal proB-type natriuretic peptide (NT-proBNP) is useful for:
         (a) Supporting the diagnosis of HF in patients with dyspnea
         (b) Determining prognosis or disease severity in acute and chronic HF
      iv. Screening for hemochromatosis, HIV, rheumatologic diseases, or amyloidosis may be reasonable in selected patients.
3. Radiology findings: Chest X-ray may demonstrate cardiomegaly or pulmonary congestion.
4. Echocardiogram: A 2-dimensional ECG with Doppler is the best single diagnostic test for the evaluation of HF. It is useful for evaluating:
   a. Left ventricular ejection fraction (LVEF)
   b. Ventricular wall motion
   c. Valvular function
   d. Decreased ventricular relaxation during diastole
5. Noninvasive (stress testing) or invasive (coronary angiography) studies may be indicated for evaluation of myocardial ischemia.

D. **Treatment**
1. Therapy:
   a. ACE-I and β blockers should be used to prevent symptomatic HF and reduce mortality.

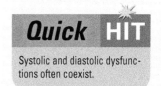

Quick **HIT**

Systolic and diastolic dysfunctions often coexist.

Cardiovascular Disorders

b. ARBs are reasonable alternatives to ACE-I unless otherwise contraindicated.

c. Diuretics and salt restriction are useful for treatment of fluid retention symptoms but have not been demonstrated to improve mortality.

d. Aldosterone receptor antagonist is indicated in patients with LVEF ≤35% to reduce morbidity and mortality.

e. A combination of hydralazine and isosorbide dinitrate may be used to reduce morbidity and mortality in African-American patients with New York Heart Association (NYHA) class III or IV systolic HF receiving optimal ACE inhibitor and β-blocker therapy.

f. Digoxin can be beneficial in decreasing hospitalizations for HF in patients with systolic HF.

g. Cardiac rehabilitation in stable patients can improve functional status, health-related quality of life, and mortality.

h. Implantable cardiac defibrillator (ICD) therapy may be recommended for primary prevention of sudden cardiac death in selected patients with LVEF <35%.

i. Cardiac resynchronization therapy may be indicated for certain patients with LVEF ≤35%.

j. Continuous intravenous inotropic support, coronary artery revascularization, mechanical circulatory support, fluid restriction, and cardiac transplantation are options for treatment of selected patients with severe HF.

2. Complications: Mortality in HF is primarily the result of sudden cardiac death or progressive pump failure.

3. Duration/prognosis: Table 8-10 shows the magnitude of benefit of drug therapies in stage C systolic HF.

4. Prevention:
   a. Treatment of hypertension and lipid disorders will lower the risk of HF.
   b. In patients with a history of MI or acute coronary syndrome, statins should be used to prevent symptomatic HF and cardiovascular events.
   c. Appropriate management of DM, obesity, tobacco use, and other CVD risk factors may lower the risk of HF.

VI. Arrhythmias

A. Diagnosis of cardiac arrhythmias may be based on rate and rhythm.

1. Rate:
   a. Bradycardia: <60 bpm
   b. Tachycardia: >100 bpm

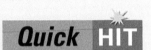

Quick HIT

Tachycardia is often a healthy, adaptive response to a physiologic stress, such as hypovolemia.

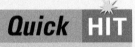

Quick HIT

Bradycardia may be a normal state (particularly in young, athletic individuals) or a desired therapeutic response to medications (such as β blockers).

TABLE 8-10	Benefits of Drug Therapies in Stage C Systolic Heart Failure			
Drug Therapy	**Relative Risk Reduction in Mortality**	**Absolute Risk Reduction in Mortality**	**Number Needed to Treat for Mortality Reduction (Over 36 mo)**	**Relative Risk Reduction in Hospitalizations for Heart Failure**
ACE-I[a] or ARB[b]	17%	3.8%	26	31%
β blocker	34%	11.1%	9	41%
Aldosterone antagonist	30%	16.7%	6	35%
Hydralazine/ nitrate[c]	43%	14.3%	7	33%

[a]Angiotensin-converting enzyme inhibitor.
[b]Angiotensin receptor blocker.
[c]Efficacy demonstrated only in African Americans.

2. Rhythm:
   a. Regular or irregular
   b. Origin of conduction impulse: sinoatrial (SA) node, atrioventricular (AV) node, other atrial source, ventricular
   c. Conduction pathway: reentrant pathway, accessory pathway (eg, Wolf–Parkinson–White syndrome)

B. **Atrial fibrillation (AF)**
   1. General characteristics:
      a. Uncoordinated atrial electrical activity results in an ECG pattern of fibrillatory atrial activity (rather than P waves) with irregular ventricular response (Figure 8-5).
      b. The most common arrhythmia in clinical practice
      c. Prevalence is 0.4% to 1.0% in the general population, but 8% in those >80 years.
      d. Causes: atrial abnormalities, hypertension, hyperthyroidism, exercise, alcohol, illicit drugs, obstructive sleep apnea, obesity
      e. Risk factors: advancing age, smoking, CAD, DM
      f. Pathophysiology:
         i. The irregular atrial activity may result in a rapid ventricular response rate, particularly if an accessory conduction pathway is present.
         ii. The lack of coordinated atrial contractions may result in stasis of blood and the formation of thrombus in the atria, leading to systemic embolic events such as ischemic stroke.
         iii. Loss of the atrial "kick" to augment filling of the left ventricle may decrease left ventricular output and precipitate or worsen HF.
   2. Clinical features:
      a. Historical findings: often asymptomatic, palpitations, dyspnea, lightheadedness, or other symptoms of decreased cardiac output
      b. Physical exam findings:
         i. Typically an irregularly irregular radial pulse or auscultated cardiac rhythm is noted.
         ii. Irregular jugular venous pulsations
         iii. Tachycardia may be present.
         iv. Rales, peripheral edema, or other signs of decreased cardiac output
   3. Diagnosis:
      a. Differential diagnosis: other causes of tachycardia (eg, atrial flutter, supraventricular tachycardia [SVT])
      b. Laboratory findings:
         i. Blood tests for electrolytes and evaluation of thyroid, renal, and hepatic function.
         ii. For acute onset: cardiac enzymes, prothrombin time (PT)/partial thromboplastin time (PTT) if considering anticoagulation

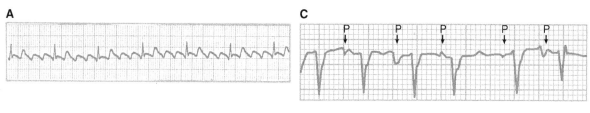

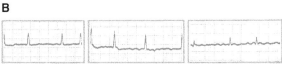

FIGURE
8-5 A: Atrial flutter: "saw tooth" appearance of the electrical atrial activity. B: Atrial fibrillation: no discernible P waves, rhythm is irregular. C: Multifocal atria tachycardia: P waves differ in appearance.

(From Wolfsthal SD. *NMS Medicine.* 7th ed. Philadelphia, PA: Lippincott Williams & Wilkins; 2012.)

c. ECG is used to make the diagnosis.

d. Echocardiogram to determine: atrial size, ventricular size and function, valvular heart disease, pericardial disease, left atrial thrombus

e. Holter monitoring may be useful in documenting episodes of paroxysmal AF.

4. Treatment: focused on rate control, rhythm control, and management of thromboembolic risk

a. Rate control—options for treatment are noted in Table 8-11.

b. Rhythm control—options for treatment are noted in Table 8-12.

c. Management of thromboembolic risk

  i. AF carries a significant risk of thromboembolic stroke (Table 8-13).

  ii. All patients with AF must be evaluated for their stroke risk, balanced against their risk of significant bleeding complications owing to anticoagulation. CHA_2DS_2-VASc are scoring systems to estimate the risk for stroke in patients with nonvalvular AF (see Table 8-13).

    (a) Oral anticoagulation is recommended score of 2 or greater.

    (b) Anticoagulation is not recommended score of 0.

    (c) For a score of 1, treatment options include no antithrombotic therapy, oral anticoagulation, or aspirin.

  iii. Anticoagulation treatment options are outlined in Table 8-14.

C. **Ventricular tachycardia/ventricular fibrillation** (Figure 8-6)

1. Approximately 50% of all CAD deaths are sudden.

2. Arrhythmias causing sudden cardiac death include ventricular tachycardia, ventricular fibrillation/flutter, and torsades de pointes.

3. Sudden cardiac death constitutes 13% of all natural deaths.

4. Acute treatment of ventricular tachycardia/fibrillation/flutter may include:

a. Cardiopulmonary resuscitation (CPR)

b. Electrical defibrillation

c. Intravenous amiodarone

d. Other advanced cardiac life support (ACLS) drugs and interventions

5. Chronic preventive treatment options for ventricular arrhythmias include:

a. Medications: β blockers, amiodarone, sotalol

b. Implantable cardioverter defibrillators

c. Surgical ablation or excision of the arrhythmogenic foci

d. In patients with ischemic CAD, revascularization procedures may decrease ventricular arrhythmias.

6. Torsades de pointes is a ventricular arrhythmia with a distinctive polymorphic twisting ECG appearance (Figure 8-7).

a. Accompanied by a markedly prolonged QT interval on ECG

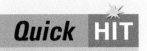

Quick HIT

Patients with atrial flutter should follow the same antithrombotic recommendations given for atrial fibrillation.

TABLE 8-11 Recommendations for Rate Control in Atrial Fibrillation	
Agent/Intervention	**Comments**
β blockers	Target is typically <80 bpm
Nondihydropyridine calcium channel blockers (verapamil, diltiazem)	May worsen heart failure
Digoxin	Works by changing vagal tone, so effective at controlling resting heart rate but not exercise-induced tachycardia
Amiodarone	Due to toxicity, typically used when other medications have not been effective
Electrical cardioversion	Indicated in the acute setting for rate control in hemodynamically unstable patients
Atrio-ventricular nodal ablation	Reasonable option when pharmacologic therapy has not been successful

TABLE 8-12	Recommendations for Rhythm Control in Atrial Fibrillation

Interventions/Medications for Conversion of Atrial Fibrillation to Sinus Rhythm

Electrical cardioversion	First choice for hemodynamically unstable patients, particularly with preexcitation pathway
	Patients may require sedation to tolerate this procedure.
	It is reasonable to repeat cardioversions in persistent AF if sinus rhythm is maintained for a reasonable period of time between procedures.
Dofetilide	
Propafenone	May be used in the outpatient setting self-administered PRN by the patient if this has been observed in the hospital setting to have been safe
Flecainide	
Ibutilide	
Amiodarone	

Interventions/Medications for Maintenance of Sinus Rhythm in Patients Who Have Converted from Atrial Fibrillation

Class IA antiarrhythmics (disopyramide, quinidine)	May prolong the QT interval
Class IC antiarrhythmics (Flecainide, propafenone)	May worsen sinus or AV node dysfunction, infranodal conduction disease, HF, CAD
Class III antiarrhythmics (amiodarone, dofetilide, dronedarone, sotalol)	May prolong the QT interval
Catheter ablation	Anticoagulation is required during and after the procedure.
	Should not be performed with the sole intent of avoiding the need for long-term anticoagulation
	Reasonable as an initial treatment strategy or as a secondary option if antiarrhythmics have not been successful
Surgical ablations (Maze procedures)	An option for selected patients with prominent symptoms not relieved with other modalities

TABLE 8-13	Stroke Risk Stratification for Patients With Nonvalvular Atrial Fibrillation

CHA_2DS_2-VASc	Scoring	CHA_2DS_2-VASc Total Score	Adjusted Stroke Rate (% per year)
		0	0
Congestive heart failure	1	1	1.3
Hypertension	1	2	2.2
Age ≥ 75 yr	2	3	3.2
Diabetes mellitus	1	4	4.0
Stroke/TIA/TE	2	5	6.7
Arterial vascular disease (prior MI, PAD or aortic plaque)	1	6	9.8
Age 65–74 yr	1	7	9.6
Female gender	1	8	6.7
Maximum score	9	9	15.2

TABLE 8-14	Options for Oral Anticoagulation in Atrial Fibrillation			
Medication (Generic)	**Brand Name**	**Mechanism**	**Comments**	**Dosing in Renal Failure**
Warfarin	Coumadin	Blocks the vitamin K– dependent synthesis of clotting factors II, VII, IX, and X	Requires adjustment of dosing to target INR of 2.0–3.0	Agent of choice in ESRD or dialysis
Dabigatran	Pradaxa	Direct thrombin inhibitor	Do not require routine monitoring of level of anticoagulation	Require dose adjustment (or omission) depending on degree of renal failure
Rivaroxaban	Xarelto	Factor Xa inhibitor	Relatively new agents compared to warfarin	
Apixaban	Eliquis	Factor Xa inhibitor		

    b. Causes: congenital long-QT syndrome, drugs or electrolyte abnormalities, advanced disease of the cardiac conduction system

    c. Treatment: IV magnesium sulfate, removal of offending drug, correction of metabolic abnormality, cardiac pacing, β blockers, and isoproterenol may be used in certain situations

D. **Supraventricular tachycardias (SVTs)** (Figure 8-8)

    1. Defined as a nonphysiologic increase in heart rate >100 bpm (typically symptoms do not develop until about 140 to 150)

    2. SVTs originate above the level of the ventricles due to disorders of impulse initiation (increased automaticity) or abnormalities of impulse conduction (reentrant pathways).

    3. Symptoms may include palpitations, fatigue, light headedness, chest discomfort, dyspnea, or syncope.

A

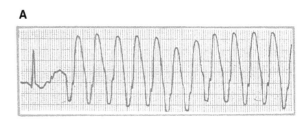

B

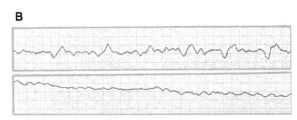

FIGURE 8-6 Ventricular tachycardia (A) and ventricular fibrillation (B).

(From Wolfsthal SD. *NMS Medicine.* 7th ed. Philadelphia, PA: Lippincott Williams & Wilkins; 2012.)

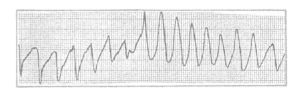

FIGURE 8-7 Torsades de pointes.

(From Wolfsthal SD. *NMS Medicine.* 7th ed. Philadelphia, PA: Lippincott Williams & Wilkins; 2012.)

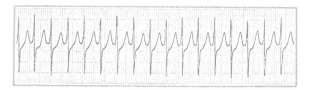

FIGURE
8-8 **Supraventricular tachycardia.**

(From Wolfsthal SD. *NMS Medicine.* 7th ed. Philadelphia, PA: Lippincott Williams & Wilkins; 2012.)

TABLE **8-15**	Differential Diagnosis of Tachycardias
Narrow Complex	**Wide Complex**
Atrial fibrillation Multifocal atrial tachycardia Atrioventricular reciprocating tachycardia Atrioventricular nonreciprocating tachycardia Atrial tachycardia	Bundle branch block with any of the causes of a narrow complex tachycardia Ventricular tachycardia Torsades de pointes

4. The differential diagnosis depends on whether the QRS complexes are *wide* (>120 ms) or *narrow* (Table 8-15).

5. In the acute setting, vagal maneuvers (cough, bearing down) or the administration of adenosine IV may slow the heart rate long enough to more easily discern the underlying rhythm.

6. Treatment options depend on the underlying abnormality and may include β blockers, nondihydropyridine calcium channel blockers, electrical cardioversion, antiarrhythmic medications, or cardiac ablation.

Cardiovascular Disorders

QUESTIONS

1. You are seeing a 60-year-old male in your office with known CAD. The greatest reduction in his relative risk for a fatal cardiovascular event will be from which one of the following medications?
   A. Ranolazine
   B. A β blocker
   C. A calcium channel blocker
   D. A long-acting nitrate preparation
   E. A thiazide diuretic

2. A 50-year-old male with a current history of smoking cigarettes presents to the Emergency Department with the new onset of chest pain and diaphoresis of 6 hours duration. To evaluate him for MI, the recommended initial serum biomarker is:
   A. Troponin
   B. Creatine phosphokinase (CPK)
   C. High-sensitivity C-reactive protein (CRP)
   D. Myoglobin
   E. Erythrocyte sedimentation rate (ESR)

3. A 65-year-old female comes to see you for a preventive health visit. She is in excellent health. She takes no medications and has no significant current or past medical problems. Her BP checked by a registered nurse at a health fair last week was 146/88 mm Hg, and is 145/86 mm Hg in your office today. You provide her with education about lifestyle changes for lowering her BP, but at her 6-week follow-up visit it is essentially unchanged, despite a 5-lb weight loss and her report that she has complied with your mutually chosen lifestyle change goals. At this point, current guidelines recommend that:
   A. You initiate treatment with an ACE-I or ARB.
   B. You initiate treatment with a β blocker.
   C. You initiate treatment with a thiazide diuretic.
   D. Pharmacotherapy is not indicated for her level of BP elevation.
   E. Pharmacotherapy is not indicated because she has most likely not complied with lifestyle changes.

4. A 59-year-old woman sees you 1 month after having sustained a NSTEMI. She brings you the results of a fasting lipid panel that was done the previous day. Your approach to the management of her lipids should be:
   A. Titrate her medication to achieve a goal LDL-C of <70 mg/dL.
   B. Use lipid-lowering medication only if lifestyle changes (weight loss, exercise, diet) are not effective in reaching her LDL-C goal.
   C. Using multiple classes of lipid lowering agents generally has a better therapeutic effect than using a single agent.
   D. Prescribe high-intensity statin therapy at a dose that would be expected to lower LDL-C an average of ≥50%.
   E. Stop statin therapy if her serum liver enzyme, ALT, goes above the upper limit of normal.

5. You are considering what diagnostic evaluation to pursue for your 45-year-old female patient with recent onset of HF with reduced ejection fraction (EF). The most frequent cause for HF with reduced EF is:

A. Valvular heart disease

B. Human immunodeficiency virus (HIV)–induced cardiomyopathy

C. Intravenous drug abuse

D. A connective tissue disorder

E. CAD

6. A 76-year-old female on dialysis for end-stage renal disease (ESRD) secondary to type 2 DM presents with recent onset of AF. The best choice of an oral anticoagulant for her is:

A. No oral anticoagulation, as her risk for stroke is low.

B. Warfarin (Coumadin)

C. Dabigatrin (Pradaxa)

D. Rivaroxaban (Xarelto)

E. Apixaban (Eliquis)

Questions

ANSWERS

1. **Answer: B.** Three β blockers (metoprolol succinate, carvedilol, and bisoprolol) have strong evidence for effectiveness in reducing relative risk for mortality in CAD.
The benefit of ranolazine, calcium channel blockers, and nitrates is primarily symptom relief. Diuretics may relieve symptoms of congestive heart failure resulting from CAD.

2. **Answer: A.** Troponin is released into the serum with myocardial cell damage and is the "gold standard" for determining acute MI. The level in the serum begins to rise 3 to 6 hours after myocardial injury, peaks at 24 to 36 hours, and remains elevated for 5 to 14 days. CPK and myoglobin are less specific markers of myocardial injury, as they are released with skeletal muscle injury as well. CRP and ESR are nonspecific markers of inflammation.

3. **Answer: D.** The 2014 JNC 8 guidelines recommend initiation of pharmacotherapy for treatment of BP in patients aged ≥ 60 years at systolic BP ≥ 150 mm Hg (previous recommendation was 140 mm Hg) or diastolic BP ≥ 90 mm Hg (unchanged from previously). Therefore, this overall healthy 65-year-old with systolic BP in the 140s should not be treated with medications. She should continue to pursue lifestyle changes, which her 5-lb weight loss suggests she has been following. A second reason that an ACE-I or ARB should not be prescribed is that they are not considered first-line antihypertensive medications for AA patients.
A second reason that β blockers should not be prescribed is that in general they are not considered to be first-line agents for initial treatment of hypertension (a change from previous recommendations).

4. **Answer: D.** The American College of Cardiology/American Heart Association guidelines, based on evidence from randomized controlled trials, recommend this approach rather than the previous strategy of determining and then treating to goal LDL-C levels. This patient with known CAD is in a high-risk group for having a recurrent CVD event; therefore treatment with a high-intensity statin is indicated. In general, the higher the risk of CVD, the greater the benefit of statin therapy. Options for high-intensity statin therapy are atorvastatin 80 mg daily or rosuvastatin 20 mg daily. Answer (E) is not correct since it is recommended that statin therapy should be discontinued if baseline ALT increases above *three times* the upper limit of normal.

5. **Answer: E.** Over 50% of cases of HF with reduced EF are secondary to cardiac muscle damage from CAD. Diagnostic options to evaluate for the presence of CAD include an ECG, an echocardiogram (to look for localized areas of reduced wall motion), a stress test, or coronary angiography. Valvular heart disease, human immunodeficiency virus (HIV)–induced cardiomyopathy, intravenous drug abuse, and connective tissue disorders such as lupus erythematosus are all causes of HF but occur less frequently than CAD.

6. **Answer: B.** The first step in deciding on treatment to reduce risk for stroke in AF is to assess the patient's level of risk. Using the CHA_2DS_2-VASc scoring (Table 8-13), this patient gets 2 points for age ≥75 years and 1 point for diabetes. Long-term oral anticoagulation is recommended for a total score of 2 or greater if no contraindications are present. This patient's score of 3 represents a 3.2% adjusted stroke rate risk per year (see Table 8-13). Treatment with oral anticoagulants will provide a relative risk reduction of 61%. The newest generation of oral anticoagulants, termed "novel oral anticoagulants" (NOACs), include dabigatran (Pradaxa), rivaroxaban (Xarelto), and apixaban (Eliquis). As a class, they have the advantage over warfarin of not requiring regular blood test monitoring of anticoagulant effect. However, since all NOACs are renally excreted to some extent, the anticoagulant effect is altered in patients with renal impairment, and warfarin (Coumadin) is still the oral anticoagulant of choice with ESRD.

DISEASES OF THE RESPIRATORY SYSTEM

9

Megan Rich • Hillary Mount

I. Bronchitis/Upper Respiratory Tract Infection

A. **General characteristics**

1. Definition: inflammation of upper respiratory airways (trachea and bronchi)
2. Epidemiology:
   a. More common in the fall and winter months
   b. According to the Centers for Disease Control and Prevention (CDC), in 2012 cough was the third most common reason for an office visit.
3. Causes:
   a. Viral causes are the most common: rhinovirus, adenovirus, respiratory syncytial virus, parainfluenza viruses, coxsackie viruses, influenza viruses, coronaviruses.
   b. Bacterial causes are less common. Think about atypical bacteria: *Chlamydia pneumoniae*, mycoplasma, and, rarely, *Bordetella pertussis*.
4. Risk factors:
   a. Age: the young and the old
   b. Chronic lung diseases like chronic obstructive pulmonary disease (COPD) or asthma
   c. Other chronic conditions like allergies or immunodeficiencies
   d. Tobacco use
   e. Other lung irritants: second-hand smoke, pollution, occupational exposures
5. Pathophysiology: irritation and inflammation of the bronchi (typically by a virus) results in swelling of the bronchial wall and mucous production

B. **Clinical features**

1. Symptoms:
   a. Principal symptom: cough, often productive
   b. Rhinorrhea
   c. Sore throat
   d. Headache
   e. Fever
   f. Malaise/fatigue
   g. In more severe cases: shortness of breath or atypical chest pain
2. Signs:
   a. Wheezing and/or rhonchi on lung auscultation
   b. Edematous and/or erythematous nasal mucosa
   c. Erythema of oropharynx
   d. Cervical adenopathy
   e. Pulse oximetry should be normal (>92% in an adult without chronic lung disease)

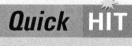

Quick HIT

Bordetella pertussis is the bacteria responsible for whooping cough.

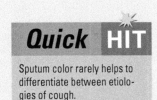

Quick HIT

Sputum color rarely helps to differentiate between etiologies of cough.

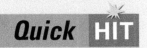

Quick HIT

The American Academy of Pediatrics (AAP) recommends against the use of over-the-counter cough and cold medications in children under 4 years old.

Quick HIT

A superimposed bacterial pneumonia should be suspected when the patient initially improves and then suddenly worsens (fever, shortness of breath, worsening cough).

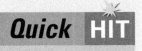

Quick HIT

Although the acute infection resolves typically within 10 days, the cough itself may last up to 3 to 4 weeks.

C. **Diagnosis**
1. Differential diagnosis:
   a. Adults: pneumonia, asthma, COPD exacerbation, allergic rhinitis, lung cancer
   b. Children: bronchiolitis, pneumonia, asthma, croup, whooping cough
2. Laboratory findings: Bronchitis is a clinical diagnosis, so there is no specific testing to confirm a patient's condition. Rather, testing is reserved for differentiating bronchitis from other diagnoses the patient might have.
   a. Complete blood count (CBC) with differential may be helpful if pneumonia is a concern.
   b. If a bacterial etiology is considered likely, test the sputum for Gram stain and culture.
   c. If whooping cough is suspected, check a culture from the nasopharynx.
3. Radiology findings: Chest X-ray is necessary only if pneumonia needs to be excluded.
4. Pulmonary function tests are not indicated in the acute diagnosis.
D. **Treatment**
1. Therapy: aimed at symptom relief, because a virus is the most likely cause
   a. Antitussive agents such as dextromethorphan
   b. Trial of albuterol in more severe cases
   c. Antipyretics and analgesics for fever or sore throat
   d. Supportive care, including rest and pushing fluids
   e. If an atypical bacterial pathogen or whooping cough is suspected, azithromycin is the preferred antibiotic. The vast majority of cases do NOT require an antibiotic.
2. Complications:
   a. Postviral pneumonia
   b. Recurrent bouts of acute bronchitis may become chronic bronchitis, part of the spectrum of diseases in COPD.
3. Duration/prognosis:
   a. Symptoms typically resolve in 7 to 10 days.
   b. Prognosis is good because this is a self-limited infection.
   c. Cough lasting more than 4 weeks may warrant additional testing such as an X-ray.
4. Prevention:
   a. As with all infectious diseases, good hand washing is paramount.
   b. Avoid lung irritants such as cigarette smoke.

II. Pharyngitis
A. **General characteristics:** inflammation of pharynx causing pain and redness
B. **Clinical features**
1. The most common presenting symptom is sore throat.
2. Associated symptoms may include cough, rhinorrhea, fever, pain with swallowing, headache, and body aches.
3. Causes:
   a. Infectious: viral (most common) or bacterial
   b. Noninfectious: chemical irritation from smoke exposure or acid reflux, postnasal drainage from allergic rhinitis, cancer
4. Risk factors:
   a. Sick contacts
   b. Environmental or seasonal allergies
   c. Medications that cause acid reflux such as bisphosphonates
C. **Diagnosis**
1. Physical exam findings:
   a. Erythema of oropharynx and tonsils
   b. Exudate can be present in both viral and bacterial pharyngitis

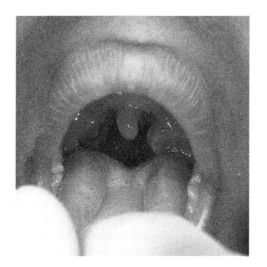

FIGURE

9-1 **Strep pharyngitis.**

(From Fleisher GR, Ludwig W, Baskin MN. *Atlas of Pediatric Emergency Medicine.* Philadelphia, PA: Lippincott Williams & Wilkins; 2004.)

  c. Cervical lymphadenopathy

  d. Strep may be associated with rash.

  e. Mononucleosis may cause hepatosplenomegaly.

 2. Differential diagnosis:

  a. Viral pharyngitis

  b. Strep pharyngitis (Figure 9-1)

  c. Mononucleosis

  d. Postnasal drip/allergic rhinitis

  e. Gastroesophageal reflux disease (GERD)

  f. Peritonsillar abscess

  g. Sexually transmitted infection such as gonococcus or acute HIV infection (for patients at risk)

  h. Oropharyngeal cancer

 3. Laboratory testing and imaging:

  a. Rapid strep test—use Modified Centor Criteria to determine if this is needed (Table 9-1)

  b. Throat culture—for confirmation as needed

  c. Monospot test or heterophile test (if suspected)

D. **Treatment**

 1. Viral pharyngitis: supportive care such as rest, fluids, analgesics, and antipyretics as needed

 2. Strep pharyngitis: antibiotics, preferably penicillin, unless the patient has an allergy. If there is an allergy, consider treatment with clindamycin.

 3. Postnasal drip: antihistamine with or without steroid nasal spray

 4. GERD: calcium carbonate tabs, H_2-blocker, or proton-pump inhibitor

III. Acute Rhinosinusitis

A. **Characteristics**

 1. Definition: inflammation of the nasal passage and paranasal sinuses

 2. Causes:

  a. Mainly owing to viruses (rhinovirus, adenovirus, influenza virus, parainfluenza)

  b. Bacterial pathogens include *S. pneumoniae, H. influenza, M. catarrhalis, S. aureus.*

Quick HIT

Strep pharyngitis is caused by Group A beta-hemolytic *Streptococcus pyogenes.*

Quick HIT

Viral infections are typically caused by adenovirus, rhinovirus, coronavirus, and other viruses, commonly causing a "cold." The exception is mononucleosis, which is typically caused by Epstein-Barr virus (EBV) or cytomegalovirus (CBV).

Quick HIT

Anterior lymphadenopathy is seen in strep throat, whereas posterior is more common with mononucleosis.

Quick HIT

Don't miss a peritonsillar abscess. Patients should have fever and deviated uvula on exam. Get a neck X-ray if this is suspected.

Quick HIT

If mono is suspected, get a CBC with differential and liver profile—you may find atypical lymphocytes and/or elevated liver enzymes.

Quick HIT

Strep throat is treated to prevent complications like rheumatic fever, not to speed the resolution of symptoms.

Diseases of the Respiratory System

TABLE **9-1** Modified Centor Criteria for Assessing Pharyngitis	
Symptom or Exam Finding	**Points**
Age:	
3–14 yr	+1
15–44 yr	0
≥45 yr	−1
Fever on exam or reported historically	+1
Tonsillar exudate on exam	+1
Tender anterior cervical lymphadenopathy	+1
Absence of cough	+1

Scoring: 0 to 1: no rapid strep test, no antibiotics
≥2: test using rapid strep method. Give antibiotics only for positive test.
Throat culture not routinely recommended to confirm negative rapid strep testing.

B. **Clinical features**
   1. Presentation:
      a. Sinus or facial pain, pressure, or congestion
      b. Rhinorrhea
      c. Toothache
      d. Possible fever
      e. Recent upper respiratory infection (URI)
   2. Physical exam:
      a. Tenderness of face overlying sinuses
      b. Rhinorrhea

C. **Diagnosis**
   1. History and exam are all that are needed to diagnose the majority of cases.
   2. Rarely, complicated cases with a concern for deeper spread of infection may require imaging and otolaryngology referral.
   3. Differential diagnosis:
      a. Allergic rhinitis
      b. Foreign body (children)
      c. Upper respiratory tract infection
      d. Dental cavities or other dental issues
      e. Otitis media (OM)

D. **Treatment**
   1. Symptomatic therapy:
      a. Analgesics (nonsteroidal antiinflammatory drugs [NSAIDs] Tylenol)
      b. Nasal saline irrigation
      c. Intranasal glucocorticoids are likely beneficial only if there is an allergic component, because evidence is mixed.
      d. Topical decongestants may provide symptom relief for viral sinusitis, but not recommended for bacterial sinusitis because they have no proven benefit.
      e. Other: Oral decongestants, antihistamines, and mucolytics (guaifenesin) have no proven benefit.
   2. Antibiotics:
      a. Indicated if worsening after 3 to 4 days, symptoms persist >10 days, the patient is immunocompromised, or there are moderate to severe symptoms at onset with a fever >101°F
      b. Amoxicillin-clavulanate is the first-line treatment.
      c. High-dose amoxicillin-clavulanate (2 g amoxicillin twice per day) is recommended for patients older than 65, recently hospitalized, immunocompromised, or in regions with *S. pneumoniae* penicillin-resistance >10%.

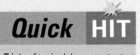

Quick HIT

Most cases of sinusitis are due to viruses and will not improve with antibiotics.

Quick HIT

Trials of topical decongestants should not extend > 3 days to avoid the risk of rebound congestion.

d. Doxycycline or fluoroquinolone can be used if the patient has a penicillin allergy.

3. Complications: recurrent sinusitis, abscess, osteomyelitis, meningitis

4. Prevention: hand hygiene, influenza vaccine, pneumoniae vaccine

IV. Infectious Otitis Media (OM)

A. **Characteristics**

1. Definition: infection of the middle ear

2. Epidemiology: There is an average of three episodes per child by 3 years old. About 80% to 90% will have at least one episode by age 3.

3. Cause: *S. pneumoniae, H. influenza, M. catarrhalis*, viruses

4. Risk factors:

   a. Recent URI

   b. Seasonal allergies

   c. Unimmunized child

   d. Daycare attendance

   e. Pacifier use past 6 months of age

   f. Sibling with a history of frequent episodes of OM

   g. Immunosuppression

   h. Craniofacial anomalies

5. Pathophysiology: eustachian tube dysfunction, often with recent URI or congestion from allergic rhinitis. Inflammation narrows and obstructs the Eustachian tube, so fluid is unable to drain, which makes it susceptible to bacterial growth and infection. As children grow, the anatomy changes, decreasing susceptibility to infection (pharyngeal muscles and palate elevate).

B. **Clinical features**

1. History: ear pain, ear pulling, fever, jaw or neck pain, decreased hearing, ear fullness, fussiness in infant

2. Physical exam:

   a. Fever

   b. Bulging, opaque, red or white tympanic membrane (TM) with decreased mobility to pneumatic pressure (Figure 9-2)

   c. Air–fluid level visible behind TM

   d. Purulent drainage if ruptured TM

   e. Conductive hearing loss by Weber test (perceived sound louder in affected ear)

C. **Diagnosis**

1. Differential diagnosis:

   a. OM with effusion

   b. Otitis externa

   c. URI

   d. Dental caries (cavities)

   e. Sinusitis

   f. Eustachian tube dysfunction

   g. Herpes zoster

2. No laboratory or radiology testing is necessary. Cultures are not helpful unless the patient is not responding to appropriate treatment.

D. **Treatment**

1. Therapy:

   a. Symptom relief: acetaminophen or ibuprofen. No evidence supports the use of decongestants or antihistamines (contraindicated in children).

   b. First-line: amoxicillin 90 to 100 mg/kg divided in twice daily dosing for 10 days

   c. If the patient is older than 6 months and has mild disease (no high fever and nontoxic appearance), it is reasonable to observe and offer a rescue prescription (a prescription to be filled if there is no improvement in 24 to 48 hours).

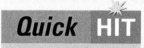

Quick HIT

Viruses, *S. pneumonia, H. influenza,* and *M. cattarrhalis* are the pathogens most likely to cause otitis, sinusitis, and bronchitis.

Diseases of the Respiratory System

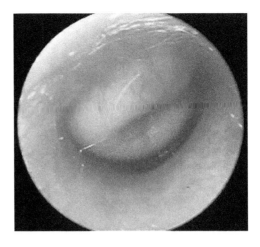

FIGURE
9-2 Acute infectious otitis media.

(Courtesy of Alejandro Hoberman, MD. Children's Hospital of Pittsburgh of UPMC. Johnson JT, Rosen CA, et al. *Bailey's Head and Neck Surgery: Otolaryngology.* 5th ed. Philadelphia, PA: Lippincott Williams & Wilkins; 2014.)

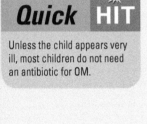

Quick HIT

Unless the child appears very ill, most children do not need an antibiotic for OM.

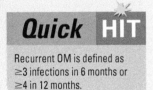

Quick HIT

Recurrent OM is defined as ≥3 infections in 6 months or ≥4 in 12 months.

d. Other options: cephalosporin or macrolide if the patient is allergic to penicillin. Treatment failures can use amoxicillin-clavulanate.
e. Tympanostomy tubes or antibiotic prophylaxis if there is recurrent disease
2. Complications: ruptured TM (often heals spontaneously within 6 weeks), mastoiditis, sinusitis, hearing loss (at risk for language delay in infants), deeper infections such as labyrinthitis or epidural abscess rare
3. Prognosis: Often improves in 48 to 72 hours, but fluid can persist for 6 to 12 weeks
4. Prevention:
    a. Recurrent disease: requires fiberoptic nasopharyngoscopy to evaluate for obstruction owing to anatomy or mass. Consider prophylactic antibiotics or tympanostomy tubes.
    b. Stay up to date on immunizations.
    c. Avoid smoke exposure.

V. Otitis Media With Effusion (Serous Otitis Media)
A. Characteristics
    1. Definition: presence of fluid in the middle ear without signs of infection
    2. Cause: slow resolution of prior infection or fluid build-up from allergic rhinitis or other causes that does not lead to infection
B. Clinical features
    1. History: ear fullness, ear popping sensation, ear itching, decreased hearing
    2. Physical exam: dull TM, visible fluid behind TM without erythema (Figure 9-3)
C. **Diagnosis:** History and exam findings. No other testing necessary.
D. **Treatment:** Observe for 12 weeks. There is no evidence to support the use of decongestants, antihistamines, or nasal corticosteroids. Refer if not resolving.

VI. Otitis Externa
A. Characteristics
    1. Definition: infection of the external ear canal
    2. Epidemiology: most commonly *S. aureus, Pseudomonas aeruginosa*
    3. Cause: swimming, minor trauma to the ear from cleaning or itching
B. Clinical features
    1. History of ear pain or itching

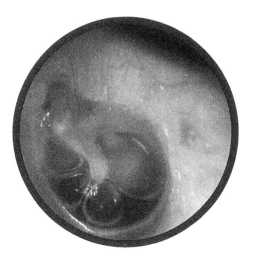

FIGURE
9-3 Serous otitis media.

(From Hawke M, Keene M, Alberti PW. *Clinical Otoscopy: A Text and Colour Atlas.* Edinburgh, Scotland: Churchill Livingston; 1984.)

2. Physical exam:
   a. Tenderness external ear and pinna
   b. Erythema of external ear
   c. Possibly external canal edema
   d. Possible purulent drainage

C. **Treatment**
   1. Topical antibiotics: neomycin/polymyxin B, ciprofloxacin, acetic acid
   2. Topical corticosteroids: hydrocortisone (available in combination with antibiotics)
   3. Analgesia: NSAIDs, acetaminophen
   4. Systemic antibiotics: if concern for malignant otitis externa (severe infection) with spread beyond external ear, immunocompromised, or diabetic patient

VII. Pneumonia

A. **General characteristics**
   1. Definition: an infection of the lower respiratory tree, generally caused by bacteria or a virus, but on occasion by a fungus
   2. Epidemiology: For those older than 65 years, there are nearly 1 million cases of pneumonia per year. Mortality rates vary depending on the severity of the infection
   3. Causes:
      a. Bacteria:
         i. Typical pathogens in the ambulatory setting include *Streptococcus pneumoniae, Haemophilus influenza, Moraxella catarrhalis*, and, less commonly, methicillin-resistant *Staphylococcus aureus* (MRSA).
         ii. Atypical pathogens: *Mycoplasma pneumoniae, Chlamydophila pneumoniae*
         iii. Concerns in hospitalized patients: MRSA, drug-resistant *S. penumoniae*, and pseudomonas
      b. Viruses: influenza A and B, respiratory syncytial virus, parainfluenza, and adenovirus
      c. Fungi: Histoplasma, Coccidioides, Blastomyces, and Cryptococcus (in endemic areas of the country)
   4. Risk factors:
      a. Age: typically, the old (65 years and older) and the young (5 years or younger)

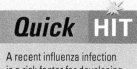

Quick HIT

A recent influenza infection is a risk factor for developing community-acquired MRSA.

Quick HIT

Legionella pneumophila is an atypical bacteria that classically causes gastrointestinal symptoms and/or hyponatremia.

Diseases of the Respiratory System

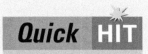

Diseases of the Respiratory System

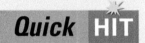

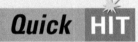

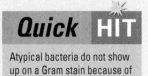

  b. Chronic lung disease: COPD, asthma, sarcoidosis, bronchiectasis
  c. Other comorbid diseases: diabetes, cancer, connective tissue diseases, heart disease, alcohol abuse, HIV infection, asplenia
  d. Tobacco use
  e. Uncontrolled gastroesophageal reflux disease causing recurrent microaspiration
  f. Medications such as proton pump inhibitors or anything that weakens the immune system (chronic steroid use, chemotherapy, tumor necrosis factor inhibitors, etc.)
5. Pathophysiology: Pneumonia is spread from person to person by contact with respiratory secretions or droplets in the air. The result is inflammation and mucous production in the lower respiratory tree, often with a systemic response (fever, myalgias).

B. **Clinical features**
1. Symptoms:
   a. Cough with purulent sputum, typically an acute finding
   b. Fever with or without rigors
   c. Upper respiratory symptoms like rhinorrhea, sore throat, nasal congestion
   d. Shortness of breath
   e. Chest pain, often pleuritic in nature
   f. Fatigue or malaise
   g. Occasional gastrointestinal symptoms like nausea, vomiting, or diarrhea
2. Signs:
   a. Bronchial breath sounds in the affected area(s)
   b. Rales in the affected area(s)
   c. Fever (temperature ≥ 100.4°F)
   d. Hypoxia (pulse oximetry ≤ 92%)

C. **Diagnosis**
1. Differential diagnosis for adults: URI, acute bronchitis, acute COPD exacerbation, pulmonary embolism (PE), allergic rhinitis, lung cancer
2. Differential diagnosis for children: URI, bronchiolitis, acute asthma exacerbation, croup, whooping cough
3. Laboratory findings:
   a. Leukocytosis on a CBC
   b. Differential with a neutrophil predominance or presence of bands
   c. Sputum Gram stain and culture may grow the bacterial pathogen.
   d. Blood culture may grow the bacterial pathogen in about 10% of cases.
   e. Rapid influenza testing or influenza culture, if suspected
   f. Legionella urinary antigen testing, if suspected (such as known exposure or severely ill)
4. Radiology findings
   a. Chest X-ray: may show consolidation, air bronchograms, or even pleural effusion (Figure 9-4)
   b. Chest computed tomography (CT): may show similar findings to the X-ray and may be helpful if trying to exclude other causes of symptoms such as lung cancer

D. **Treatment**
1. Therapy:
   a. Antibiotics are geared toward the most likely bacterial pathogen.
      i. Adults less than 65 years old AND with no chronic conditions can be treated for atypical pathogens with azithromycin.
      ii. Adults 65 years or older, or adults of any age who have comorbidities, should be empirically treated for drug-resistant *S. pneumoniae* with 1 of 2 regimens:
         (a) High-dose amoxicillin plus azithromycin
         (b) Respiratory fluoroquinolone such as levofloxacin or moxifloxacin

      iii. Children should be treated for drug-resistant *S. pneumoniae* with high-dose amoxicillin.

    b. Supportive care with antipyretics, rest, and fluids

    c. Supplemental oxygen as needed

2. Complications:

    a. Sepsis or septic shock

    b. Empyema: a purulent pleural effusion, essentially an extension of the infected lung

    c. Lung abscess: a walled-off area of infection within the lung

    d. Hospitalization

        i. Use the CURB-65 or PORT scoring systems to help determine which adult patients require admission to the hospital (Table 9-2).

        ii. Hypoxia and inability to tolerate oral medications are other reasons to hospitalize.

    e. Respiratory failure

    f. Death

3. Duration/prognosis:

    a. With timely treatment, improvement is usually seen within a few days.

    b. Antibiotics should be continued for a minimum of 5 days, but not longer than 8 days.

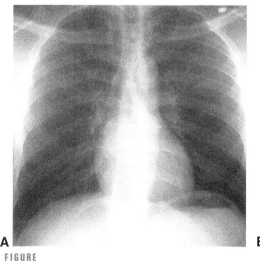 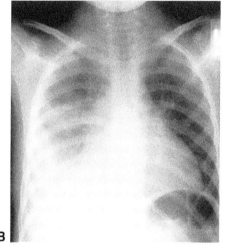

A   B

FIGURE 9-4 **Chest X-ray depicting pneumonia.**

(From Fleisher GR, et al. *Textbook of Pediatric Emergency Medicine.* 5th ed. Philadelphia, PA: Lippincott Williams & Wilkins; 2005.)

TABLE 9-2	CURB-65 Criteria for Pneumonia Severity

Factor	Points
Confusion	1
Uremia (BUN ≥ 20)	1
Elevated **R**espiratory rate (≥30 breaths/min)	1
Low **B**lood pressure (systolic < 90, diastolic ≤ 60)	1
Age ≥ **65** years	1

Scoring: 0 to 1: Mortality rate of 0.7% to 2.1%, able to treat in ambulatory setting
≥ 2: Mortality rate of 9.2% or greater, treat patient in hospitalized setting

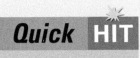

Quick HIT

Kids who have diseases that put them at risk for pneumococcal infections may require the 23-valent "adult" version of the pneumococcal vaccine.

4. Prevention:
   a. Immunizations for adults:
      i. Pneumococcal vaccine: typically given at age 65 starting with the 13-valent pneumococcal conjugate vaccine and followed by the 23-valent pneumococcal polysaccharide vaccine 1 year later; may be given earlier for patients with a qualifying condition (such as diabetes or COPD)
      ii. Influenza: recommended annually for all adults
   b. Immunizations for children:
      i. Pneumococcal vaccine: covers the 13 most common strains and is typically given at ages 2 months, 4 months, 6 months, and 15 months
      ii. Influenza: starting at 6 months of age and then given annually

VIII. Asthma

A. **Characteristics**
   1. Definition: a disorder of airway hypersensitivity characterized by intermittent airway obstruction that is reversible with bronchodilator therapy
   2. Epidemiology: prevalence 8.4%; estimated 25.7 million people with 7 million <18 years old
   3. Genetics: complex and not fully determined
   4. Risk factors:
      a. Tobacco smoke: smoking, second-hand exposure to tobacco smoke (including prenatal exposure)
      b. Family history
      c. History of atopy (seasonal allergies, allergic rhinitis, atopic dermatitis)
      d. Indoor and outdoor pollutants or irritants
   5. Pathophysiology: chronic inflammation owing to underlying hyperresponsiveness of airways that leads to intermittent airway obstruction

B. **Clinical features**
   1. History: dyspnea, wheezing, cough (especially nighttime), chest pain or tightness, symptoms worsened by specific triggers (exercise, smoke exposure, allergies, reflux, etc.)
   2. Physical exam: can be normal exam if no acute exacerbation, wheezing typically high-pitched, decreased breath sounds, increased respiratory effort

C. **Diagnosis**
   1. Differential diagnoses:
      a. COPD
      b. Cystic fibrosis
      c. GERD
      d. Acute coronary syndrome
      e. Bronchiolitis or other respiratory infection
      f. Anatomic airway narrowing
      g. Pulmonary embolism
      h. Anxiety disorder
   2. No labs or imaging tests are typically necessary.
   3. Pulmonary function testing with spirometry:
      a. Obstructive lung disease: forced expiratory volume 1/forced vital capacity (FEV_1/FVC) ratio < 0.7
      b. FEV_1 < 80% of the normal expected value calculated for patient's age, gender, and other factors
      c. Severity of illness partially determined by FEV_1 percentage of expected normal
      d. Reversibility: FEV_1 improvement with bronchodilator (at least 15%)
   4. Peak flow:
      a. Useful for monitoring disease at home once diagnosis is made (patients >5 years old)
      b. Determine "personal best" when symptoms are well-controlled.
      c. When symptoms of exacerbation start can monitor percent decrease from personal best to determine severity

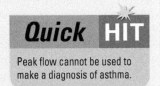

Quick HIT

Peak flow cannot be used to make a diagnosis of asthma.

D. **Treatment**
1. Therapy:
    a. Initially based on disease severity (Table 9-3)
    b. Adjustments based on disease control (Figure 9-5)
    c. Goals are to reduce impairment in function and reduce risk of exacerbations.
    d. Requires regular monitoring with asthma assessment tools (questionnaires) to determine if increase in therapy required.
2. Medications:
    a. Short-acting beta agonist (SABA) as needed for immediate symptoms relief
    b. Inhaled glucocorticoids in gradually increased doses for long-term control of disease
    c. Additional therapies:
        i. Long-acting beta agonists (LABA)
        ii. Leukotriene receptor antagonists
        iii. Theophylline
3. Acute exacerbation:
    a. Oral glucocorticoids with duration determined by disease response
    b. Frequent, regular bronchodilator therapy
    c. Hospital admission
        i. Severe disease (<40% predicted peak flow)
        ii. Hypoxia
        iii. Inability to self-manage
4. Complications:
    a. Hospitalization
    b. Respiratory failure requiring intubation
    c. Bronchiectasis
    d. Death if respiratory failure prior to seeking medical care
5. Prognosis:
    a. Children often have resolution of disease
    b. Asthma in adolescence highly correlated with persistence into adulthood
    c. Progressive loss of lung function in minority of patients if resistant disease or poorly controlled
6. Prevention:
    a. Avoid or minimize triggers
    b. Vaccinations: pneumonia and annual influenza
    c. Asthma action plan
        i. Details a self-management plan for the patient
        ii. Includes regular medication instructions and plan for when symptoms worsen
        iii. Often based on percent decline in peak flow as well as symptoms

IX. Chronic Obstructive Pulmonary Disease

A. **Characteristics**
1. Definition:
    a. A progressive disease of airflow limitation, often because of chronic inflammation in response to noxious inhaled stimuli
    b. Chronic bronchitis is defined as a chronic productive cough for 3 months present in two successive years.
2. Epidemiology:
    a. >6% of the U.S. population is affected.
    b. >120,000 deaths annually
3. Cause: About 80% of patients have a history of tobacco abuse. Other causes include occupational or environmental exposures, or family history.

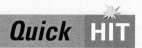

Quick HIT

Asthma is diagnosed by an obstructive pattern on spirometry with an FEV_1 <80% predicted that is *reversible* with bronchodilator therapy.

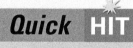

Quick HIT

LABA should not be used in asthma without an inhaled steroid.

Diseases of the Respiratory System

Diseases of the Respiratory System

TABLE 9-3 Classification of Asthma Disease Severity and Treatment Recommendations

Classification of Asthma Severity (5–11 yr of Age)

Components of Severity		Intermittent	Persistent		
			Mild	Moderate	Severe
Impairment	Symptoms	≤2 d/wk	>2 d/wk but not daily	Daily	Throughout the day
	Nighttime awakenings	≤2x/mo	3–4x/mo	>1x/wk but not nightly	Often 7x/wk
	Short-acting β₂-agonist use for symptom control (not prevention of EIB)	≤2 d/wk	>2 days/week but not daily	Daily	Several times per day
	Interference with normal activity	None	Minor limitation	Some limitation	Extremely limited
	Lung function	• Normal FEV₁ between exacerbations • FEV₁ >80% predicted • FEV₁/FVC >85%	• FEV₁ ≥ 80% predicted • FEV₁/FVC >80%	• FEV₁ = 60%–80% predicted • FEV₁/FVC = 75%–80%	• FEV₁ >30% predicted • FEV₁/FVC <75%
Risk	Exacerbations requiring oral systemic corticosteroids	0–1/yr (see note)	≥2/yr (see note) →		
			Consider severity and interval since last exacerbation. Frequency and severity may fluctuate over time for patients in any severity category. Relative annual risk of exacerbations may be related to FEV₁.		
Recommended Step for Initiating Therapy		Step 1	Step 2	Step 3, medium-dose ICS option, or step 4	
(See Figure 9-6 for treatment steps.)		In 2–6 wk, evaluate level of asthma control that is achieved, and adjust therapy accordingly.		Consider short course of oral systemic corticosteroids	

EIB, exercise-induced bronchospasm; FEV₁, forced expiratory volume in 1 second; FVC, forced vital capacity; ICS, inhaled corticosteroids.

From NHLBI: Guidelines for the Diagnosis and Management of Asthma (EPR-3), https://www.nhlbi.nih.gov/health-pro/guidelines/current/asthma-guidelines

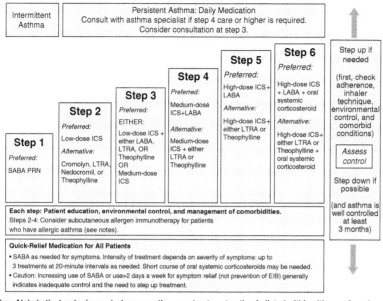

Intermittent Asthma	Persistent Asthma: Daily Medication Consult with asthma specialist if step 4 care or higher is required. Consider consultation at step 3.

Step 1
Preferred:
SABA PRN

Step 2
Preferred:
Low-dose ICS
Alternative:
Cromolyn, LTRA, Nedocromil, or Theophylline

Step 3
Preferred:
EITHER:
Low-dose ICS + either LABA, LTRA, OR Theophylline
OR
Medium-dose ICS

Step 4
Preferred:
Medium-dose ICS+LABA
Alternative:
Medium-dose ICS + either LTRA or Theophylline

Step 5
Preferred:
High-dose ICS+ LABA
Alternative:
High-dose ICS+ either LTRA or Theophylline

Step 6
Preferred:
High-dose ICS + LABA + oral systemic corticosteroid
Alternative:
High-dose ICS+ either LTRA or Theophylline + oral systemic corticosteroid

Step up if needed
(first, check adherence, inhaler technique, environmental control, and comorbid conditions)

Assess control

Step down if possible
(and asthma is well controlled at least 3 months)

Each step: Patient education, environmental control, and management of comorbidities.
Steps 2-4: Consider subcutaneous allergen immunotherapy for patients who have allergic asthma (see notes).

Quick-Relief Medication for All Patients
• SABA as needed for symptoms. Intensity of treatment depends on severity of symptoms: up to 3 treatments at 20-minute intervals as needed. Short course of oral systemic corticosteroids may be needed.
• Caution: Increasing use of SABA or use>2 days a week for symptom relief (not prevention of EIB) generally indicates inadequate control and the need to step up treatment.

Key: Alphabetical order is used when more than one treatment option is listed within either preferred or alternative therapy. ICS, inhaled corticosteroid; LABA, inhaled long-acting beta2-agonist; LTRA, leukotriene receptor antagonist; SABA, inhaled short-acting beta$_2$-agonist

FIGURE
9-5 Assessing asthma disease severity and adjusting control.

(From NHLBI: Guidelines for the Diagnosis and Management of Asthma (EPR-3), https://www.nhlbi.nih.gov/health-pro/guidelines/current/asthma-guidelines.)

4. Risk factors:
    a. Tobacco use (especially a >10 to 15 pack year history)
    b. Occupational exposures—dust or chemical inhalants
    c. Environmental exposures—indoor and outdoor; cooking fumes if poor ventilation in developing countries, etc.
    d. Poor lung development (low birth weight, frequent respiratory infections in childhood)
    e. Atopy
    f. Family history
5. Pathophysiology: chronic inflammation involving airways. Exact pathology may vary because patients have different combinations of emphysema, chronic bronchitis, and asthma.

B. **Clinical features**
1. History: Consider diagnosis in patients >40 with any of the following:
    a. Chronic cough
    b. Dyspnea that is persistent or progressive (Table 9-4)
    c. Chronic sputum production
    d. History of tobacco use, environmental exposure, or occupational exposures
    e. Family history of COPD
    f. Wheezing
2. Physical exam:
    a. Normal unless there is acute exacerbation or severe disease
    b. Acutely, the patient can have decreased air movement, wheezes, rhonchi, increased respiratory effort with pursed lip breathing, and prolonged expiratory phase.

C. **Diagnosis**
1. Differential diagnosis:
    a. Asthma
    b. Congestive heart failure
    c. Interstitial lung disease
    d. Allergies
    e. Tuberculosis or fungal infection

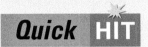

Quick HIT

COPD is diagnosed by spirometry showing an obstructive pattern and decreased FEV$_1$ that is NOT reversible with bronchodilator therapy.

f. Sarcoidosis

g. α-1 antitrypsin deficiency

2. Laboratory findings:

   a. Not necessary for a diagnosis of COPD

   b. Check α-1 antitrypsin levels if the patient is <45 years old, has a family history, or is a nonsmoker.

   c. Radiology: chest X-ray (CXR) useful for excluding other diagnoses, but often normal until advanced disease (hyperinflation)

3. Pulmonary function testing required for diagnosis:

   a. FEV$_1$/FVC < 0.70 that is not reversible with bronchodilator

   b. FEV$_1$ helps determine severity (Table 9-5).

D. **Treatment**

1. Management of stable COPD is based on category of disease severity (Table 9-6).

2. Other therapies:

   a. Smoking cessation support (nicotine replacement, counseling, etc.)

   b. Oxygen (if oxygen saturation equal or less than 88%)

   c. Pulmonary rehabilitation if group B, C, or D

   d. Phosphodiesterase inhibitor (roflumilast)

   e. Theophylline

   f. Lung volume reduction surgery

   g. Lung transplantation

3. Acute exacerbations:

   a. Defined by three main symptoms: increased sputum production, increased dyspnea, and/or increased sputum purulence

   b. Often associated with wheezing, rhonchi, or decreased air movement from baseline exam

   c. Oral steroids—prednisone 40 mg for 5 days (unless severe flare or chronic steroid user)

   d. Regular inhaler or nebulizer treatments with short-acting bronchodilator

   e. Antibiotics are indicated if two or three main symptoms are present (see **a**).

      i. Macrolide if low risk (age < 65, FEV$_1$ > 50% predicted, <3 exacerbations per year, no cardiac disease)

      ii. Respiratory fluoroquinolone if complicated or risk factors

TABLE 9-4	mMRC: Modified Medical Research Council Dyspnea Scale
Grade	**Choose the One Best Response to Describe Your Shortness of Breath.**
0	"I only get breathless with strenuous exercise"
1	"I get short of breath when hurrying on the level or walking up a slight hill"
2	"I walk slower than people of the same age on the level because of breathlessness or have to stop for breath when walking at my own pace on the level"
3	"I stop for breath after walking about 100 yards or after a few minutes on the level"
4	"I am too breathless to leave the house" or "I am breathless when dressing"

TABLE 9-5	GOLD Classification of Airway Obstruction			
Patients With	**Mild**	**Moderate**	**Severe**	**Very Severe**
FEV1/FVC <0.7	FEV1: ≥80% GOLD 1	FEV1: 50%–79% GOLD 2	FEV1: 30%–49% GOLD 3	FEV1: <30% GOLD 4

TABLE 9-6	Management of Stable COPD is Based on Category of Disease Severity								
Patient Class	**Characteristics**	**GOLD Class**	**Exacerbations per Year**	**CAT**	**mMRC**	**Treatment Nonpharm**	**Treatment Pharm 1st line**	**Treatment Pharm Alternative**
A	Low risk Fewer symptoms	1–2	≤1 and no hospitalization	<10	0–1	Smoking cessation, physical activity, flu and pneum vaccine	SAMA prn Or SABA prn	SABA and SMA Or LAMA Or LABA
B	Low risk More symptoms	1–2	≤1 and no hospitalization	≥10	≥2	Smoking cessation, physical activity, flu and pneum vaccine, Pulm Rehab	LAMA Or LABA	LAMA And LABA
C	High risk Fewer symptoms	3–4	≥2 or hospitalization	<10	0–1	Smoking cessation, physical activity, flu and pneum vaccine, Pulm Rehab	ICS + LABA Or LAMA	LAMA and LABA Or LAMA and PDE4-inh Or LABA and PDE4-inh
D	High risk More Symptoms	3–4	≥2 or hospitalization	≥10	≥2	Smoking cessation, physical activity, flu and pneum vaccine Pulm Rehab	ICS + LABA And/or LAMA	ICS + LABA and LAMA Or ICS+LABA and PDE4-inh Or LAMA and LABA Or LAMA and PDE4-inh

CAT, COPD Assessment Test; ICS, inhaled corticosteroid; LABA, long-acting beta agonist; LAMA, long-acting muscarinic antagonist; PDE4-inh, phosphodiesterase-4 inhibitors; SABA, short-acting beta agonist; SAMA, short-acting muscarinic antagonist. http://www.catestonline.org/index.htm.

Diseases of the Respiratory System

4. Complications: bullae, pneumothorax, prolonged steroids can cause osteo-porosis, increased infections
5. Prognosis: BODE (body mass index, airflow obstruction, dyspnea, and exercise capacity) index gives a 4-year survival estimate.
6. Prevention:
   a. Smoking cessation
   b. Treatment of comorbid conditions
   c. Removal of triggers (allergens, environmental exposures, etc.)
   d. Vaccinations: influenza, pneumococcal
   e. Pulmonary rehabilitation

X. Pulmonary Embolism
A. **General characteristics**
1. Definition: a thrombotic event in the pulmonary venous vasculature
2. Epidemiology:
   a. In the United States, first-time occurrences appear in about 100 people for every 100,000.
   b. Affects men and women equally
   c. Asians and Latinos are less likely to develop veno-thromboembolism than Caucasians or African Americans.
   d. Increasing incidence with increasing age
3. Causes:
   a. Genetic predisposition: also called thrombophilia or hypercoagulable state. Common conditions include:
      i. Factor V Leiden
      ii. Protein C or S deficiency
      iii. Antithrombin III deficiency
      iv. Prothrombin mutation
      v. Antiphospholipid antibody syndrome
   b. Acquired states developed in adulthood:
      i. Cancer
      ii. Surgery
      iii. Pregnancy
4. Risk factors:
   a. Active cancer
   b. Recent surgery (in past 30 days)
   c. Previous PE or deep vein thrombosis (DVT)
   d. Pregnancy
   e. Thrombophilic state
   f. Medications such as estrogen
      i. Oral contraceptive pills
      ii. Hormone replacement therapy
   g. Bed-bound functionally
5. Pathophysiology:
   a. Virchow triad creates conditions right for clot formation: venous stasis, endothelial damage, hypercoagulability.
   b. A piece of thrombosis located within the deep vessels in the leg breaks off and gets lodged in the pulmonary vasculature (i.e., embolization).

B. **Clinical features**
1. Symptoms:
   a. Cough with or without hemoptysis
   b. Shortness of breath
   c. Pleuritic chest pain
   d. Occasionally low-grade or tactile fevers
   e. Symptoms of DVT may be present: unilateral leg swelling or redness, calf pain.
2. Signs:
   a. Abnormal vital signs such as tachycardia or tachypnea. Low pulse oximetry is also possible.
   b. Heart and lung exams are often unremarkable.

c. Signs of DVT: unilateral lower extremity edema and/or erythema, and calf tenderness

C. **Diagnosis**
1. Differential diagnosis for adults:
   a. Pneumonia
   b. Acute COPD exacerbation
   c. Acute coronary syndrome
   d. Pericarditis
   e. Lung cancer
   f. Tuberculosis
2. Laboratory findings:
   a. Elevated D-dimer: a negative D-dimer can rule out a PE in patients with a low or moderate pretest probability. A positive or elevated D-dimer requires further testing (i.e., chest CT). Use the Well's score to determine a patient's pretest probability. For those who are at low or moderate risk, order a D-dimer. For those at high risk, proceed to chest CT (Table 9-7).
   b. Leukocytosis, typically mild if present at all
   c. Lab testing for common thrombophilic conditions as needed
3. Radiology findings:
   a. CXR: frequently without abnormal findings.
   b. Chest CT: Given with IV contrast, this can evaluate for PE. PE will be manifested as filling defects.
   c. Ventilation–perfusion (V/Q) scan: a radioactively tagged agent is injected into the blood, while a similarly tagged gas is inhaled into the lungs. The scan looks for a mismatch between blood flow and aeration. When a PE is present, there is diminished circulation in that part of the lung.

D. **Treatment**
1. Therapy:
   a. Anticoagulation: injectable varieties
      i. Unfractionated heparin: given as a continuous infusion
      ii. Low-molecular-weight heparin: given as subcutaneous injection
   b. Anticoagulation: oral varieties
      i. Newer anticoagulants such as dabigatran (Pradaxa), apixaban (Eliquis), and rivaroxaban (Xarelto) are considered the first-line treatment for PE.
      ii. Warfarin (Coumadin) is a second-line option. It has no set dose and requires frequent monitoring with prothrombin time (PT)/international normalized ratio (INR).
   c. Duration of anticoagulation treatment:
      i. The first occurrence is treated for 3 months.
      ii. A second occurrence requires lifelong treatment.

TABLE 9-7 Well's Score for Pulmonary Embolism

Factor	Points
Suspected DVT	3
PE is the most likely diagnosis	3
Tachycardia	1.5
Immobilized > 3 d or surgery in past 4 wk	1.5
Hemoptysis	1
Known malignancy	1
Previous history of DVT or PE	1.5

Scoring: 0 to 1: Low-risk pretest probability
2 to 6: Moderate pretest probability
>6: High pretest probability

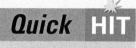

Quick HIT

Hampton hump is the radiologic finding of a wedge-shaped opacity suggestive of pulmonary infarct.

Quick HIT

Underlying lung disease can limit the diagnostic accuracy of V/Q scans, but this testing may be a good alternative for those patients with a contraindication to chest CT.

Quick HIT

Low-molecular-weight heparins have unpredictable metabolism in patients with poor kidney function (CrCL less than 30) or morbid obesity (weight over 150 kg).

Quick HIT

The goal of INR for patients being treated for PE with warfarin is 2 to 3. Novel oral anticoagulants like dabigatran and rivaroxaban do not require INR monitoring.

Quick HIT

Warfarin can be reversed by giving vitamin K, but the newer oral drugs cannot.

Diseases of the Respiratory System

2. Complications:
   a. Arrhythmia, such as pulseless electrical activity (PEA) arrest
   b. Pulmonary infarct
   c. Pulmonary hypertension
   d. Death
3. Duration/prognosis:
   a. The blood clot itself is broken down and resorbed by the body in a matter of weeks to months.
   b. Mortality rates depend on the risk factors/clinical picture.
4. Prevention:
   a. Prophylaxis with low-molecular-weight heparin or dabigatran in high-risk patients
      i. After orthopedic surgeries
      ii. During pregnancy for patients with thrombophilic conditions
      iii. Admissions to the ICU
   b. Avoid prescribing estrogen-containing medications to high-risk patients (such as a known history of previous blood clot or thrombophilic condition, OR women over the age of 35 and smoking).
   c. Lifelong anticoagulation for patients with recurrent events or certain thrombophilic conditions (such as lupus anticoagulant or antithrombin III deficiency)

QUESTIONS

1. A 5-year-old otherwise healthy female is brought to the office by her mother for sore throat and fever up to 102.3°F last night. She has no other symptoms. On exam, she is currently afebrile. Her oropharynx is erythematous and a tonsillar exudate is noted. The next BEST step in management of this patient is:

   A. Order a throat culture
   B. Order rapid strep testing
   C. Order a CBC with differential and liver profile
   D. Treat empirically for streptococcal infection
   E. Treat empirically for viral pharyngitis

2. A 67-year-old male with a past history of hypertension and diabetes comes to the office for the new onset of cough, productive of yellow sputum. He reports tactile fevers and chills, feeling winded when walking around the house, and general malaise. He denies chest pain or weight loss. His only other significant history is prior tobacco use, which he ceased 15 years before. His vital signs include a temperature of 100.1, heart rate of 81, and respirations of 20 with a normal BP. His oxygen saturation is 97% on room air. Upon auscultation, you note harsh breath sounds and rales at his left lung base but no wheezing or rhonchi. His most likely diagnosis is:

   A. COPD exacerbation
   B. PE
   C. pneumonia
   D. acute bronchitis
   E. lung neoplasm

3. A 45-year-old healthy nonsmoking female presents to the emergency department with sharp, pleuritic chest pain and shortness of breath for the past 12 hours. Chest pain is not worsened by exertion and is not altered by position changes. She reports a mild cough, no hemoptysis, and no fevers, chills, or weight change. On exam, she appears anxious. Her heart rate is 115, respirations 24, and oxygen saturation 93% on room air. Auscultation of the chest reveals a rapid but regular heart rate and clear lungs. There is no edema or erythema of her legs. Considering the most likely diagnosis, the next BEST step in the workup is to order:

   A. D-dimer
   B. B-type natriuretic peptide (BNP)
   C. Cardiac enzymes
   D. Chest X-ray
   E. Chest CT scan
   F. Ventilation–perfusion scan
   G. Echocardiography

4. A 6-year-old male is brought to the office by his father for a follow-up appointment 2 weeks after an episode of acute OM. He is still feeling itching and discomfort with his right ear, but denies fever or other concerns. Exam reveals a dull TM with a small amount of fluid visible behind the TM. The next BEST step in management is:

   A. Refer for placement of tympanostomy tube
   B. Prescribe amoxicillin 80 to 90 mg/kg/day for 10 days
   C. Prescribe topical ciprofloxacin otic drops twice per day
   D. Follow-up in 8 to 10 weeks
   E. Refer for otolaryngology specialty evaluation

5. A 12-year-old female with a history of mild persistent asthma presents for a regular follow-up. She currently has no complaints. She has been having dyspnea 3 to 4 days/week requiring her to use her rescue inhaler (inhaled short-acting beta agonist or SABA). She describes nighttime cough 2 to 3 times/month. She has had no flares requiring oral steroids in the past 6 months. Her exam is normal. Your next BEST step in management is:

    A. Refill the SABA and schedule follow-up in 3 months
    B. Review her asthma action plan, refill SABA, and follow up in 3 months
    C. Add an oral glucocorticoid to her regimen
    D. Change her inhaler prescription to a nebulizer formulation
    E. Add a low-dose inhaled glucocorticoid
    F. Add a leukotriene modifier

6. A 52-year-old male with a history of smoking presents for a follow-up appointment for exertional dyspnea worsening over the past 3 months. He has no history of heart problems or family history of cardiac or pulmonary disease. He denies fever, weight loss or gain, cough, chest pain, or any other symptoms. Your initial testing including chest X-ray is normal. He presents today to follow-up after his pulmonary function testing. His results show an $FEV_1/FVC = 0.6$ with a prebronchodilator $FEV_1 = 52\%$ predicted and a postbronchodilator $FEV_1 = 55\%$ predicted. You diagnose him with:

    A. Asthma
    B. Interstitial lung disease
    C. Further testing is needed to determine diagnosis
    D. COPD
    E. Sarcoidosis
    F. Congestive heart failure
    G. Pulmonary embolism

Questions

ANSWERS

1. **Answer: B.** This patient may have streptococcal pharyngitis (strep throat). The next step for diagnosis is to consult the Centor criteria. She has at least 3 of the Centor criteria (fever, tonsillar exudate, absence of cough, but there was no mention of lymphadenopathy). According to the CDC guidelines and the Centor criteria, those patients with 2 or more points should go on to get rapid strep testing in the office. If positive, she should be empirically treated with an antibiotic such as penicillin. Throat cultures are not routinely used to confirm or exclude strep pharyngitis. A CBC with differential and liver enzyme testing would be helpful if mononucleosis was considered most likely. As previously stated, empiric treatment for strep pharyngitis would be indicated only if her rapid strep testing result was positive. If the patient had less than 2 points by Centor criteria, then treating her empirically for a virus is indicated. This would include supportive care measures such as rest, drinking fluids, and using analgesics/antipyretics as needed.

2. **Answer: C.** This patient most likely has pneumonia. Although any of the diagnoses in the answer list could present as cough with or without shortness of breath, his description of symptoms includes an acute onset, fevers, and chills. Recall that older adults may not manifest fevers or leukocytosis with the robustness of younger patients. Finally, he has focal findings on his lung exam, and bronchial breath sounds are a classic finding of pneumonia. Although he is a former smoker, this is not likely a COPD exacerbation given the focal lung findings and the lack of wheezing. Pulmonary embolism can cause low-grade fevers as well but typically is associated with chest pain and tachycardia. PE rarely produces focal lung findings on exam. Acute viral bronchitis can cause a productive cough but should have diffuse wheezing on exam. Lung neoplasms typically do not present acutely and often have associated weight loss. Again, abnormal lung findings on exam are not common.

3. **Answer: A.** The most likely diagnosis for this patient is a PE. The next step in the diagnosis of PE depends on the likelihood of the patient having a PE. A Well's score determines this likelihood. This particular patient's Well's score is 4.5 points (she received points for tachycardia and for PE being the most likely diagnosis) giving her a moderate pretest probability. For low or moderate risk of PE, a D-dimer is the next best step. If negative, PE would be ruled out. If positive, a chest CT (or, if CT is contraindicated, a ventilation–perfusion scan) would be needed to confirm the diagnosis. A BNP can be helpful when congestive heart failure (CHF) exacerbation is suspected because the BNP is frequently elevated in this scenario. However, this patient did not have signs or symptoms of CHF (no weight gain, no edema in her legs or crackles in her lungs, no cardiac history). Cardiac enzymes or biomarkers are useful when acute coronary syndrome is suspected. Although she has chest pain, this patient has few risk factors for underlying coronary artery disease (no PMHx of diabetes or hypertension, nonsmoker, <55 years old, female). A chest X-ray could be useful for confirming a suspect pneumonia. Again, her presentation (no fevers or chills) and normal respiratory exam findings do not support pneumonia as the most likely diagnosis. A chest CT scan given with contrast can evaluate for PE or a pulmonary neoplasm. Although PE is suspected in this case, her moderate pretest probability means a D-dimer should be ordered first. The same is true for ventilation–perfusion scan. Echocardiography is often part of the workup for patients with CHF, pericarditis, or coronary artery disease.

4. **Answer: D.** Monitoring for resolution up to 12 weeks is appropriate. If pain or symptoms worsen, then you would suspect complications and consider reevaluation or referral. However, if truly no erythema and mild symptoms related to the presence of fluid, then it is reasonable to observe up to 12 weeks. Oral antibiotics are indicated in OM. Topical antibiotics would be indicated for otitis externa.

5. **Answer: E.** In assessing her disease severity, she would be considered mild persistent (symptoms >2 days/week, nighttime awakenings 3 to 4 times/month) (see Tables 9-3 and 9-4). Addition of an inhaled glucocorticoid is the correct next step with close follow-up in 2 to 6 weeks to ensure this adequately controls her disease (symptoms should be less than or equal to 2 days in a month, < or = 2 nighttime awakenings per month, no interference with activity level). Asthma action plans are important in the management of asthma and should be completed with all patients. Oral steroids are not necessary if there is no concern for an acute exacerbation. There is no difference in nebulizer versus adequately administered inhaler treatments. Leukotriene modifiers are reasonable alternatives if not tolerating or patient prefers to avoid low-dose inhaled glucocorticoids, but these would not be first line.

6. **Answer: D.** COPD is suspected in patients with progressive dyspnea and may be accompanied by chronic cough and a history of smoking. Initial evaluation should include an exam and chest X-ray. Pulmonary function testing will reveal an obstructive pattern on spirometry based on $FEV_1/FVC < 0.7$. The FEV_1 is not improved with bronchodilator use as it would be in asthma. Interstitial lung disease may have chest X-ray abnormalities, and spirometry results vary but often show a restrictive pattern (decreased FVC, normal or increased FEV_1/FVC, and normal or decreased FEV_1). Pulmonary embolism usually does not present with a 3-month course and spirometry would be normal. He has no other signs or symptoms of CHF.

I. Nausea and Vomiting

A. **Definitions**
1. Nausea: a sensation of uneasiness in the stomach, which requires conscious awareness and cerebral function
2. Vomiting: emesis, the forceful emptying of stomach. This is not just a more severe degree of nausea; it is mediated by separate pathways.

B. **Pathophysiology**
1. Central nervous system (CNS): Nausea has distinct neural pathways from emesis, and different triggers.
2. Emesis is controlled by the chemoreceptor trigger zone (CTZ) and vomiting center (VC) in the brain.
3. The CTZ lacks a blood–brain barrier (BBB), allowing toxins to directly activate it via dopamine 2 receptors.
4. Peripheral signals in the gut detect stomach contents and gastric stretch via serotonin triggering emesis.

C. **Approach**
1. Address causes.
2. Address consequences.
3. Treat causes.

D. **Causes**
1. Acute:
   a. Infectious: especially gastrointestinal (GI) illnesses, but also systemic, sepsis
   b. Endotoxic: food poisoning, ingestion of toxins
   c. Non-GI infections
   d. Postoperative: from anesthetic agents or surgical complications
   e. Neurologic:
      i. Vertigo and nystagmus triggering nausea = vestibular neuritis (labyrinthitis)
      ii. Motion sickness
      iii. Intracranial pressure (tumor or bleed): Neurogenic vomiting may be positional, projectile, or associated with other neurologic signs.
   f. Chemotoxic:
      i. Central: Consider toxins, direct stimulation from CTZ as outside BBB.
      ii. Gastric irritants: may not be relieved with emesis compared with obstructive process (medications, alcohol, marijuana)
   g. Endocrine: abrupt cessation of corticosteroids owing to adrenal insufficiency
2. Chronic:
   a. CNS: mass effect from tumor, abscess, bleed
   b. Pregnancy: typically first trimester
   c. Gut dysmotility (gastroparesis), related to chronic endocrine issues (eg, diabetes mellitus [DM])

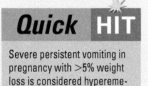

Quick HIT

Severe persistent vomiting in pregnancy with >5% weight loss is considered hyperemesis gravidarum.

Nutritional and Digestive Disorders

   d. Inflammatory/irritative: nonsteroidal anti-inflammatory drugs (NSAIDs), chemotherapeutic agents, other medications
   e. Outlet obstruction:
      i. Nausea relieved (even temporarily) by emesis—refer to surgery
      ii. Severe constipation can lead to nausea
   f. Psychological: bulimia, depression, anxiety
E. **Treatment:**
   1. Eliminate offending agents as far as possible.
   2. Diet modification; promote optimal bowel hygiene
   3. Medications:
      a. Migraine-related: dopamine antagonist (prochlorperazine)
      b. Vestibular:
         i. Histamine antagonist: promethazine
         ii. Anticholinergic: scopolamine patch or pretravel benzodiazepine
      c. Pregnancy:
         i. Dietary ginger, vitamin B_6
         ii. Histamine antagonist: promethazine
      d. Postoperative:
         i. Serotonin (5HT3) antagonists (eg, ondanestron)
         ii. Dopamine antagonist: prochlorperazine
      e. Palliative care: subcutaneous somatostatin analogs like octreotide
      f. Gastroparetic:
         i. Optimize diabetic control and neurologic function.
         ii. Methotrexate: 10 mg every 4 to 6 hours
         iii. Erythromycin
      g. Psychological:
         i. Psychological support
         ii. Conscious breathing, stress reduction
   4. Integrative methods:
      a. Acupuncture, ginger, guided imagery, progressive muscle relaxation, music therapy
      b. There is some evidence for benefit for nausea/vomiting in patients on chemotherapy.

II. Dyspepsia, Gastroesophageal Reflux Disease, Peptic Ulcer Disease

A. **Definitions**
   1. Dyspepsia: one or more episodes of postprandial fullness, early satiation, or epigastric pain/burning
   2. Gastroesophageal reflux disease (GERD): reflux of stomach contents into the esophagus leading to symptoms or complications
   3. Peptic ulcer disease (PUD): an ulcer in the gastric or duodenal wall that extends through the muscularis mucosa
B. **Pathophysiology**
   1. Parietal cells in the gastric mucosa produce acid for proteolysis.
   2. Nonorganic dyspepsia: 75% (no cause identified after diagnostic evaluation)
   3. Organic finding in 25%
      a. GERD
      b. Inflammation of esophagus, stomach, or duodenum
      c. Ulcer of stomach or duodenum
      d. GI malignancy
      e. Drug induced (eg, NSAIDs, aspirin, bisphosphonates)
      f. Biliary
C. **Diagnosis**
   1. History: postprandial fullness, early satiation, epigastric pain or burning, retrosternal burning pain, regurgitation, medication history
   2. Exam: usually normal except for possible epigastric tenderness
   3. Labs: complete blood count (CBC), comprehensive metabolic panel (CMP), *Helicobacter pylori*

4. Diagnostic testing:
   a. Radiologic: Barium swallow may diagnose disease but is insufficient for confirmation.
   b. Endoscopic: allows visualization and pathologic confirmation (biopsy)
   c. ECG: if there is a possible cardiac cause

D. **Treatment**
1. Lifestyle.
   a. Weight loss
   b. Nonrestrictive clothing
   c. Meal timing: Allow 3 hours after meal before reclining.
   d. Recumbency: elevate the head of the bed with 5-inch lifts, tilt, not bend centrally
   e. Smoking cessation
   f. Avoid extra pillows because they may increase gastric pressure.
2. Diet modification:
   a. Eliminate irritants: caffeine, alcohol, NSAID/aspirin, specific food/additives.
   b. Support digestion with adequate whole foods, fiber.
   c. Adequate hydration
   d. Enzymes: fresh papaya (papain), pineapple (bromelain), or supplement
3. Psychological: stress reduction, emotional support network
4. Microbiome: probiotics—*Lactobacillus acidophilus* interferes with *H. pylori* epithelial cell adhesion and may inhibit growth, inhibiting ulcer formation.
5. Pharmaceutical:
   a. Nonorganic disease
      i. Antacids, calcium carbonate
      ii. Histamine 2 blockers (ranitidine, famotidine)
      iii. Proton pump inhibitors (omeprazole, lansoprazole, etc.)
      iv. Cytoprotectants (sucralfate): mucosal protective agent binds to the ulcer crater, forms a protective coating
      v. Treating *H. pylori*: Eradication reduces recurrence of PUD to 10%, ongoing infection may have 50% to 80% recurrence.
   b. Organic disease
      i. Prolonged antacid regimen
      ii. Surveillance for malignant potential

III. Diarrhea

A. **Characteristics**
1. Definition:
   a. Nonformed stool with increased fluid content
   b. Severe diarrhea is defined as ≥4 fluid stools per day for more than 3 days.
   c. Functional diarrhea: limited to the waking hours, large and semi-formed, progressively looser throughout the day
2. Pathophysiology:
   a. Incomplete colonic absorption of water from the intestinal lumen
      i. Decreased electrolyte absorption or excessive electrolyte secretion
      ii. Osmotic retention of water in the lumen
   b. Reduction of net water absorption by even 1% is sufficient to cause diarrhea.
3. Causes:
   a. Acute:
      i. Infectious
         (a) Viral: probably most common, rarely tested clinically, self-limited (under 2 weeks)
         (b) Bacterial: typically most severe, from various foods or contaminated water
         (c) Toxin: enterotoxigenic *E. coli*, staph toxin
         (d) Protozoal: giardia, entamoeba

ii. Dietary history:

    (a) Symptoms within 6 hours: ingestion of preformed toxin (eg, *Staphylococcus aureus* or *Bacillus cereus*)

    (b) Symptoms start at 8 to 16 hours: *Clostridium perfringens*

    (c) Symptoms start at >16 hours: viral or bacterial infection (eg, enterotoxigenic or enterohemorrhagic *E. coli*)

    (d) Diarrhea that progresses to fever, headache, muscle aches, and stiff neck suggest infection with *Listeria monocytogenes*, especially in pregnancy.

    (e) Osmotic: Check consumption of carbohydrates, sorbitol-sweetened juices.

b. Persistent:

  i. Chronic low-grade infections

  ii. Postenteritis syndrome: symptoms beyond the typical 14-day resolution, occasionally follows acute illness, enzymatic deficiency proposed

  iii. Delayed healing of intestinal mucosa, host factors zinc or vitamin A deficiency, malnutrition prolong duration of diarrhea

c. Chronic:

  i. Dietary

    (a) Food intolerances: lactose, sorbitol, specific food irritant, gluten (intolerance)

    (b) Candies or gums with osmotic potential, sorbitol

    (c) Autoimmune processes: gluten sensitivity (celiac)

  ii. Laxative history: use or abuse

  iii. Cholerheic diarrhea: post cholecystectomy, drainage of bile salts into small bowel with limited ileal reabsorption

  iv. Ileal resection and osmotic effect of bile salts in colon

B. **Diagnosis**

1. Rule out extracellular volume depletion (decreased skin turgor, orthostatic hypotension).

2. Fever and peritoneal signs are clues to infection with an invasive enteric pathogen.

3. Exposure/travel history

4. Laboratory studies:

  a. Serum electrolytes, CBC, liver function tests (LFTs), albumin for protein status

  b. Stool testing

    i. Fecal leukocytes (WBC) of limited usefulness

    ii. *Clostridium difficile*: patients with a history of hospitalization

    iii. Lactoferrin: marker for fecal WBC, test is more specific, less variation in lab processing

  c. Endoscopy: for severe symptoms that are not improving

C. **Treatment**

1. Good hand washing, hygiene, and public health measures

2. Rehydration: Use over-the-counter rehydration solution.

3. Eliminate triggers (eg, food sensitivities).

4. BRAT (bananas, rice, applesauce, toast) diet:

  a. Boiled starches and cereals (potatoes, noodles, rice, wheat, oats) with salt; crackers, bananas, soup, and boiled vegetables

  b. Avoid foods with high fat content until gut function returns to normal.

5. Secondary lactose malabsorption is common after infectious enteritis, and can last for several weeks to months.

6. Medications:

  a. Antibiotics: specific to organism (eg, for *C. difficile*, oral metronidazole or vancomycin)

  b. Probiotics: reduce stool frequency and duration of persistent diarrhea

  c. Bulking agents: fiber

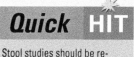

Stool studies should be reserved for those with severe or prolonged symptoms.

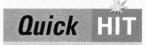

Most cases of diarrhea in the United States are self-limited.

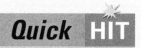

Loperamide can cause rebound constipation, particularly in young adults and children.

Nutritional and Digestive Disorders

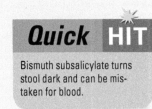

d. Motility agents
   i. Loperamide: initially, then after each unformed stool
   ii. Diphenoxylate: may increase risk of hemolytic uremic syndrome (HUS) in *E. coli*
   iii. Bismuth subsalicylate
e. Micronutrients: replace K and Zn
7. Psychological:
   a. Address anxiety.
   b. Consider factitious diarrhea: laxative abuse

IV. Constipation
A. **Characteristics**
   1. Definition:
      a. Common: refers to difficult or infrequent passage of stool
      b. Medical: fewer than three spontaneous, complete bowel movements (BMs) per week
   2. Epidemiology:
      a. Most common intestinal complaint in the United States
      b. Adult prevalence of 15% to 20% of population
      c. Rare in non-Westernized cultures with a much higher dietary fiber intake
      d. Common in pediatric population, may be related to behavioral issues, toilet training
   3. Pathophysiology:
      a. Some biorhythms are present with optimal evacuation in AM.
      b. Typically after a meal (gastrocolic reflex)
      c. Slow transit of food (95%)
      d. Less often pelvic floor dysfunction, prolapse or denervation (neuro issues)
   4. Clinical contributors:
      a. Dietary: diet low in insoluble fiber, insufficient fluid intake
      b. Neurologic: central or peripheral
      c. Metabolic: DM, thyroid disease
      d. Outlet delay: pelvic floor weakness, neurologic/dyssynergy
      e. Pharmaceutical/Iatrogenic: narcotics, calcium, iron, calcium channel blocker, antibiotics, etc.
B. **Diagnosis**
   1. Diet diary
   2. Lab testing:
      a. Thyroid assessment
      b. Lead levels in children
      c. UA/culture as constipation can trigger urinary track infection
      d. Stool testing for digestive markers, dysbiosis
   3. Imaging:
      a. Radiologic: plain films can detect megacolon or megarectum (Hirschsprung's in children). Plain films cannot distinguish ileus from mechanical obstruction.
      b. Avoid barium if perforation is suspected.
   4. Endoscopic: Colonoscopy can investigate obstruction.
   5. Anorectal manometry to verify internal and external anal sphincter tone and intrarectal pressure during defecation
C. **Treatment**
   1. Eliminate triggers
      a. Avoidance of cow's milk may improve colon transit
      b. Food antigens and immune activation are known to affect gastric motility.
      c. Medications: iron, antacids
   2. Diet
      a. Hydration: Increase water intake; 1.5 to 2 L of water daily.
      b. Fiber: Increase dietary fiber (optimal 25 g or more).
      c. Probiotics aid digestion.

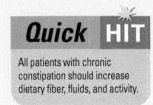

3. Medications
    a. Magnesium supplement (titrate dose to BM frequency, too much magnesium will lead to diarrhea)
    b. Stool softeners: docusate, mineral oil, glycerin suppository
    c. Osmotic agents
       i. Poorly absorbed or nonabsorbable sugars, saline laxatives, cause intestinal water secretion
       ii. Polyethylene glycol (PEG), synthetic disaccharides: lactulose/sorbitol, milk of magnesia, magnesium citrate, juice (apple juice)
       iii. Side effect: Excessive use causes diarrhea.
    d. Laxatives: (Senna) increases motility; can cause habituation
    e. Bulk-forming laxatives: psyllium, methylcellulose, polycarbophil (fiber supplements)
4. Behavioral
    a. Daily physical activity, jogging, and/or running most beneficial
    b. Biofeedback for pelvic floor toning or retraining
    c. Reward systems, charting BM for kids
5. Severe constipation may require multimodal approach and/or manual disimpaction.

V. GI/Rectal Bleeding

A. **Characteristics**
  1. Definition: gross or occult loss of heme into the bowel lumen
    a. Bright red blood per rectum (BRBPR) or hematochezia: usually associated with a lower GI bleed
    b. Melena: dark tarry stools that contain partially digested blood and are usually associated with an upper GI bleed
  2. Causes:
    a. Need to rule out cancer, typically an occult presentation.
    b. Consider inflammatory process (inflammatory bowel disease).
    c. Diverticulosis: 40% of bleeding presentations, usually painless
    d. Ischemic process can result in mucosal compromise and vascular breakdown.
    e. Hemorrhoids: leading cause
    f. Small bowel source: may be difficult to detect
B. **Clinical presentation**
  1. Historical findings:
    a. Use of aspirin, NSAIDs, or anticoagulant
    b. History of liver disease, coagulopathy
    c. Site of the bleed is hinted by texture/color.
       i. Bright red: lower colon
       ii. Black/tarry: upper GI tract
    d. Emesis: coffee grounds: partly digested heme or frank blood
  2. Physical exam findings:
    a. Signs of anemia: pale mucus membranes
    b. Volume depletion from acute losses
       i. Stable with minimal symptoms: patient education, arrange treatment as outpatient
       ii. Unstable with dropping BP, tachycardia, weakness: send patient to the emergency room
    c. Hemorrhoids (varicose veins around the anus)
       i. Internal or external
       ii. Risk factors: constipation/straining, portal hypertension, prolonged sitting or standing, pregnancy, obesity, anal intercourse
C. **Diagnosis**
  1. Labs: fecal occult blood test (FOBT), CBC, coagulation factors (international normalized ratio/prothrombin time)
  2. Nasogastric tube in the hospital

3. Endoscopy
    a. Anoscopy: an office-based procedure that can find hemorrhoids, fissures, anal mass
    b. Upper endoscopy: looking for the site of bleeding or malignancy
    c. Sigmoidoscopy or colonoscopy
4. Bleeding scan (radionuclide)
5. Arteriography/CT arteriogram
6. Exploratory laparoscopy in extreme cases

D. **Treatment**
1. Upper GI bleed (depends on cause):
    a. Remove offending agents (aspirin [ASA], NSAID)
    b. Observation if not acute
    c. Serial CBCs
    d. Antacid regimen
    e. Mucosal support
    f. Referral if chronic signs/symptoms or unstable
    g. Lifestyle/diet modification
2. Lower GI bleed (depends on cause):
    a. Observation
    b. Serial CBCs
    c. Referral if chronic signs/symptoms, age over 50, or unstable
    d. Lifestyle/diet modification: fiber (dietary and supplementation), hydration, weight loss
    e. Topical care: Sitz baths for hemorrhoids, evacuation of thrombus, Intra-anal analgesics, lidocaine, hydrocortisone
    f. Address source of bleed: hemorrhoid banding, surgical hemorrhoidectomy, colon resection for persistent colonic source of bleed, arterial embolization

VI. Irritable Bowel Syndrome

A. **Characteristics**
1. Definition: GI disorder consisting of chronic abdominal pain and altered bowel habits without identified trigger
2. Epidemiology:
    a. The most common GI diagnosis, and the reason for about 30% of referrals to gastroenterologists
    b. Prevalence in North America estimated at 10% to 15% of the population
    c. 2:1 ratio female to male
    d. The second highest cause of work absenteeism after the common cold

B. **Clinical features.** Historical findings include:
1. Variety of complaints: crampy sensation, variable intensity, periodic exacerbations
2. Location and character of the pain can vary widely.
3. Severity of pain ranges from mildly annoying to crippling.
4. May worsen with eating and emotional stress
5. Defecation often provides some relief.
6. Altered bowel function:
    a. Diarrhea is dominant (IBS-D):
        i. Frequent loose stools of small to moderate quantity
        ii. Occasionally fecal urgency, fecal incontinence
        iii. Sensation of incomplete voiding
        iv. Half of IBS patients report mucus discharge with stools.
    b. Constipation is dominant (IBS-C):
        i. Infrequent evacuation: days to months
        ii. Intervals of normal or loose bowel function
        iii. Pellet-like, dry BM

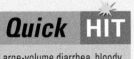

Quick HIT

Large-volume diarrhea, bloody stools, nocturnal diarrhea, and greasy stools are *not* associated with IBS and suggest an organic disease.

7. Red flags: These features do NOT support a benign process.
   a. Pain associated with anorexia, malnutrition, or weight loss
   b. Pain that is gradually worsening, or awakens the patient from or interferes with sleep
   c. Large-volume diarrhea, bloody stools, nocturnal diarrhea, and greasy stools

C. **Diagnosis:** IBS is a diagnosis of "exclusion"
   1. Diagnose based on Rome IV criteria: recurrent abdominal pain at least 1 day/week over the last 3 months and two or more of the following:
      a. Related to defecation
      b. Associated with a change in stool frequency
      c. Associated with a change in stool form/appearance
   2. Improvement with stress modification
   3. Improvement with dietary modification
   4. Lab testing
      a. Stool culture: There is little role for culture except in cases of significant diarrhea, or possible *Giardia* exposure.
      b. Celiac testing: IgA to tissue transglutaminase Ab, conflicting results
   5. Dietary elimination trials: gluten, dairy
   6. Colonoscopy, sigmoidoscopy with biopsy

D. **Treatment**
   1. Education, reassurance
   2. Diet modification:
      a. Food diary: journaling of foods eaten, symptoms experienced, emotional details
      b. Reduce gas-forming foods: cruciferous, legumes
      c. Reduce alcohol, caffeine, lactose
      d. Low FODMAP (fermentable oligosaccharides, disaccharides, monosaccharides, and polyols) diet: simple sugar avoidance
      e. Trial of gluten avoidance: 14- to 21-day elimination, IgA transglutaminase testing BEFORE elimination if needed
      f. Fiber: soluble psyllium for IBS-C, insoluble methylcellulose; start low and go slow to reduce irritation from bulk
      g. Food allergy testing: not well studied and individual food elimination trials may be more useful
   3. Medications:
      a. IBS-C PEG
      b. Bile acid sequestrants: cholestyramine, colestipol (side effects: gas, etc.)
      c. Antispasmodics: dicyclomine or hyoscyamine
      d. Antidepressants: tricyclic antidepressants or selective serotonin reuptake inhibitors
      e. Antibiotics: may warrant a 2-week trial of rifaximin
      f. Probiotics: limited evidence, trial warranted in history of frequent or prolonged antibiotic use
   4. Behavior modification and psychological support

VII. Inflammatory Bowel Disease (IBD)

A. **Crohn disease**
   1. Characteristics:
      a. Mean onset at 15 to 35 years old
      b. More common in people of European ancestry.
      c. Can affect *any* part of intestinal tract (mouth to anus):
         i. 40% terminal ileum and cecum
         ii. 30% only small bowel
         iii. 25% just large bowel
         iv. Rarely stomach, mouth, esophagus
   2. Clinical features:
      a. Usually (nonbloody) diarrhea, nausea, vomiting
      b. Malabsorption and weight loss
      c. Abdominal pain, classically right lower quadrant

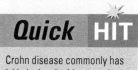

Quick HIT

Crohn disease commonly has "skip lesions" with areas that are free of disease between patches of disease.

Nutritional and Digestive Disorders

    d. Can have fever and malaise

    e. Extraintestinal symptoms in 15% to 20% of the time (eye inflammation, ankylosing spondylitis, arthritis, oral ulcers, gallstones, kidney stones)

    f. Nutritional considerations

      i. Malabsorption of B vitamins (especially B_{12}) and vitamin D

      ii. Impaired permeability caused by inflammation may allow absorption of allergenic or toxic matter.

      iii. Terminal ileal disease reduces reabsorption of bile acids affecting enterohepatic circulation, contributing to cholelithiasis.

      iv. Increased oxalate absorption contributing to kidney stones

      v. Growth retardation from chronic malnutrition in pediatric ages

    g. Impaired immune function, 70% of body's lymph tissue associated with gut, gut-associated lymphoid tissue

  3. Diagnosis:

    a. Endoscopy (sigmoidoscopy/colonoscopy): focal ulcerations adjacent to normal areas, skip areas of involvement, rectum is often lesion free

    b. Barium enema: may be normal early

    c. Abdominal CT: useful in evaluating extent of disease and in evaluating for small bowel involvement

    d. Pathology:

      i. Aphthous ulcers, patchy skip lesions, cobblestone appearance, pseudopolyps

      ii. *Transmural*: findings through the bowel wall from mucosa to serosa

  4. Treatment:

    a. Nutritional support

      i. Supplementation of various nutrients is key.

      ii. Address side effects of various Rx medications (steroids, etc.).

    b. Medications

      i. Sulfasalazine (active compound is mesalamine, 5-ASA): useful when colon is involved; blocks prostaglandin release, reduce inflammation

      ii. Metronidazole when 5-ASA not effective

      iii. Systemic steroids (prednisone) for acute exacerbations

      iv. Immunosuppressants (azathioprine, 5-mercaptopurine, newer immune modulating drugs)

      v. Bile acid sequestrants (colestipol, cholestyramine) to bind bile for patients with terminal ileal disease

      vi. Antidiarrheal meds with caution

      vii. Pain medications for chronic pain with comprehensive care planning

    c. Surgical

      i. Bowel resection frequently required eventually

      ii. Segmental resections of most diseased portions of bowel

      iii. Recurrence after surgery is high, 50% after 10 years

      iv. Indicated for small bowel obstruction (SBO), fistula, perforation, disabling pain

    d. Complications

      i. Fistulae between colon and other portions of intestines, bladder, vagina, or skin

      ii. Anorectal disease with fissures, abscesses

      iii. Bowel obstruction

      iv. Malignancy from colon and small bowel tumors (less common than in ulcerative colitis [UC])

B. **Ulcerative colitis**

  1. Characteristics:

    a. May occur at any age, but commonly in adolescence or young adulthood

    b. Distribution:

      i. Entirely colonic and always involves the rectum

      ii. Large bowel may be involved to various extents.

        (a) Rectum alone in 10%

        (b) Rectum and left colon in 40%

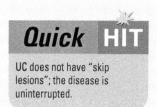

(c) Rectum, left and right colon in 25%

(d) Pancolitis in 25%

   iii. Small bowel is not typically involved, but the disease may reach the terminal ileum ("backwash ileitis").

2. Clinical features:

  a. Bloody diarrhea (hematochezia)

  b. Abdominal pain

  c. Small frequent BM

  d. Fever, anorexia

  e. Tenesmus (rectal spasms)

  f. Extraintestinal symptoms (similar to Crohn's: eye involvement, arthritis, skin lesions, jaundice)

3. Diagnosis:

  a. Stool cultures, *C. difficile*, and ova and parasites: to rule out infection

  b. Fecal leukocytes: not specific to UC but support inflammatory process if present

  c. Colonoscopy needed to assess extent of disease

  d. Pathology: *nontransmural* involvement, only mucosa and submucosa

  e. CT scan of abdomen and pelvis: may demonstrate bowel wall thickening, may be normal early in the disease

4. Treatment:

  a. Nutritional

    i. Exacerbations may require total parenteral nutrition (TPN).

    ii. Address side effects of prescription medications.

  b. Medications

    i. Corticosteroids for acute flare ups

    ii. Sulfasalazine (active component is 5-ASA, mesalamine)

    iii. Immunosuppressive agents: not effective for acute attacks

  c. Surgical

    i. Surgical resection may cure.

    ii. Total colectomy for severe disease, perforation, obstruction, hemorrhage, cancer

  d. Complications

    i. Gross or occult blood loss

    ii. Electrolyte imbalance from diarrhea

    iii. Strictures

    iv. Sclerosing cholangitis: may not parallel bowel disease, may not be prevented with surgical resection

    v. Nutritional

      (a) Growth retardation from malabsorption

      (b) Iron deficiency

      (c) Specific nutrient malabsorption: B vitamins

      (d) Electrolyte loss

    vi. Colon cancer: risk parallels extent and duration of disease, higher rates than with Crohn's

    vii. Cholangiocarcinoma, half of bile duct cancers are in patients with UC

    viii. Narcotic abuse risks from chronic pain treatment

    ix. Psychological distress from chronic illness, pain

C. **Celiac disease (celiac sprue, gluten enteropathy)**

1. Characteristics:

  a. Inflammatory bowel changes related to hypersensitivity to gluten protein contained in wheat, barley, and rye.

  b. Immune-mediated disorder of the small intestine in which gluten is identified as a foreign Ag; the immune response damages the mucosal lining

  c. Can start in infants upon introduction of solids and cereals or not until later in life (age 10 to 40)

   d. Genetics: 95% have HLA DQ2 or HLA DQ8 mutations; occurs in 10% of first-degree relatives
   e. Patients with trisomy have double the risk of having celiac disease.
2. Clinical features:
   a. Bloating, diarrhea, and weight loss
   b. Children: can have failure to thrive (FTT), delayed growth, irritability, vomiting, constipation, large stools, edema, frequent respiratory infections
   c. Adults: may be asymptomatic or have diarrhea, weight loss, bloating, gas pain, stool changes
   d. Extraintestinal symptoms:
      i. Malabsorption of vitamin D = rickets, osteomalacia
      ii. Malabsorption of iron: anemia
      iii. Joints: other autoimmune overlapping with rheumatoid arthritis or nonautoimmune arthropathies
      iv. Hormonal: amenorrhea, infertility
      v. Skin: dermatitis herpetiformis
3. Diagnosis:
   a. Endoscopy: proximal small bowel with villous flattening, inflammatory changes
   b. Serology for IgA tissue transglutaminase (TTG) or antiendomysial Ab; antigliadin testing less reliable
   c. Gluten elimination diet can be helpful in diagnosis.
   d. Small intestinal biopsy via endoscopy
   e. HLA haplotype to establish risk for offspring
   f. Follow-up biopsy after strictly gluten-free diet for 3 to 6 months
4. Treatment:
   a. Strict adherence to zero-gluten diet (nutrition consult is helpful)
   b. Nutritional recovery, supplement of specific nutrients: B complex, fat-soluble vitamins
   c. Immunosuppressant therapy with corticosteroids may be needed.
   d. Dapsone for associated dermatitis herpetiformis, although in time it will resolve on its own with a gluten-free diet

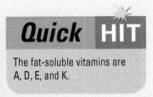

Quick HIT

The fat-soluble vitamins are A, D, E, and K.

VIII. Failure to Thrive (FTT)

A. **Definition**
   1. An inability to maintain growth or weight and bodily composition
   2. Encompasses findings of physical frailty, disability, and impaired neuropsychiatric function
   3. Pediatric: weight loss, developmental delay, psychosocial impairment, and regression of social skills
   4. Adult: weight loss (5% over 2 years) or malnourishment, weakness, cognitive decline, loss of ADLs, inability to stand from a chair five times without using arms to push up, impaired immunity

B. **Risk factors**
   1. BMI < 22 in community-based elders was associated with an increased 1-year mortality risk.
   2. Underweight is associated with poorer functional status.

C. **Causes**
   1. Medical history:
      a. Oral impairments: poor oral health, impaired saliva, dry mouth, changes in taste, difficulty chewing/swallowing
      b. Malignancy: lung, breast, hematologic, GI, GU, ovarian, prostate, hepatobiliary
      c. GI: hypochlorhydria, early satiety, chronic constipation, PUD, dysmotility, cirrhosis, bacterial overgrowth, chronic pancreatitis, ischemic bowel, celiac disease
      d. Cardiac: congestive heart failure, coronary artery disease, unstable angina

e. Pulmonary: chronic obstructive pulmonary disease, interstitial lung disease, bronchiectasis, chronic infection, aspiration pneumonia

f. Infectious: TB, subacute bacterial endocarditis, recurrent bladder infections

g. Neurologic: dementia, cerebrovascular accident, Parkinson, motor neuropathies

h. Endocrine: DM2, adrenal insufficiency, hyperparathyroidism, hyper/hypothyroidism

i. Nutritional: deficiency of thiamine, vitamin B_{12}, vitamin D, vitamin C, zinc

j. Renal: uremia, nephrotic syndrome

k. Psychiatric: depression, bereavement, alcoholism, mania, psychosis

2. Rheumatologic: chronic pain, polymyalgia rheumatica, giant-cell arteritis

3. Iatrogenic: medications including beta blockers, medications that interfere with nutrient absorption, anticholinergics, CNS suppressants, chemotherapeutics

4. Socioeconomic: poor support system, decreased sense of purpose, drug and alcohol abuse

D. **Clinical features:** The following should be checked to help determine cause:

1. Weight/height/BMI, pediatric growth curves

2. Dental: edentulous, ill-fitting dentures

3. Swallow: impaired by dry mouth, hydration

4. Vision and hearing

5. Foot abnormalities, pain

6. Joint restrictions, pain

7. Balance issues, fall risk

8. Tremor, incoordination

9. Labs: based on history and exam

E. **Treatment:** based on underlying cause

IX. Liver, Gallbladder, Pancreas Disease

A. **Gallbladder disease**

1. Characteristics:

a. There is a marked variation in gallstone prevalence between different ethnic populations.

b. Incidental gallstones only 15% to 25% will become symptomatic in 10 to 15 years.

c. Rome criteria for pain of biliary origin:

i. Located in the epigastrium and/or right upper quadrant

ii. Recurrent, but occurs at variable intervals (not daily)

iii. Lasts at least 30 minutes

iv. Builds up to a steady level

v. Severe enough to interrupt daily activities or lead to an emergency department visit

vi. Not relieved by BM, postural changes, or antacids

d. Types of stones

i. Cholesterol: associated with metabolic disease, pregnancy, oral contraceptive pills, cystic fibrosis, cirrhosis, Crohn's

ii. Pigmented stones

(a) Black: hemolysis (sickle cell disease, thalassemia, alcohol cirrhosis)

(b) Brown: biliary infection

2. Clinical features:

a. May be asymptomatic

b. Colicky pain often associated with meal

c. Biliary obstruction

i. Typically located right upper quadrant or epigastrium

ii. Classically after eating meal containing fat or at night

iii. Boas sign: biliary pain referred to right scapula

iv. Can result in cholecystitis with prolonged blockage of cystic duct

d. Cholecystitis: inflammation of the gallbladder, often associated with stone disease, biliary sludge

3. Diagnosis:
   a. Labs: bilirubin, alk phos, LFT
   b. Right upper quadrant ultrasound: high sensitivity and specificity for stones over 2 mm
   c. CT scan and MRI can also identify
   d. HIDA scan with CCK (cholecystokinin): to look at gallbladder function

4. Treatment:
   a. Diet modification: low-fat diet
   b. Gradual weight loss, sudden weight loss can trigger more stones.
   c. Surgical referral for possible cholecystectomy
   d. NSAIDs have been shown to be helpful for pain.
   e. If not a surgical candidate: oral dissolution therapy with ursodeoxycholic acid

B. **Liver disease (cirrhosis)**
   1. Characteristics:
      a. Definition: chronic liver disease with fibrosis, architectural distortion, nodularity, disruption of hepatocyte function
      b. Causes
         i. Drug: alcohol, methotrexate, acetaminophen, macrodantin
         ii. Obstructive: gallstones, cholestasis
         iii. Metabolic: nonalcoholic steatohepatitis, hemochromatosis, Wilson's
         iv. Infectious: hepatitis B and C (rarely A)
         v. Autoimmune
   2. Diagnosis:
      a. Labs: bilirubin (direct, indirect), alk phos, LFTs
      b. Right upper quadrant ultrasound: small nodular or fibrotic liver
      c. CT scan and MRI: small, nodular liver
      d. Liver biopsy: usually needed to confirm diagnosis/cause
      e. Paracentesis: collection of ascetic fluid for pressure reduction or diagnosis
   3. Treatment:
      a. Abstinence from EtOH
      b. Avoidance of triggers: acetaminophen (APAP)
      c. Lactulose to prevent reabsorption of ammonia (NH_3)
      d. Minimize protein in diet if NH_3 levels warrant.
      e. Antibiotic prophylaxis to prevent peritonitis
      f. Diuretics for ascites
      g. Interferon Tx for viral Hep B, C
      h. Liver transplantation (to be on transplant list, 6 months of sobriety)
      i. Chelating agents (penicillamine) if copper overload
      j. Phlebotomy for iron excess

C. **Pancreatitis**
   1. Characteristics:
      a. Acute onset of persistent, severe, epigastric pain, frequently radiating to the middle back
      b. Can be acute or chronic
      c. Incidence of acute pancreatitis is 5 to 35 per 100,000 people.
      d. Higher incidence in women due to a higher prevalence of gallstones
      e. Causes:
         i. Alcohol: 30% acute pancreatitis in the United States
         ii. Gallstones: 35% to 40%
         iii. Hypertriglyceridemia: TG > 1,000 mg/dL can trigger attack
         iv. Hypercalcemia
         v. Drug induced: rare outside of alcohol, but many medications have been implicated
         vi. Infections/toxins: usually rare

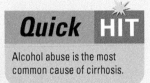

Quick HIT

Alcohol abuse is the most common cause of cirrhosis.

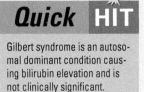

Quick HIT

Gilbert syndrome is an autosomal dominant condition causing bilirubin elevation and is not clinically significant.

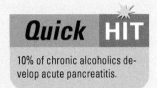

Quick HIT

10% of chronic alcoholics develop acute pancreatitis.

Nutritional and Digestive Disorders

(a) Viruses: mumps, coxsackie, hep B, CMV, VZV, HSV, HIV

(b) Bacteria: mycoplasma, legionella, leptospira, salmonella

(c) Fungi: aspergillus

(d) Parasites: toxoplasma, cryptosporidium, ascaris

(e) Venom of arachnids and reptiles

vii. Trauma

viii. Idiopathic: 15% to 25%

ix. Inherited: considered in patient with strong family history, or younger age ($<$35 years)

2. Clinical features:

a. Epigastric pain

b. Acute or persistent, severe, epigastric pain often radiating to the back

c. Stool changes: steatorrhea (fatty stools): loose, greasy, foul-smelling stools that are difficult to flush

3. Diagnosis:

a. Differential diagnosis: PUD, biliary obstruction, pseudocysts, pancreatic carcinoma, pancreatic duct stricture, stones

b. Serum lipase and/or amylase three times the upper limit of normal in acute pancreatitis

c. Fecal elastase testing is the test of choice for chronic pancreatic exocrine dysfunction.

d. Plain radiograph: may see ileus

e. Ultrasound: Bowel gas can obscure the pancreas, but ultrasound can identify gall/duct stones that may be causative.

f. Abdominal CT or MRI: focal or diffuse enlargement of the pancreas, necrosis may be seen

g. Endoscopic retrograde cholangiopancreatography and magnetic resonance cholangiopancreatography : used to evaluate for choledocholithiasis

4. Complications:

a. Nutritional: unable to digest complex foods, malabsorption of fat-soluble vitamins, vitamin B_{12}

b. Chronic pain syndromes that can lead to addictions

c. Infection and abscess in and around the pancreas

d. Pancreatic pseudocysts

e. Pancreatic cancer

f. Diabetes: end-stage endocrine pancreatic disease

5. Treatment:

a. Alcohol avoidance

b. Smoking cessation

c. Small meals

d. Pancreatic enzyme replacement therapy, lipase replacement

e. Restrict fat intake if steatorrhea, generally intake of 20 g/day or less

f. Supplement medium chain triglycerides (MCT)

g. Pain control

h. Treat any underlying cause

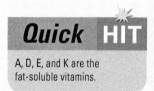

Quick HIT

A, D, E, and K are the fat-soluble vitamins.

Nutritional and Digestive Disorders

QUESTIONS

1. A 48-year-old male has a history of ulcerative colitis. He is at increased risk for which of the following **EXCEPT**?
   A. Crohn disease
   B. Depression
   C. Colon cancer
   D. Heart disease

2. A 63-year-old male has been on omeprazole for GERD for the past 10 years. Which of the following is he at increased risk for?
   A. Hypokalemia
   B. Gastric carcinoma
   C. Osteoporosis
   D. Diverticulitis

3. A 33-year-old female presents with a 6-week history of epigastric to right upper quadrant (RUQ) abdominal pain. It is worse after eating a meal. Her weight has decreased 10 pounds over the last month owing to being afraid to eat because of the pain. She does not have any bowel or bladder changes. She has tried taking Tums but that does not seem to help. Which test is the most likely to give you the correct diagnosis?
   A. Right upper quadrant ultrasound
   B. Abdominal XR
   C. Upper endoscopy (EGD)
   D. Lipase

4. A 37-year-old female complains of on and off diffuse crampy abdominal pain that has lasted over a year. She has intermittent times of diarrhea and constipation. She denies blood in her stool but occasionally has mucus. She has not had any fevers and has not traveled outside the United States in several years. She has tried elimination diets including gluten and lactose without improvement. She had a normal colonoscopy about 6 months ago. What is her most likely diagnosis?
   A. Crohn's
   B. Parasitic infection
   C. Irritable bowel syndrome
   D. Somatic symptom disorder

ANSWERS

1. **Answer:** A. Patients with UC are at higher risk for depression, colon cancer, and heart disease. This should be kept in mind when discussing preventative services with the patient. He is not at increased risk for developing Crohn disease.

2. **Answer:** C. Long-term use of PPIs such as omeprazole increases the risk of osteoporosis, hypomagnesemia, *H. pylori* infection, *C. difficile* infection, renal failure, and gastric polyps. It does not increase the risk of the others listed.

3. **Answer:** A. The patient presentation is suspicious for gallbladder disease and a RUQ U/S is the best test to evaluate for this. An abdominal XR is nonspecific and is not likely to help in this patient. The EGD could be useful if the U/S is normal to look for ulcers or other causes, but it is more invasive and would not be the first-line test. The presentation is also more consistent with gallbladder disease. Lipase is helpful in the diagnosis of pancreatitis which is less likely in this patient.

4. **Answer:** C. This patient meets Rome IV Criteria for IBS including abdominal pain lasting >3 months, change in stool frequency, and change in stool form or appearance. The lack of red flags and the normal colonoscopy makes Crohn's unlikely. She does not have any risk factor for a parasitic infection which would be extremely rare. Her symptoms better fit IBS, so this rules out somatic symptom disorder.

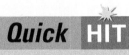

Most gonorrhea infections are asymptomatic.

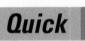

Urethral Gram stain is sensitive for a gonorrheal infection in symptomatic men but not in women.

Anyone positive for gonorrhea should also be screened for chlamydia, syphilis, and HIV.

Those with gonorrheal infections are often coinfected with chlamydia.

All sexual partners of a patient with gonorrhea or chlamydia need to be treated.

Abstain from sexual activity for 7 days after a single dose or until completion of 7-day course.

I. Sexually Transmitted Infections (STIs) and Vaginitis

A. Gonorrhea
1. General characteristics:
   a. *Neisseria gonorrhea* (gram-negative diplococci)
   b. Can affect the mucous membranes of the cervix, uterus, fallopian tubes, urethra, mouth, throat, eyes, and anus
2. Clinical features:
   a. Dysuria, increased vaginal discharge, irregular vaginal bleeding
   b. Rectal discharge, anal pruritus, anal bleeding
   c. Pharyngitis
3. Diagnosis:
   a. Urine or endocervical/vaginal swab for PCR
   b. Urine or endocervical/vaginal swab for culture
4. Treatment:
   a. Uncomplicated:
      i. Ceftriaxone IM × 1 + azithromycin 1 g PO × 1
      ii. Cefixime PO × 1 + doxycycline 100 mg PO × 7 days
   b. Disseminated:
      i. Hospitalization
      ii. Ceftriaxone IV then cefixime PO
   c. Abstinence until therapy is complete and symptoms resolved
5. Complications: pelvic inflammatory disease (PID), infertility

B. Chlamydia
1. General characteristics:
   a. *Chlamydia trachomatis* (gram-negative cocci or rod)
   b. Most frequently reported bacterial STI in the United States
2. Clinical features:
   a. Often asymptomatic
   b. Cervicitis: increased vaginal discharge, endocervical bleeding
   c. Urethritis: pyuria, dysuria, frequency
   d. Proctitis: rectal pain, discharge, bleeding
   e. Conjunctivitis
3. Diagnosis: urine or vaginal/endocervical swab PCR
4. Treatment:
   a. Azithromycin: 1 g orally, single dose
   b. Doxycycline: orally for 7 days
5. Complications: PID, Fitz–Hugh–Curtis syndrome (perihepatitis, infertility, chronic pelvic pain).

C. Human papilloma virus (HPV)
1. General characteristics:
   a. There are more than 40 serotypes.
   b. Serotypes 16 and 18 cause 70% cervical cancer.
   c. Serotypes 6 and 11 cause 90% of genital warts.

   d. Can also cause vulvar, vaginal, anal, and oropharyngeal cancers
   e. Screening:
      i. Routine Pap smear from 21 to 65 years old
      ii. Concomitant HPV testing if 30 to 65 years old
2. Treatment:
   a. Most infections will resolve without treatment.
   b. There is treatment for the virus itself.
   c. HPV vaccine: approved for boys and girls age 11 to 26 years
   d. Treat abnormal pap smear per guidelines.

D. **Trichomonas**
1. General characteristics: *Trichomonas vaginalis* (protozoan parasite)
2. Clinical features:
   a. 70% are asymptomatic
   b. Vaginal discharge that is thin and clear to yellow/green
   c. Dysuria
   d. Pruritus
3. Diagnosis:
   a. Wet prep (Figure 11-1) showing mobile flagellated protozoan
   b. Gold standard is a culture.
4. Treatment:
   a. Metronidazole 2 g orally, single dose, or 500 mg orally twice a day for 7 days
   b. Treat all sexual partners.

E. **Herpes simplex**
1. Clinical features:
   a. Most cases are asymptomatic.
   b. One or more vesicles on the genitals/mouth/rectum
   c. Vesicles break and leave painful ulcers that take 2 to 4 weeks to heal.
   d. First outbreak:
      i. Longer duration of lesions
      ii. Increased viral shedding
      iii. Systemic symptoms: headache, fever, myalgias
   e. Recurrent outbreak:
      i. Common particularly in the first year
      ii. Prodrome of tingling/burning hours to days before outbreak
      iii. Shorter duration and less severe
2. Diagnosis:
   a. Viral culture is the gold standard.
      i. Requires collection of a sample from the base of the vesicle
      ii. Low sensitivity but high specificity
   b. Antibody testing only indicates prior infection.

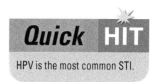

Quick HIT

HPV is the most common STI.

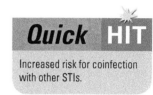

Quick HIT

Increased risk for coinfection with other STIs.

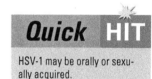

Quick HIT

HSV-1 may be orally or sexually acquired.

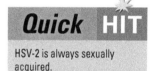

Quick HIT

HSV-2 is always sexually acquired.

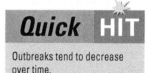

Quick HIT

Outbreaks tend to decrease over time.

Gynecologic Disorders

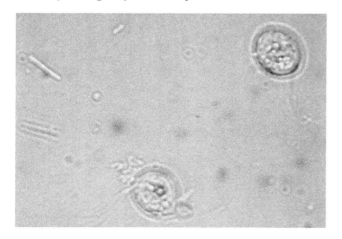

FIGURE
11-1 *Trichomonas vaginalis.* **Note the four flagella (1,000×).**

(From Mundt L, Shanahan K. *Graff's Textbook of Urinalysis and Body Fluids.* 2nd ed. Philadelphia, PA: Lippincott Williams & Wilkins; 2011.)

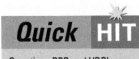

Over time, RPR and VDRL decrease and can become negative even if untreated.

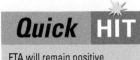

FTA will remain positive following treatment.

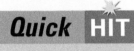

Treatment at more advanced stages will not repair damage that has already been done.

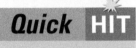

Hepatitis B virus can survive outside the body for 7 days.

3. Treatment:
   a. Initiate treatment within 1 day of prodrome or lesion.
   b. Acyclovir, famciclovir, valacyclovir
   c. Suppressive therapy reduces outbreaks by 70% to 80%.
   d. Severe/hospitalization requires IV acyclovir.

F. **Syphilis**
   1. General characteristics:
      a. *Treponema pallidum* (spirochete)
      b. Detected by dark field microscopy
      c. Average time from infection to symptoms is 21 days.
   2. Clinical features: Table 11-1
   3. Diagnosis:
      a. Nontreponemal test
         i. VDRL and RPR
         ii. Not specific
      b. Treponemal test
         i. Fluorescent treponemal antibody absorption test (FTA-ABS), treponema pallidum antibody (TP-PA)
         ii. Detects antibody specific for syphilis
   4. Treatment:
      a. First-degree, second-degree, and early latent: single dose of IM penicillin
      b. Late latent or unknown: three doses of IM penicillin

G. **Hepatitis B**
   1. General characteristics:
      a. DNA virus
      b. Transmitted through sexual activity or as a blood-borne pathogen
      c. 15% to 25% of patients die prematurely from cirrhosis or liver cancer
   2. Clinical features:
      a. 30% to 50% of patients have symptoms that begin an average of 90 days after exposure.

TABLE 11-1 Stages of Syphilis			
Stage	**Primary Lesion**	**Other Symptoms**	**Duration**
Primary	Single painless chancre at site of infection		3–6 wk Will progress if not treated
Secondary	Nonpruritic rash on skin and mucous membranes (Condyloma lata)	Fever, LAD, pharyngitis, hair loss, HA, weight loss, myalgias, fatigue	
Late (tertiary)		Cardiovascular: ascending aorta dilation, aortic valve regurgitation, coronary artery narrowing, and thrombosis Gummas: can involve skin, bones and internal organs	
Latent		Ataxia, paralysis, numbness, blindness, dementia, death	Early latent = infection within 12 mo Late latent = infection >12 mo ago
Neurosyphilis		Asymptomatic HA, altered mental status, movement disorders	Can occur at any stage

b. Symptoms: fever, fatigue, anorexia, nausea, vomiting, abdominal pain, dark urine, clay colored stools, joint pain, jaundice

c. 95% of adults DO NOT become chronically infected

3. Diagnosis: Table 11-2

4. Treatment:

a. Acute infection: supportive care

b. Chronic infection: adefovir, interferon α-2b, pegylated interferon, lamivudine, entecavir, telbivudine

c. Vaccination for prevention: three-dose series

H. **Pelvic inflammatory disease (PID)**

1. General characteristics:

a. Ascension of infection from cervix/vagina to upper genital tract

b. Polymicrobial: gonorrhea, chlamydia, *Ureaplasma urealyticum*, *Mycoplasma genitalium*, bacterial vaginosis (BV), endogenous microorganisms

2. Clinical features:

a. Lower abdominal/pelvic pain

b. Increased vaginal discharge

c. Irregular menses

d. Fever

e. Cervical motion tenderness (CMT)

f. Dysuria

3. Diagnosis:

a. Physical exam: CMT, friable cervix, vaginal discharge

b. Wet prep and cultures for specific infections

4. Treatment: Table 11-3

a. If no improvement on oral regimen in 72 hours, change to parenteral route.

b. Treatment should be for at least 14 days totally.

I. **Vaginitis/vaginosis**

1. General characteristics:

a. Candidiasis (yeast infection): usually *Candida albicans*

b. BV: *Gardnerella vagininalis, Mycoplasma hominis, Bacteroides, Peptostreptococcus*

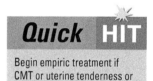

Begin empiric treatment if CMT or uterine tenderness or adnexal tenderness.

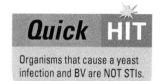

Organisms that cause a yeast infection and BV are NOT STIs.

Gynecologic Disorders

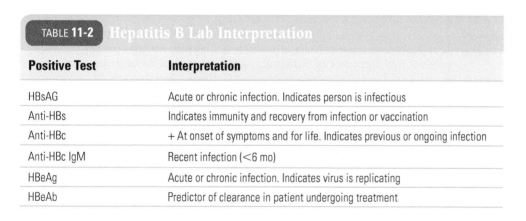

TABLE **11-2**	Hepatitis B Lab Interpretation
Positive Test	**Interpretation**
HBsAG	Acute or chronic infection. Indicates person is infectious
Anti-HBs	Indicates immunity and recovery from infection or vaccination
Anti-HBc	+ At onset of symptoms and for life. Indicates previous or ongoing infection
Anti-HBc IgM	Recent infection (<6 mo)
HBeAg	Acute or chronic infection. Indicates virus is replicating
HBeAb	Predictor of clearance in patient undergoing treatment

TABLE **11-3**	Antibiotic Regimens for Treatment of PID
Parenteral regimen A	Cefotetan or cefoxitin + doxycycline
Parenteral regimen B	Clindamycin + gentamycin
Alternative parenteral regimen	Ampicillin/sulbactam + doxycycline
Oral regimen A	Ceftriaxone + doxycycline ± metronidazole
Oral regimen B	Cefoxitin + probenecid + doxycycline ± metronidazole

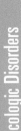

2. Clinical features:
   a. Vulvar/vaginal pruritus
   b. Vaginal discharge
      i. Yeast: thick, white, curd-like
      ii. BV: thin, gray, fishy odor
3. Diagnosis: KOH wet prep (Figure 11-2)
4. Treatment:
   a. Yeast: oral or topical antifungals
   b. BV: metronidazole

II. Menstrual Problems

A. Premenstrual syndrome (PMS)/premenstrual dysphoric disorder (PMDD)
   1. Definition:
      a. PMS: a collection of symptoms during the luteal phase (1 week before menses)
      b. PMDD: more severe and debilitating symptoms that affect relationships and social/occupational realms
   2. Clinical features: Table 11-4
   3. Diagnosis: clinical diagnosis, *must* have a symptom-free period (day 6 to 10)

> **Quick HIT**
>
> Absence of a symptom-free period indicates an underlying psychiatric disorder.

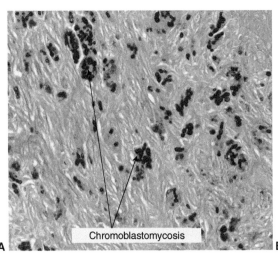

Chromoblastomycosis

A   B

FIGURE 11-2 A: Vaginal secretions of candidiasis exhibit branching pseudohyphae and tiny, budding yeasts on a microscopic examination of vaginal secretions. B: Bacterial vaginosis.

(**A** from Edwards L, Lynch PJ. *Genital Dermatology Atlas.* 2nd ed. Philadelphia, PA: Lippincott Williams and Wilkins; 2011. **B** from McGarry KA, Tong IL. *The 5-Minute Consult Clinical Companion to Women's Health.* 2nd ed. Philadelphia, PA: Lippincott Williams & Wilkins; 2013.)

TABLE 11-4 Symptoms Associated With PMS/PMDD
Abdominal bloating
Breast tenderness/fullness
Cramps/abdominal pain
Fatigue
Headache
Weight gain
Anger/irritability
Anxiety
Change in appetite
Change in libido
Depressed mood
Feeling out of control
Change in sleep
Withdrawal from usual activities

4. Treatment:
   a. Nonpharmacologic: cognitive behavioral therapy (CBT)
   b. Pharmacologic: oral contraceptive pill (OCP), selevtive serotonin reuptake inhibitor (SSRI)

B. **Dysmenorrhea**
  1. Definition: painful cramps that occur with menstruation
  2. Clinical features:
   a. Primary:
     i. Onset 6 to 12 months after menarche
     ii. Duration of 8 to 72 hours
     iii. Lower abdominal/pelvic pain with or without radiation to the back and legs, diarrhea, nausea, vomiting
     iv. NO underlying pathology
   b. Secondary:
     i. Suspect in older women who have no prior history
     ii. Results from underlying pelvic pathology such as endometriosis, adenomyosis, leiomyomata, PID
  3. Diagnosis:
   a. Primary: H&P, laparoscopy if etiology remains unknown
   b. Secondary: transvaginal ultrasound, beta-human chorionic gonadotropin, complete blood count, erythrocyte sedimentation rate, pap smear
  4. Treatment:
   a. NSAIDs
   b. Hormonal contraception (OCP, Depo-Provera, Nexplanon, Mirena)

C. **Menorrhagia**
  1. Definition: abnormally heavy or prolonged bleeding
  2. Clinical features:
   a. Soaking >1 pad/tampon per hour for several hours
   b. Need to use double protection (pad and tampon)
   c. Frequent changing of protection at night
   d. Bleeding >7 days
   e. Large clots
   f. Need to restrict regular activities
   g. Symptoms of anemia
  3. Causes: endometriosis, fibroids, cervical polyps
  4. Diagnosis: pap smear, ultrasound, endometrial biopsy, hysteroscopy
  5. Treatment:
   a. OCP/oral progestins
   b. D&C
   c. Endometrial ablation
   d. Hysterectomy

D. **Amenorrhea**
  1. General characteristics:
   a. Primary: failure to reach menarche
     i. Evaluate if no pubertal development by age 13, no menarche by 5 years after breast development, or no menarche by age 15.
     ii. Usually a chromosomal irregularity (Turner syndrome) or anatomic abnormality (mullerian agenesis)
   b. Secondary: cessation of previously regular menses for 3 months or previously irregular menses for 6 months
     i. Pregnancy
     ii. Polycystic ovarian syndrome (PCOS), hypothalamic, primary ovarian insufficiency
  2. Diagnosis and management: Figures 11-3 and 11-4

E. **Dysfunctional uterine bleeding**
  1. Definition: irregular uterine bleeding in the absence of recognizable pelvic pathology, general medical disease, or pregnancy (Figure 11-5)
  2. General characteristics:
   a. Usually anovulatory bleeding
   b. Rule out other cause

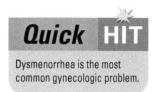

Quick HIT

Dysmenorrhea is the most common gynecologic problem.

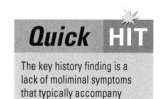

Quick HIT

The key history finding is a lack of moliminal symptoms that typically accompany ovulation.

Gynecologic Disorders

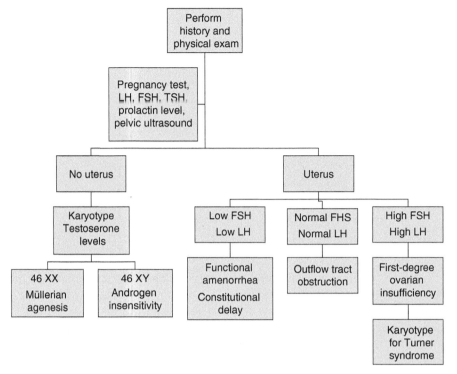

FIGURE 11-3 Approach to the diagnosis and management of primary amenorrhea.

3. Clinical features: obesity, androgen excess (hirsutism, acne), galactorrhea, visual field defects, ecchymosis, or purpura
4. Diagnosis: Table 11-5
5. Complications: iron-deficiency anemia, endometrial adenocarcinoma, infertility
6. Treatment: OCP, progestin, D&C, endometrial ablation

F. **Endometriosis**
   1. General characteristics:
      a. Presence of endometrial tissue outside of the uterine cavity
      b. Estrogen-dependent disease
      c. Highest incidence in patients 25 to 29 years old
   2. Clinical features: infertility, dysmenorrhea, ovarian cyst, dyspareunia, abdominal/pelvic pain, IBS
   3. Diagnosis:
      a. Usually clinical
      b. Transvaginal ultrasound
      c. Confirmed by laparoscopy
   4. Treatment:
      a. NSAIDs
      b. OCP
      c. Medroxyprogesterone
      d. Laparoscopic ablation
      e. Excision of endometrioma

G. **Polycystic ovarian syndrome (PCOS)**
   1. General characteristics:
      a. Menstrual dysfunction
      b. Anovulation
      c. Hyperandrogenism
      d. Metabolic syndrome
   2. Clinical features: obesity, acne, hirsutism, acanthosis nigricans, hypertension

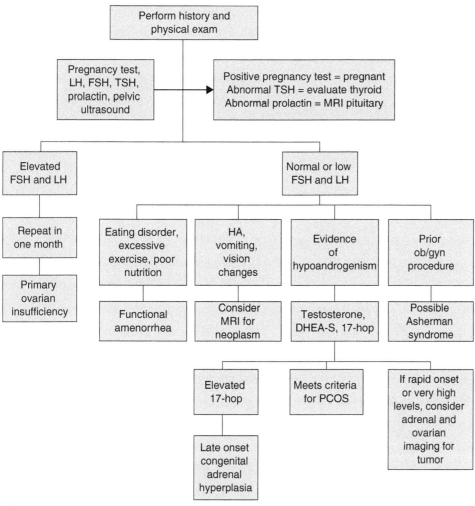

FIGURE
11-4 Approach to the diagnosis and management of secondary amenorrhea. DHEA-S, dehydroepiandrosterone sulfate; FSH, follicle-stimulating hormone; LH, luteinizing hormone; TSH, thyroid-stimulating hormone; 17-hop, 17-hydroxyprogesterone.

Constant, non-cycling estrogen levels → Endometrial proliferation → Endometrium outgrows the blood supply → Irregular bleeding

FIGURE
11-5 Etiology of DUB.

TABLE 11-5	Workup for DUB

Pap smear
STI screen
Pregnancy test
CBC
TSH
Prolactin level
LFTs
Von Willebrand disease
Endometrial biopsy
Pelvic ultrasound

3. Diagnosis:
   a. Labs:
      i. TSH, prolactin, testosterone, DHEA-S, FSH/LH to rule out other causes of oligomenorrhea
      ii. HbA$_{1c}$, lipids to look for comorbid conditions
   b. Requires two of the following:
      i. Oligo or anovulation
      ii. Clinical/laboratory evidence of hyperandrogenism
      iii. Polycystic ovaries on ultrasound
4. Treatment: Table 11-6

III. Menopause

A. **Definition:** permanent cessation of menses
B. **Diagnosis**
   1. Amenorrhea for 12 months
   2. Increased FSH, decreased estradiol
C. **Perimenopausal and menopausal signs/symptoms** (Table 11-7) can occur up to 6 years before and last for several years after the diagnosis.
D. **Treatment**
   1. Hormone replacement therapy (HRT) is the most effective treatment for vasomotor symptoms (Tables 11-8 and 11-9).
   2. Alternative medications for vasomotor symptoms: SSRI/serotonin norepinephrine reuptake inhibitor (SNRI), clonidine, gabapentin
E. **Complications:** osteoporosis, increased risk for CAD, decreased quality of life

IV. Breast Disorders

A. Mastalgia
   1. Definition: breast pain
   2. General characteristics:
      a. Cyclic: related to the menstrual cycle; diffuse, bilateral, radiates to axilla
      b. Noncyclic: not related to the menstrual cycle
         i. Trauma, chest wall pain, nerve pain
         ii. Medications: OCP, HRT, SSRI, haldol, spironolactone, digoxin

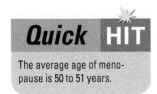

Quick HIT

The average age of menopause is 50 to 51 years.

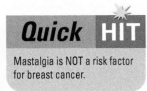

Quick HIT

Mastalgia is NOT a risk factor for breast cancer.

TABLE 11-6 Treatment of PCOS	
Treatment	**Result**
Lifestyle modification (diet/exercise)	Weight loss, ↓BP, ↓BS, ↓lipids
OCP	Regulate menses, ↓androgen production
Metformin	↑Insulin sensitivity, ↓androgens
Clomid	Improves fertility
Benzoyl peroxide, retinoids	Improves acne
Spironolactone	↓Androgens, improves hirsutism

TABLE 11-7 Perimenopausal and Menopausal Signs/Symptoms
Hot flashes
Insomnia
Weight gain
Mood changes/depression
Irregular menses
Vaginal atrophy
Dyspareunia

TABLE **11-8**	Goals of HRT

Relief of vasomotor symptoms
Reduce risk of unwanted pregnancy
Avoid irregular menstrual cycles
Preserve bone density
Improve quality of life

TABLE **11-9**	Contraindications to HRT

Undiagnosed vaginal bleeding
Severe liver disease
Pregnancy
Venous thrombosis
Personal history of breast cancer

3. Diagnosis:
   a. Imaging is usually not needed.
   b. If there is focal pain, obtain imaging.
      i. Under 30 years old: ultrasound
      ii. Over 30 years old: ultrasound and mammogram
4. Treatment: NSAIDs, danazol

B. **Nipple discharge**
1. General characteristics:
   a. Physiologic
      i. Bilateral, multiple ducts, associated with nipple stimulation
      ii. Bilateral milky discharge appropriate during pregnancy, lactation, and up to 1 year postpartum or after cessation of breastfeeding
      iii. Not pregnant/lactating = galactorrhea
   b. Pathologic: spontaneous, unilateral, bloody, serous, clear, or associated with a mass
2. Etiology:
   a. Galactorrhea: prolactinoma, hypothyroidism, medications (Table 11-10)
   b. Pathologic: intraductal papilloma, duct ectasia, carcinoma, infection
3. Diagnosis:
   a. Labs: pregnancy test, prolactin level, TSH
   b. Imaging: mammogram, ultrasound, MRI brain (prolactinoma)
4. Treatment:
   a. Galactorrhea: bromocriptine, cabergoline
   b. Pathologic: surgery

C. **Mastitis**
1. General characteristics:
   a. Localized, painful inflammation of the breast
   b. Flu-like symptoms: fever, malaise, myalgias
   c. Most commonly occurs in lactating women.
2. Risk factors: nipple fissures, blocked milk ducts
3. Etiology: usually *Staphylococcus aureus*
4. Treatment:
   a. Improve breastfeeding technique.
   b. Adequate draining of breast milk
   c. Antibiotics (Table 11-11)
5. Complication: abscess

D. **Fibrocystic breast disease**
1. General characteristics:

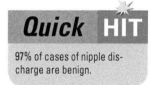

Quick **HIT**

97% of cases of nipple discharge are benign.

Gynecologic Disorders

TABLE **11-10**	Medications That Cause Galactorrhea

Methyldopa
Reserpine
Verapamil
Antipsychotics
Cimetidine
Metoclopramide
OCP
MAOI
SSRI
TCA
Codeine
Heroin
Methadone
Morphine

TABLE **11-11**	Antibiotics for Mastitis

Amoxicillin-clavulanate
Cephalexin
Ciprofloxacin
Clindamycin
Dicloxacillin
Trimethoprim/sulfamethoxazole

    a. Fibroadenoma: most common cause of mass in women under 25 years old

    b. One in three women between the ages of 35 and 50 years will have breast cysts.

  2. Clinical features:

    a. Single, firm, rubbery, smooth, mobile, painless mass

    b. Usually 1 to 5 cm

    c. Ultrasound can distinguish cystic from solid lesions.

  3. Treatment: cyst-aspiration, follow-up exam

E. Breast cancer

  1. General characteristics:

    a. The second most commonly diagnosed cancer in women

    b. The second leading cause of cancer death in women

    c. 1% of breast cancer occurs in men

    d. 8% are hereditary: BRCA1 and BRCA2

    e. Risk factors: Table 11-12

  2. Clinical features:

    a. Mass: solitary, discrete, hard

    b. Nipple discharge: spontaneous, bloody

    c. Erythema, edema, retraction of skin/nipple

  3. Diagnosis:

    a. Mammography

      i. Screening: appropriate for asymptomatic women

      ii. Diagnostic: used if patient has any signs or symptoms of cancer

    b. Ultrasound

      i. Differentiates solid from cystic mass

      ii. Not used for screening

    c. Biopsy

      i. Fine needle aspiration (FNA) with or without ultrasound guidance

      ii. Core biopsy

      iii. Excisional biopsy

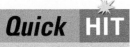

Quick HIT

Screening mammogram should be performed every 1 to 2 years in patients 50 to 75 years old. For patients 40 to 49 years old, screening is based on individual risk factors.

    d. Histochemical testing
        i. Estrogen receptors
        ii. Progesterone receptors
        iii. HER2/neu
    e. Staging
        i. T—tumor size
        ii. M—metastasis
        iii. N—lymph node involvement
4. Types of breast cancer: Table 11-13

TABLE 11-12	Risk Factors for Breast Cancer

Age > 50
Prior history of breast cancer
Family history
Early menarche (<12)
Late menopause (>50)
Nulliparity
Age >30 at first birth
Obesity
High socioeconomic status
Atypical hyperplasia on biopsy
Ionizing radiation exposure

TABLE 11-13	Types of Breast Cancer

Type	Frequency	Invasive	Characteristics	Prognosis
Ductal carcinoma in situ (DCIS)	20%	No	"Pre–breast cancer"	Good
Lobular carcinoma in situ		No	• Atypical cells found in lobules of milk-producing glands • 7- to 11-fold increased risk of developing an invasive cancer	
Invasive ductal carcinoma	80% of all invasive breast cancers	Yes	• Starts in milk ducts then invades through the wall into surrounding fatty tissue • Can metastasize	Varies by stage
Invasive lobular carcinoma	10%	Yes	• Starts in lobules then invades surrounding fatty tissue • Can metastasize	Varies by stage
Inflammatory	1%–3%	No	• Cancer cells block the lymph vessels in the skin • "peau de orange"	Poor
Paget disease of the breast	1%	Possibly	• Begins in ducts and spreads to skin of the nipple and areola • Skin appears crusted, scaly, red • Associated with DCIS or invasive ductal carcinoma	Varies by number of tumors and invasiveness
Phyllodes tumor	Very rare	No	• Tumor develops in stroma of breast • Usually benign but can be malignant	

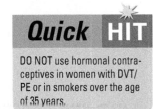

5. Breast cancer treatment
   a. Varies based on type and staging
   b. Surgery: breast conserving (lumpectomy), mastectomy
   c. Adjuvant therapy: chemotherapy, radiation, tamoxifen, trastuzumab

V. Contraception: Table 11-14

TABLE 11-14	Comparison of Contraceptive Methods		
Type	**Hormonal**	**Protect Against STD**	**Failure Rate (%)**
Condom	No	Yes	3–14
Natural family planning	No	No	4–25
OCP	Yes	No	0.1–5
Depo-Provera	Yes (progestin only)	No	0.3
NuvaRing	Yes	No	1–3
Nexplanon	Yes	No	0.2–1.1
IUD	Paragard—No Mirena—Yes	No	0.1–0.6
Female sterilization	No	No	0.8–3.7
Vasectomy	No	No	0.1

QUESTIONS

1. A 24-year-old G0P0 female with a BMI of 31 presents to the office with complaints of acne and dark hair on her upper lip. She also has irregular menses with LMP 3 months ago. Workup is most likely to reveal:
   A. Low TSH
   B. High prolactin level
   C. High testosterone level
   D. Low blood sugar
   E. High FSH

2. An 18-year-old female is complaining of increased thin vaginal discharge with a slight odor. She has had three sexual partners and consistently used condoms. KOH wet prep shows clue cells. Which of the following medications should be prescribed?
   A. Ceftriaxone
   B. Doxycycline
   C. Acyclovir
   D. Metronidazole
   E. Azithromycin

3. Which of the following is a risk factor for breast cancer?
   A. Low socioeconomic status
   B. Multiparity
   C. Early menopause <50
   D. Mastalgia
   E. Early menarche, <12

4. A 27-year-old G2P2 female presents with complaints of pain and redness of her left breast for the past few days. She is breastfeeding her 4-month-old daughter. She does not take any medications. She also admits to feeling more run down and achy over the past few days. Appropriate treatment would include:
   A. Avoid breastfeeding from the left breast.
   B. Prescribe dicloxacillin.
   C. Use ice pack on left breast.
   D. Order diagnostic mammogram of left breast.
   E. Refer her to a gynecologist.

ANSWERS

1. **Answer: C.** High testosterone level. This patient has PCOS which is characterized by menstrual dysfunction secondary to anovulation, hyperandrogenism, and metabolic syndrome. There is not a specific etiology for PCOS and other causes of menstrual dysfunction must be excluded. Therefore, answers A, B, and E are incorrect as they would indicate an organic etiology for her irregular menses. A hallmark of PCOS is obesity and metabolic syndrome, so these patients typically have elevated blood sugar, making answer D incorrect.

2. **Answer: D.** Metronidazole. This patient has bacterial vaginosis (BV). Symptoms typically include a thin gray-white discharge with a musty or fishy vaginal odor. Risk factors for BV include smoking, new/multiple sexual partners, use of spermicides, and vaginal douching. BV is NOT an STD. Diagnosis is often confirmed in the office by finding clue cells on a KOH wet prep. Ceftriaxone is the antibiotic of choice for gonorrhea which is caused by Neisseria gonorrhea. Most patients are asymptomatic. Diagnosis is by urine or vaginal swab. Doxycycline and azithromycin are typically used to treat Chlamydia which is caused by the bacteria Chlamydia trachomatis. Again, most patients are asymptomatic and diagnosis is by urine or vaginal swab. Acyclovir is an anti-viral medication used to treat the Herpes Simplex Virus (HSV). HSV can present orally or on the genitals. It is characterized by painful blisters which can recur.

3. **Answer: E.** Early menarche, < 12. Increased estrogen and unopposed estrogen exposure are considered risk factors for breast cancer. The longer a woman is ovulating and experiencing menses, the more estrogen she is exposed to; therefore, early menarche and late menopause are risk factors for breast cancer. A higher socioeconomic status is a risk factor for breast cancer. However, patients with a lower socioeconomic status often present or are diagnosed at a later stage and tend to have a more complicated course and poorer prognosis. Multiparity decreases overall exposure time to estrogen and so decreases the risk for breast cancer. Mastalgia is simply breast pain and is not a risk factor for breast cancer.

4. **Answer: B.** Prescribe dicloxacillin. This patient has mastitis. Mastitis is localized painful inflammation and infection of the breast. It is most often seen in breastfeeding/lactating women. It is often accompanied by flu-like symptoms. Risk factors include nipple fissures and blocked milk ducts. Dicloxacillin is one of many antibiotics that can be used to treat mastitis. Other nonpharmacologic treatments include continued breastfeeding/adequate drainage of the breast, improved breastfeeding techniques, nipple/breast skin care, and hot/wet compresses. A diagnostic mammogram would be an inappropriate test to order for this patient. Diagnosis is clinical and treatment can be initiated by the patient's PCP. Referral to a gynecologist could be done if the diagnosis was uncertain but would delay treatment and possibly increase the risk for complications including a breast abscess.

RENAL, URINARY, AND MALE REPRODUCTIVE SYSTEM

Ronald Reynolds

I. Renal Failure/Insufficiency

A. **Acute kidney injury**
1. Characteristics:
   a. Diminished renal function that appears in a short period of time
   b. Common in hospitalized patients and often has multiple causes including dehydration, hypovolemia, and medications
2. Clinical features: There are often no symptoms or physical findings with acute kidney injury.
3. Diagnosis:
   a. Definition: increase in serum creatinine by 0.3 mg/dL in a 48-hour period OR increase in serum creatinine to equal or greater than 1.5 times baseline within 7 days
   b. Associated laboratory findings often include elevated blood urea nitrogen (BUN) and potassium.
   c. Differential diagnosis includes interstitial nephritis, characterized by eosinophils in the urine.
4. Treatment:
   a. Therapy is always directed at treating the underlying cause—such as fluids for dehydration or hypovolemia, improving congestive heart failure (CHF), stopping medications, etc.
   b. Complications: electrolyte abnormalities, fluid retention, excess edema, infections, etc.
   c. Prognosis depends on cause and duration, but chronic kidney disease is a common result.

B. **Chronic kidney disease**
1. Characteristics:
   a. Diminished renal function over a prolonged period of time
   b. Frequently a result of long-term poorly controlled diabetes and hypertension
2. Clinical features:
   a. There are often no symptoms or physical findings of chronic renal disease.
   b. Causes are multifactorial including long-term kidney damage from diseases like diabetes and hypertension, intrinsic disorders of the kidney, and postrenal causes like benign prostatic hyperplasia (BPH).
3. Diagnosis:
   a. Definition: glomerular filtration rate (GFR) < 60 mL/minute/1.73 m^2 OR kidney damage as evidenced by either albuminuria, urine sediment abnormalities, electrolyte or other abnormalities due to tubular disorders, abnormal histology, abnormal structure detected by imaging, or history of kidney transplant
   b. Associated laboratory findings often include elevated BUN and potassium.
   c. An early sign of chronic kidney disease is microalbuminuria, defined as between 30 and 300 mg of albumin excreted in a 24-hour period.

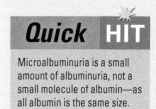

Quick HIT

Microalbuminuria is a small amount of albuminuria, not a small molecule of albumin—as all albumin is the same size.

163

4. Treatment:
   a. Therapy is directed at treating the underlying cause—such as better diabetic and hypertension control.
   b. ACE inhibitors are frequently employed to improve glomerular filtration.
   c. Complications: electrolyte abnormalities, fluid retention, excess edema, infections
   d. Prognosis depends on cause and duration, but end-stage renal disease requiring dialysis or transplantation is a common result.

II. Kidney Stones (Nephrolithiasis)

A. **Characteristics**
   1. Stones of various composition that form within the kidney and pass down the ureter
   2. The majority of stones contain calcium and will appear on X-ray.
   3. Causes: hypercalciuria, hyperoxaluria, polycystic kidney disease. Concentrated urine is a very frequent cofactor.
   4. Stones generally start from crystals that coalesce.
   5. When a stone traverses the ureter, there are three common places for it to get stuck—entrance into the ureter, pelvic brim, and ureterovesical junction.
   6. Kidney stones affect 19% of men and 9% of women by age 70.

B. **Clinical features**
   1. The presence of a kidney stone in the kidney generally causes no symptoms.
   2. As a stone passes down the ureter, it is common for it to get stuck and block urine flow.
   3. Renal colic is an intense visceral pain that starts in the costovertebral angle and rotates around the flank, into the groin, and down into the testicle or labia.
   4. During renal colic, the patient has severe pain that comes in waves. The patient is often pale and constantly moves trying to find a comfortable position.
   5. The abdominal exam is usually normal during renal colic.

C. **Diagnosis**
   1. Hematuria, either gross or microscopic, is an almost universal finding.
   2. Plain X-ray will sometimes see a stone, but phleboliths can be confusing.
   3. Helical computed tomography (CT) without contrast is used to identify presence, location, and size of suspected stones.

D. **Treatment**
   1. Stones that are ≤ 5 mm in size generally spontaneously pass within a few days.
   2. Narcotics are usually necessary for the pain of renal colic.
   3. Medical expulsive therapy with tamsulosin, calcium channel blockers, and/or nonsteroidal anti-inflammatory drugs (NSAIDs) may help with stone passage but data is mixed.
   4. Stones >5 mm generally require urologic intervention—including ureteral stenting to relieve hydronephrosis, basket retrieval, intraureteral laser lithotripsy, or extracorporeal shockwave lithotripsy.
   5. Urine should be strained to retrieve the stone, which is sent for stone analysis to determine its composition.
   6. Increasing fluid intake will reduce the recurrence of stones.

III. Urinary Tract Infection

A. **Cystitis**
   1. Characteristics:
      a. Bacterial infection within the bladder, causing inflammation of the bladder wall
      b. Much more common in women owing to a shorter urethra
      c. Cause is an ascending infection, generally of bowel flora.
      d. Most common organisms: *Escherichia coli, Staphylococcus saprophyticus, Klebsiella, Enterococcus, Pseudomonas, Serratia,* and *Proteus*
      e. Risk factors in women are intercourse, bacterial vaginosis, and infrequent urination.

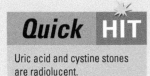

Quick HIT

Uric acid and cystine stones are radiolucent.

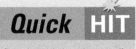

Quick HIT

Once formed, there is no medical way to "dissolve" a kidney stone.

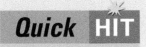

Quick HIT

The pain of renal colic is caused by acute hydronephrosis distending the kidney capsule.

Renal, Urinary, and Male Reproductive System

2. Clinical features:
   a. Symptoms: urgency, frequency, dysuria, nocturia, suprapubic pain, low back pain
   b. Physical exam: suprapubic pain and lack of costovertebral angle (CVA) tenderness/warmth
3. Diagnosis:
   a. Differential diagnosis: urethritis caused by gonorrhea or chlamydia, and vulvitis characterized by external dysuria
   b. A clean-catch midstream urinalysis often shows positive leukocyte esterase and possibly positive nitrites on dipstick (Table 12-1).
   c. Microscopy will show many white blood cells (WBCs) and bacteria.
   d. If there are many WBCs but no bacteria, urethritis is more likely.
   e. Urine culture will typically show greater than 100,000 organisms per mL, but even 1,000 organisms per mL is diagnostic in symptomatic patients.
4. Treatment:
   a. Uncomplicated cystitis in women is treated with a 3-day course of oral antibiotics.
   b. Longer courses do not have higher efficacy, but cause higher chance of vaginal yeast infection.
   c. Preferred antibiotics include trimethoprim–sulfamethoxazole, nitrofurantoin, or fosfomycin—based on local resistance patterns.
   d. Nitrofurantoin causes less resistance in native bowel flora, but does not penetrate tissue to treat an occult pyelonephritis or prostatitis.
   e. Men are treated with a minimum of 7- to 10-day course of trimethoprim–sulfamethoxazole or ciprofloxacin.
   f. Daily cranberry consumption can reduce the frequency of recurrent cystitis in high-risk patients.
   g. Asymptomatic bacteriuria is not treated because it leads to antibiotic-resistant organisms and does not change outcomes.

B. **Pyelonephritis**
1. Characteristics:
   a. Bacterial infection within the tissue of the kidney
   b. Generally unilateral
   c. Cause is an ascending infection from ureteral reflux of a bladder infection
   d. Hematogenous pyelonephritis is much less common.
2. Clinical features:
   a. Symptoms: urgency, frequency, dysuria, nocturia, suprapubic pain, low back pain from the associated cystitis, in addition to unilateral flank pain and fever
   b. Physical exam: suprapubic tenderness *and* CVA tenderness and palpable warmth
   c. The patient is generally febrile and appears ill.
3. Diagnosis:
   a. Differential diagnosis: musculoskeletal back pain, which does not include fever and urinary symptoms
   b. Clean-catch midstream urinalysis: positive leukocyte esterase and possibly positive nitrites on dipstick
   c. Microscopy will show many WBCs and bacteria PLUS WBC casts.
   d. Urine culture will show greater than 100,000 organisms per mL.

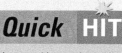

Quick HIT

It is unusual for a patient with uncomplicated cystitis to be febrile.

Quick HIT

Female patients need to be clearly taught how to obtain a clean-catch midstream specimen so as not to contaminate the specimen with vaginal secretions.

Quick HIT

Relying on just the dipstick findings without doing office microscopy will miss vaginal contamination, urethritis, and occult pyelonephritis.

Quick HIT

Cranberry juice does not treat cystitis once it has developed.

Quick HIT

Call your local hospital microbiology lab to find out the resistance patterns of local *Escherichia coli*.

Quick HIT

Recurrent urinary tract infections (UTIs) caused by *Proteus* are often associated with stone disease.

Renal, Urinary, and Male Reproductive System

TABLE 12-1	Urinary Pathogens That Reduce Urinary Nitrate to Nitrite in 4 Hours of Bladder Incubation
Nitrite-forming organisms	*E. coli, Klebsiella, Proteus*
Organisms that do not form nitrite	*S. saprophyticus, Enterococcus, pseudomonas*

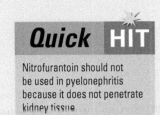

4. Treatment:
   a. A very ill patient, especially one who is nauseated or vomiting, should be admitted for intravenous antibiotics.
   b. Outpatient management generally starts with an intramuscular (IM) injection of ceftriaxone.
   c. Preferred oral antibiotics to follow include either trimethoprim–sulfamethoxazole, ciprofloxacin, or levofloxacin—based on local resistance patterns.
   d. Urosepsis and perinephric abscesses can occur from pyelonephritis.

IV. Hematuria

A. **Characteristics**
   1. Definitions:
      a. Gross hematuria: bloody colored urine with intact red cells on microscopy
      b. Microscopic hematuria: normal-appearing urine with more than three intact red cells per high-power field on microscopy
   2. Causes are numerous, including sources in the kidney, ureter, bladder, prostate, and urethra. Microscopic hematuria may run in families.
   3. The primary concern with hematuria is to rule out a malignant cause.

B. **Clinical features**
   1. Most frequently, hematuria is asymptomatic. If the patient has ureteral colic, stone disease is most likely the cause. Men with perineal pain might have prostatitis.
   2. Physical exam is usually unremarkable. Edema might suggest glomerulonephritis.

C. **Diagnosis**
   1. Diagnosis is made with urine microscopy—do not rely on the dipstick alone.
   2. Myoglobinuria: Urine dipstick shows blood, but microscopy does not reveal intact red blood cells (RBCs).
   3. Glomerulonephritis: associated proteinuria and abnormally shaped RBCs
   4. Urine cytology can be useful if positive, but should not be relied on to rule out malignancy.
   5. If a transient benign cause such as urinary tract infection or menstruation is found and the hematuria resolves, no further workup is indicated.
   6. Workup of persistent hematuria includes abdominal and pelvic CT imaging with and without contrast.
   7. In patients >35, smokers, and those with irritative voiding symptoms, cystoscopy is needed to evaluate the bladder mucosa.

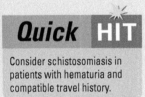

D. **Treatment**
   1. Treatment of microscopic hematuria is directed at its identified cause.
   2. Refer to nephrology in patients with proteinuria and abnormal RBCs.

V. Proteinuria

A. **Characteristics**
   1. Proteinuria is generally detected on urine dipstick. It needs to be quantified.
   2. Classification of protein in the urine:
      a. Microproteinuria—urine total protein loss 150 to 499 mg/24 hours
      b. Clinical proteinuria—urine total protein loss 500 to 999 mg/24 hours
      c. Heavy proteinuria—urine total protein loss 1,000 to 4,500 mg/24 hours
      d. Nephrotic range proteinuria > 4,500 mg/24 hours
   3. Proteinuria can be evaluated with spot urine/creatinine ratios, but 24-hour urine collection is most accurate.
   4. Risk factors: diabetes, prolonged hypertension, intrinsic renal diseases
   5. Transient proteinuria is common with exercise and dehydration.

B. **Clinical features**
   1. Patients with proteinuria are generally asymptomatic.
   2. Proteinuria does not cause any physical findings unless there is hypoalbuminemia with resultant edema from nephrotic range proteinuria.

C. Diagnosis
1. Diagnosis is based on 24-hour urine collection and quantifying proteinuria.
2. Urine sediment needs to be evaluated on microscopy to look for associated findings of renal disease such as casts and dysmorphic RBCs.
3. Chemistries including electrolytes, BUN, creatinine, glucose, and serum proteins should be measured. Estimation of creatinine clearance should be done.
4. There is no need for imaging.
D. Treatment
1. Therapy is directed at the underlying cause, but generally includes prescription of an angiotensin-converting-enzyme inhibitor (ACE-I).
2. Unless transient or microproteinuria, patients are usually referred to a nephrologist.

VI. Urinary Incontinence
A. Characteristics
1. Definition: involuntary loss of urine
2. Stress incontinence: happens during coughing, sneezing, stepping down hard
   a. Frequent in women
   b. Seldom in men unless they have had a prostatectomy
   c. Associated with having had a child and with estrogen deficiency
3. Urge incontinence: happens with involuntary detrusor contraction (in men, this is associated with BPH)
4. Mixed incontinence: a combination of both stress and urge incontinence
B. Clinical features
1. Ask about involuntary loss of urine with coughing, sneezing, and physical activity.
2. Inquire whether there have been any recent urinary tract infections.
3. Physical exam findings include skin excoriation in the genital or vulvar area.
C. Diagnosis
1. Clinical diagnosis, exclude UTI
2. A dipstick urinalysis to exclude hematuria and infection
3. Imaging is not needed.
4. Specialists may use urodynamic testing, but this is not necessary for the diagnosis.
D. Treatment
1. Stress incontinence:
   a. Absorptive undergarments
   b. Pelvic floor muscle exercises such as Kegels
   c. Surgery, including urethral bulking agents and urethral sling, may be helpful
2. Urge incontinence:
   a. Bladder training exercises to gradually increase the bladder capacity
   b. Anticholinergics, but caution must be exercised in men with BPH, because this can cause urinary retention, and in the elderly because of multiple side effects

VII. Prostate Disease
A. Prostatitis
1. Characteristics
   a. Three distinct subtypes: acute bacterial prostatitis, chronic bacterial prostatitis, and prostatodynia/chronic pelvic pain
   b. Acute bacterial prostatitis is usually caused by the same organisms that cause cystitis—*Escherichia coli, Klebsiella, Proteus, Pseudomonas*, etc.
   c. Chronic bacterial prostatitis may be caused by the same organisms as acute prostatitis, but organisms that cause sexually transmitted infections (STIs) such as chlamydia, gonorrhea, and trichomonas may also be causes.
   d. Prostatodynia is not of bacterial origin, and its etiology is poorly understood.
   e. Common problem in older men

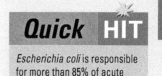

***Quick* HIT**

Escherichia coli is responsible for more than 85% of acute prostatitis.

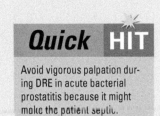

Quick HIT

Avoid vigorous palpation during DRE in acute bacterial prostatitis because it might make the patient septic.

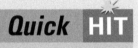

Quick HIT

Alpha blockers have a very quick response by relaxing prostatic smooth muscle. 5-α reductase inhibitors take longer but will significantly reduce prostatic volume with time.

2. Clinical features:
   a. Symptoms: suprapubic, perineal, and genital pain. Acute prostatitis may be accompanied by fever, constitutional symptoms, and both irritative and obstructive voiding symptoms
   b. Acute prostatitis often has a boggy prostate on digital rectal examination (DRE).
   c. Chronic prostatitis and prostatodynia cause a tender prostate on DRE.
3. Diagnosis:
   a. Classic symptoms accompanied by prostate tenderness on DRE
   b. Urinalysis (UA) in both acute and chronic bacterial prostatitis usually show WBCs and bacteria.
   c. Differential diagnosis includes urethritis and cystitis.
4. Treatment:
   a. Bacterial forms of prostatitis are treated with antibiotics.
   b. Acute prostatitis is treated with ciprofloxacin, levofloxacin, or trimethoprim–sulfamethoxazole. Very ill patients may require inpatient IV antibiotics.
   c. Chronic prostatitis is treated with longer courses of the same antibiotics, but azithromycin, doxycycline, and/or metronidazole may be added.
   d. Alpha blockers may reduce symptoms in chronic prostatitis.
   e. Prostatodynia is difficult to treat, and there is no clearly superior treatment.

B. **Benign prostatic hypertrophy**
1. Characteristics:
   a. Nonmalignant enlargement of the prostate gland
   b. Driven by androgens, especially dihydrotestosterone
2. Clinical features:
   a. Urinary hesitancy, straining, slow urine stream, incomplete voiding, dribbling, and nocturia
   b. Increased incidence of UTI
   c. In severe cases, BPH can cause urinary retention and renal failure.
3. Diagnosis:
   a. Obstructive lower urinary tract symptoms with an enlarged prostate on DRE
   b. Urinalysis and serum renal panel should be done.
   c. PSA is not indicated unless there is a concern for cancer.
   d. Imaging is not necessary. Urodynamics are optional.
4. Treatment:
   a. Initial treatment is usually medical:
      i. Alpha blocker: doxazosin or tamsulosin
      ii. 5-α reductase inhibitor: finasteride or dutasteride
   b. Surgery for refractory cases: transurethral resection, vaporization, or incision of the prostate
   c. Herbal remedies such as saw palmetto have no objective evidence of efficacy.

C. **Prostate cancer**
1. Characteristics:
   a. Adenocarcinoma originating within the glands of the prostate
   b. Spreads locally and tends to metastasize to bone
   c. Second leading cause of cancer-related death among men
   d. Widespread use of prostate-specific antigen (PSA) screening has not changed the mortality rate.
   e. Most prostate cancer diagnosed by PSA screening is Gleason score 6, associated with an indolent course even without treatment.
   f. The underlying cause of prostate cancer is not understood.
2. Clinical features:
   a. Prostate cancer may cause no symptoms until late in its course, because it tends to start peripherally in the gland and not cause urinary obstruction.
   b. A hard mass may be palpated within the prostate on DRE.

3. Diagnosis:
   a. The United States Preventive Services Task Force (USPSTF) recommends against PSA for prostate cancer screening. There is a draft recommendation making it a category C recommendation for men 55-69.
   b. DRE has a very low sensitivity and specificity for prostate cancer.
4. Treatment:
   a. Options include watchful waiting, PSA monitoring, radioactive seed implantation, external beam radiation, radical prostatectomy, and physical and chemical castration.
   b. Bone metastasis of prostate cancer may be treated with radiation, testosterone suppression, and/or bisphosphonates.
   c. Prostate cancer treatment frequently causes incontinence, impotence, and/or difficulty with sexual functioning.
   d. Prognosis is very good with Gleason score of 6 and diminishes with higher grades.

VIII. Erectile Dysfunction

A. **Characteristics**
   1. Definition: persistent inability to attain or maintain an erection satisfactory for intercourse
   2. Incidence increases with age, and affects up to three-fourths of men over age 75.
   3. Strongly associated with smoking, hypertension, atherosclerosis, and diabetes
   4. Causes are multifactorial, usually involving both physical and emotional factors.
   5. A normal erection requires testosterone, cerebral arousal, nerve transmission to the penis, adequate arterial inflow to the erectile bodies, and reduced venous outflow of the erectile bodies. Disruption of any of these can produce erectile dysfunction.

B. **Clinical features**
   1. History should include details of the onset and time course, associated medical problems, medications, presence or absence of nocturnal tumescence, problems within the relationship with partner(s), and whether this only happens with certain partners.
   2. Physical exam is often normal. Small testicular size might suggest inadequate testosterone.

C. **Diagnosis**
   1. Erectile dysfunction (ED) is a clinical diagnosis, based primarily on the patient's history.
   2. All patients should have a glucose or A_{1c}, lipid panel, and morning testosterone level.
   3. Testosterone levels over 230 ng/dL do not cause erectile dysfunction.
   4. Differential diagnosis: premature ejaculation and anorgasmia caused by SSRIs

D. **Treatment**
   1. Lifestyle modification such as quitting smoking and losing weight are often effective.
   2. Treat contributing medical problems such as diabetes or hypogonadism.
   3. If practical, discontinue causative medications.
   4. Phosphodiesterase 5 (PDE5) inhibitors: Sildenafil, vardenafil, and tadalafil enhance erectile function with sexual stimulation.
   5. Alternative medications include intraurethral and intracavernosal injections of prostaglandins.
   6. If medications are ineffective or not tolerated, vacuum erection devices and penile implants are an option.

IX. Enuresis

A. **Characteristics**
   1. Definition: intermittent involuntary urinary incontinence at least twice weekly while sleeping in children > 5 years old
      a. Primary enuresis: no period of being dry for more than 6 months
      b. Secondary enuresis: there has been a period of being dry for more than 6 months

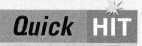

Quick HIT

Simply ordering a PSA is likely to set off a cascade of diagnostic testing and treatment that is more likely to hurt than help the patient, because 50% of patients treated for prostate cancer experience impotence and/or incontinence, and most would have had an indolent course without treatment.

Quick HIT

If a man loses an erection during intercourse, the fear that it will happen again often causes distraction that leads to further erectile dysfunction.

Quick HIT

Relationship discord is a frequent contributor, and needs to be discovered and addressed.

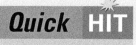

Quick HIT

A substantial majority of men treated with PDE5 inhibitors will "get their confidence back" and be able to stop the medication after a few months.

Renal, Urinary, and Male Reproductive System

2. Between the ages of 5 and 9, boys are affected twice as often as girls.
3. Proposed causes include high evening fluid consumption, overactive bladder, genetics, low nocturnal antidiuretic hormone (ADH) production, sleep disorders including obstructive sleep apnea and, constipation.

B. **Clinical features**
1. History should include how often this occurs, estimation of volume, how deep a sleeper the child appears to be, whether there is associated snoring, history of parental enuresis, and an understanding of how this is handled by the child and parent, including punishments, rewards, and whether the child is involved in cleaning the bed.
2. A diary should be kept for a few weeks to document the problem.
3. Physical exam should include checking the upper airway for signs of obstruction such as tonsillar hypertrophy, and abdominal exam palpating for bladder distension and fecal impaction.

C. **Diagnosis**
1. Clinical diagnosis
2. Dipstick urinalysis to rule out diabetes and infection
3. No imaging studies are necessary.

D. **Treatment**
1. Simple advice includes an understanding that this is "no one's fault," addressing any coexisting constipation, stopping caffeine consumption, reducing late evening fluid intake, and voiding at bedtime.
2. Enuresis alarms are the mainstay of treatment and can be quite effective.
3. Nightly desmopressin can be effective if an enuresis alarm has not produced substantial change within 3 months.
4. If no other treatment is effective, imipramine may be used.

QUESTIONS

1. A 35-year-old man presents with acute onset of right flank pain that radiates into the right groin and down to the right testicle. He has never had pain like this before, and it is the most intense pain he has ever experienced. On examination, he is constantly moving, appears pale, and has a soft, nontender abdomen. Urinalysis is remarkable for 4+ blood on dipstick and too numerous to count RBCs per high-power field on microscopy. A noncontrast CT shows a 4-mm calcified stone at the right ureterovesical junction and a right hydronephrosis. The next best intervention for this patient is:
   A. Trimethoprim/sulfamethoxazole
   B. IV infusion of 1 L of normal saline
   C. Extracorporeal shock wave lithotripsy
   D. Tamsulosin
   E. Transurethral stone basket procedure

2. A 26-year-old previously healthy woman presents with 4 days of urgency, frequency, and dysuria. She has been trying to self-treat with 32 oz of cranberry juice daily. In the last 24 hours, she has developed chills and sweats, and her right midback has become tender. On examination, she appears mildly ill, and has both suprapubic and right flank pain on palpation. Urinalysis shows 3+ leukocyte esterase and negative nitrites. Microscopy shows 30 to 50 WBCs per high-power field and occasional WBC casts. Appropriate management of this patient includes:
   A. 1 g of intramuscular ceftriaxone
   B. Prescription of nitrofurantoin
   C. Advice to continue drinking the cranberry juice
   D. Immediate hospitalization
   E. CT scan of the abdomen and pelvis

3. Two weeks ago, you were troubled to find 3+ blood on the urine dipstick of a 58-year-old female smoker who was newly diagnosed with hypertension and started on lisinopril 10 mg daily. The dipstick did not show proteinuria. Microscopic urinalysis showed 10 to 15 RBCs per high-power field. A urine culture at that time showed no growth. She remains asymptomatic. Today, her blood pressure is under good control, and a repeat dipstick urinalysis shows 2+ blood. Appropriate management today includes:
   A. An excretory urogram (intravenous pyelogram [IVP])
   B. Nephrology consultation
   C. Prescription of trimethoprim–sulfamethoxazole
   D. CT scan of the abdomen and pelvis with and without contrast
   E. Urgent cystoscopy

4. A 39-year-old G2P2 woman presents with a 2-year history of urinary incontinence that requires her to wear a pad daily. She loses urine when she coughs, sneezes, or steps down hard. When she feels the need to void, she is able to make it to the bathroom. An office dipstick and microscopic urinalysis is unremarkable. Speculum and bimanual pelvic exam are normal. Your first step in the management of this patient is:
   A. Referral to an urologist
   B. Prescription for intravaginal estrogen cream
   C. Fitting her for a pessary
   D. Teaching her Kegel exercises
   E. Prescription for long-acting tolterodine

5. A 36-year-old married male patient presents with erection problems. He has fathered three children and reports previously normal sexual functioning. Three months ago, he was having intercourse with his wife and lost his erection. Since that time he reports normal libido and episodes of nocturnal tumescence, but has on multiple occasions been unable to have an erection satisfactory for intercourse with his wife. He reports no marital discord or infidelity. At his last visit, you prescribed sildenafil 50 mg to be taken 1 hour before intercourse, and he now reports that his sexual functioning is "back to normal." Your long-term prognosis is that he will:

   A. Need ever-increasing doses of sildenafil to maintain normal erectile function

   B. Eventually need an implantable penile prosthesis

   C. Need to stay on the same dose of sildenafil indefinitely

   D. Likely be able to stop sildenafil once he "gets his confidence back"

   E. Probably soon develop hypogonadism and need testosterone replacement

6. A 7-year-old male child presents to your office with nightly bedwetting that has persisted throughout his life. His parents have unsuccessfully tried to restrict his fluid for 2 hours before bedtime. He has been wearing diapers to bed, but these sometimes leak through. His parents feel uncomfortable allowing him to sleep over at a friend's house because of this and ask your help in solving the problem. His father did not become dry until he was 9 years old. Your examination reveals a soft abdomen without palpable bladder or stool, and normal Tanner stage I external genitalia. An office dipstick urinalysis is unremarkable. Your first step in management of this patient is:

   A. Setting up a reward/punishment system for staying dry at night

   B. Having his parents purchase a bed alarm system

   C. Prescription of trimethoprim–sulfamethoxazole

   D. Prescription of nasal desmopressin spray

   E. Prescription of nightly imipramine

ANSWERS

1. **Answer: D.** This patient has classic right ureteral colic with a stone that is stuck at the ureterovesical junction. Stones that are < 5mm are very likely to pass without surgical intervention. The patient is in severe pain and exhibiting a vagal response by his pale appearance. The pain is caused by ureteral spasm around the stone, creating an acute hydronephrosis that stretches the kidney capsule. Tamsulosin is an alpha-blocker that will likely relieve some of the ureteral spasm that is blocking the ureter, and may allow the stone to pass. A prescription of trimethoprim–sulfamethoxazole would not be appropriate because there is no indication of infection here. A normal saline infusion is not likely to provide any direct benefit for pain or passing of the stone. Lithotripsy and stone basket procedures are not indicated for this small stone because it should pass spontaneously.

2. **Answer: A.** This patient has a right pyelonephritis, and history suggests that she started with a cystitis. Negative nitrites on urinalysis do not preclude bacterial infection because many urinary pathogens do not reduce nitrate. She is ill, but will likely respond to outpatient management. It is helpful to start antibiotic treatment of the pyelonephritis with parenteral antibiotics, and intramuscular ceftriaxone will provide bactericidal levels that will last 24 hours. She does not appear ill enough to require hospitalization. If she was having difficulty with oral intake, she would warrant admission. A CT scan of her abdomen and pelvis will not add any information to her current management, but could be useful to identify a perinephric abscess or stone disease if she does not rapidly respond to treatment. Cranberry juice may reduce the incidence of cystitis, but has no role once infection has developed. Nitrofurantoin is an inappropriate choice of antibiotic for pyelonephritis because it develops almost no tissue level. This patient should be seen back in 24 hours, and an oral antibiotic such as trimethoprim–sulfamethoxazole should be started if she is improving. A urine culture sent on the first day will guide appropriate antibiotic selection.

3. **Answer: D.** Microscopic hematuria needs expedient evaluation. It is appropriate on the first visit to check for infection with a urine culture and to repeat a urinalysis to determine if the microscopic hematuria is persistent. At this visit, it is clear that the patient does not have an infection and has persistent microscopic hematuria. CT scan of the abdomen and pelvis with and without contrast can identify renal and ureteral tumors as well as stone disease. An IVP had been used frequently in the past to evaluate microscopic hematuria, but provides much less information than the CT scan. Urinalysis findings do not suggest glomerulonephritis, so nephrology consultation is not indicated. There is no evidence of infection, so trimethoprim–sulfamethoxazole is not indicated. If the CT scan does not identify a cause of the microscopic hematuria, cystoscopy should be done to evaluate the bladder mucosa of this smoker, who may have a bladder tumor. Cystoscopy is not indicated before the CT scan.

4. **Answer: D.** This patient has stress urinary incontinence. Wearing a pad daily identifies this as a significant problem and needs to be taken seriously. She does not exhibit urge incontinence, and infection is unlikely with her negative urinalysis. Kegel exercises have a good likelihood of improving her symptoms. It is appropriate to start with pelvic floor exercises before intervening surgically. There is no reason to suspect that this patient has estrogen deficiency, so intravaginal estrogen is not indicated. It may be helpful in a patient with atrophic vaginitis and urge incontinence. She does not need urology referral presently, but might benefit from this for a urethral sling if she does not respond to Kegel exercises. Tolterodine has no role in stress incontinence. If she has pelvic organ prolapse that is changing her vesicourethral angle, a pessary could be helpful.

5. **Answer: D.** Erectile dysfunction is very common and often results from a single episode of losing an erection during intercourse. Any sort of physical or mental distraction, or drug/alcohol intake can lead to detumescence. Once this happens, the patient may fear that it will happen again—and this performance anxiety interferes with normal sexual arousal, creating a cycle of erectile dysfunction. The fact that this patient has normal libido and nocturnal tumescence reassures that he has normal underlying sexual functioning. Once the appropriate dose of sildenafil is identified, it is not likely to change with time. Erectile dysfunction does not lead to hypogonadism. This patient's normal libido and nocturnal tumescence is strong evidence that he does not have hypogonadism presently. After a few months of sildenafil use, the majority of men will stop obsessing about the possibility of another episode of losing their erection during intercourse. At this point, most men are able to stop the medication and maintain normal sexual functioning. Implantable penile prostheses are a last resort for men who do not respond to any medical intervention.

6. **Answer: B.** Primary enuresis is a common problem, and frequently runs in the family. It is frequent for parents to try simple measures such as reducing fluid intake before bedtime. Unfortunately, it is also common for parents to try to inappropriately punish the child for the bedwetting. It is always important to exclude urinary infection and constipation as the cause of enuresis. A bed alarm system has a very high likelihood of helping. Bed alarms are reasonably inexpensive and their use is generally curative. Reward and punishment systems are not likely to be successful. There is no sign of infection in this patient, so trimethoprim–sulfamethoxazole is not indicated. If the patient does not respond to a bed alarm, desmopressin may be prescribed. However, tablets are the appropriate dosage form because overdoses are common with nasal spray and can lead to hyponatremia. Imipramine would be a third-line choice here.

13 PREGNANCY, CHILDBIRTH, AND PUERPERIUM

Montiel T. Rosenthal • Elizabeth Weage

I. Pregnancy: Prenatal Care

A. **Confirmation of pregnancy**
 1. Qualitative urine or serum beta-human chorionic gonadotropin (β-hCG) test with or without quantitative serum β-hCG)
 2. Ultrasound, depending on the gestational age
 3. Doppler fetal heart tones by 10 to 14 weeks

B. **Initial prenatal visit**
 1. Patient history: Elicit reproductive and previous obstetric, past medical, medications, allergy, immunization, surgical, infectious exposure, social, family, and occupational histories. Screen for domestic violence.
 2. Initial prenatal exam: physical exam, including pelvic examination (note size of uterus, cervical lesions, shape of pelvis). Fundal height should be ±2 cm of gestational age after 19 weeks' gestation (Table 13-1).
 3. Initial prenatal labs: complete blood count (CBC), blood type and Rh factor, blood antibody screen, hepatitis B surface antigen, syphilis cascade/rapid plasma reagin/venereal disease research laboratory (RPR/VDRL), HIV, rubella IgG, urinalysis, urine culture, pap smear/cervical cytology/HPV typing per screening guidelines, gonorrhea, chlamydia, urine drug screen, hemoglobin electrophoresis, 25-hydroxy vitamin D level, thyroid-stimulating hormone (TSH), Hgb A_{1c} (if at risk for occult Type II diabetes mellitus [DM])
 4. Initial prenatal assessment:
  a. Determine estimated gestational age and date of delivery using:
   i. Pregnancy calculator apps
   ii. Pregnancy wheel
   iii. Naegele's rule: [(Last menstrual period + 1 year) – 3 months] + 7 days = estimated delivery date
  b. Determine the patient's risk stratification based on pregnancy-related and comorbid factors.
  c. Prescribe daily prenatal vitamins.

TABLE 13-1 Anatomical Markers That Predict Gestational Age	
Gestational Age in Weeks	**Fundal Height and Anatomical Marker**
12	Above pelvic brim
20–22	Umbilicus
36	Xiphoid process
>37	Fundal height generally starts to decrease as fetus begins descent into pelvis

d. Orient to after-hours contact information and basic reasons to call (vaginal bleeding, loss of fluid, decreased fetal movement, contractions >5/hr).

e. The Edinburgh Postnatal Depression Scale (EPDS) has been validated for use during pregnancy. A score of greater than 10 indicates additional intervention is necessary.

C. **Sequencing of prenatal visits**

1. Prenatal visits should occur every 4 weeks until 28 weeks, then every 2 weeks. Weekly or biweekly visits may be indicated by maternal complications and need for more frequent testing and monitoring.

2. Consider more frequent visits for younger mothers or those for whom there may be a psycho/social concern.

3. Subsequent prenatal visit labs/vaccinations (Table 13-2):

a. 1-hour (50 g) glucose challenge test (GCT)

    i. Nonfasting screen for gestational diabetes

    ii. Glucola 50 g consumed within 5 minutes

    iii. Venous blood glucose sampling 1 hour after start of test

    iv. Results:

        (a) >200 mg/dL: gestational diabetes

        (b) 140 to 200 mg/dL: perform fasting 3-hour glucose tolerance test (GTT)

b. 3-hour glucose (100 g) tolerance test (3-hr GTT): gestational diabetes diagnosed with any of the following:

    i. Fasting > 95 mg/dL

    ii. 1 hour > 180 mg/dL

    iii. 2 hours > 155 mg/dL

    iv. 3 hours > 140 mg/dL

c. Group B streptococcal (GBS) screen:

    i. Streptococcal bacteria can cause neonatal meningitis, sepsis, bacteremia, pneumonia, or urinary tract infection (UTI).

    ii. Screen with a rectovaginal culture or PCR probe at 35 to 37 weeks gestation if there is no history of a previous infant affected by GBS or prior GBS infection this pregnancy (ie, UTI with GBS).

    iii. If the patient is allergic to penicillin, order clindamycin sensitivities as there is increasing clindamycin resistance.

d. Immunizations:

    i. Influenza: given at any point during pregnancy as indicated by season and availability

    ii. Tdap: administered each pregnancy. The optimal time to immunize for maximal protective benefit to the fetus is 27 to 36 weeks. Should also be offered to anyone who will be actively involved in childcare.

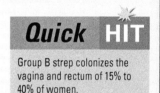

Quick HIT

Group B strep colonizes the vagina and rectum of 15% to 40% of women.

TABLE **13-2** Sequence of Tests and Vaccinations After Initial Prenatal Visit	
Gestational Age (Weeks)	**Testing/Vaccinations Recommended**
Any	Influenza (when available)
16–21	Maternal quad screen
18–22	Level 1 (anatomy scan) ultrasound
24–28	GCT, Hgb/Hct, Rh antibody (if Rh neg)
28	Rhogam (if Rh −), syphilis[a], STD screen[b]
27–36	Tdap
35–37	GBS screen

[a]If in endemic area.
[b]If STD noted earlier in pregnancy.

iii. Live vaccinations such as measles, mumps, and rubella (MMR) should not be administered during pregnancy. If prenatal testing reveals lack of immunity to rubella, MMR should be given to the mother postpartum before discharge from the hospital.

D. **Antenatal surveillance and genetic screening**
1. α-fetoprotein (AFP):
   a. AFP is a globulin produced by the fetal yolk sack, liver, and gastrointestinal (GI) tract.
   b. Maternal serum AFP is measured at 15 to 20 weeks.
   c. Higher maternal serum AFPs are associated with neural tube defects.
2. First trimester maternal serum: levels of pregnancy-associated plasma protein-A (PAPP-A) and β-hCG, which is combined with an ultrasound measurement of nuchal translucency (at 11 to 13 weeks) and sometimes to look for absence of nasal bone (11 to 14 weeks)
3. Quadruple (Quad) test: AFP, unconjugated estriol (uE3), hCG, and inhibin A. Screen for trisomy 21 and 18 as well as open neural tube defects (at 16 to 21 weeks)
4. Cell-free fetal DNA: maternal blood sample required, fetal DNA is isolated and evaluated for aneuploidy and gender as early as 10 weeks
5. Amniocentesis: sampling of amniotic fluid with a transabdominal approach. Indications include genetic testing, assessment for fetal lung maturity, neural tube defects
6. Chorionic villus sampling: if done, usually performed at 9 to 14 weeks' gestation

E. **Imaging and other testing during pregnancy**
1. Ultrasound: the most common form of visual assessment of the female reproductive tract as well as the anatomy of the fetus
   a. Transvaginal ultrasound can visualize an intrauterine pregnancy when β–hCG is >1,500.
   b. Transabdominal ultrasound can visualize an intrauterine pregnancy when β–hCG is >6,000.
2. Nonstress test (NST):
   a. A combination of fetal heart rate monitoring as well as tocometry, reflecting the development of the fetal sympathetic nervous system by 28 weeks
   b. A fetus that is not sleeping, is acidotic or neurologically depressed will manifest short accelerations of the heart rate above baseline.
   c. Indications: gestational hypertension (HTN), chronic HTN, medication-controlled gestational or pre-pregnancy diabetes, history of fetal demise, intrauterine growth restriction (IUGR), decreased fetal movement after 28 weeks, oligohydramnios, postterm pregnancy, or other serious maternal illness
   d. Reactive or satisfactory NST:
      i. >32 weeks' gestation: accelerations above the baseline of at least 15 bmp for a length of at least 15 seconds, occurring at least two times in 20 to 40 minutes
      ii. 28 to 32 weeks' gestation: accelerations above the baseline of at least 10 bmp for a length of at least 10 seconds, occurring at least two times in 20 to 40 minutes
3. Amniotic fluid index (AFI):
   a. Ultrasound measurement of amniotic fluid surrounding the fetus
   b. The sum of the largest vertical pocket of fluid (without fetal parts) in each of four abdominal quadrants
   c. Normal, 10 to 20 cm
   d. Severe oligohydramnios, < 5 cm
   e. Polyhydramnios, > 20 cm
4. Umbilical artery Doppler velocimetry: detailed Doppler ultrasound to follow-up suspected IUGR
5. Level II ultrasound: a face-to-face perinatology consult using ultrasound to look for fetal anatomical anomalies noted on a previous ultrasound where a serious fetal anomaly was suspected

6. Fetal MRI: used in antenatal diagnosis of fetal neural tube defects, structural cardiac anomalies, or suspected neoplasm

7. Other more invasive measures of evaluating a pregnancy include amniocentesis and cordocentesis.

F. **Vaginal bleeding**

1. Differential diagnosis: ectopic pregnancy, threatened abortion, partial placental/chorionic plate separation, trauma, cervicitis, venereal warts, trichomonas, placenta previa, implantation bleeding, or cervical varices

2. Testing: speculum exam, wet prep/KOH, CBC, Rh factor and antibody screen, serial quantitative β–hCGs, ultrasound, Kleihauer–Betke screen

G. **Anticipatory guidance and common discomforts of pregnancy**

1. Ideal weight gain: based on the pre-pregnancy maternal BMI (Table 13-3)

2. Nausea and vomiting:

   a. Common complication of pregnancy

   b. Generally self-limited

   c. Emergency when the pregnant woman is dehydrated or has hyperemesis gravidarum

   d. Treatment: diet modification, Zofran, Phenergan, H_1 blockers, ginger, vitamin B_6, Reglan, acupuncture, and/or hypnosis

3. Back pain:

   a. Common during the 3rd trimester as weight increases and lordosis of the lower back increases in response

   b. Pregnancy belts, exercise balls used appropriately, and gentle yoga stretching can offer relief.

   c. Prenatal massage, ice/heat, and acetaminophen are safe.

4. GERD:

   a. Exacerbated by relaxation of gastric sphincter from hormone changes

   b. Reduced room for the stomach owing to fetal growth

   c. Treatment: frequent small meals, stay upright for 2 hours after eating, calcium antacids, sucralfate, H_2 blockers, proton pump inhibitors, and avoidance of spicy/greasy foods

5. Swelling of feet:

   a. Often related to physiologic hemodynamic changes of pregnancy

   b. Decreased return of blood from lower extremities owing to compression of vena cava by the fetus

   c. Can be a warning sign of preeclampsia, and important to evaluate for proteinuria and hypertension

   d. Treatment: limit dietary sodium, elevation of legs, hydration, and use of compression stockings

6. Pelvic pain:

   a. Round ligament pain:

      i. Sharp, stabbing pain radiating into the groin

      ii. May be unilateral or bilateral

      iii. Starts during the 2nd trimester with stretching of the round ligament

TABLE **13-3** Recommended Weight Gain in a Singleton Pregnancy	
Pre-pregnancy Maternal Weight	**Recommended Weight Gain**
Underweight, BMI <18.5	28–40 lb
Normal Weight, BMI 18.5–24.9	25–35 lb
Overweight, BMI 25–29.9	15–25 lb
Obese, BMI >30	11–20 lb

iv. Exacerbated by climbing stairs or getting out of a car

v. Treatment: acetaminophen, core muscle strengthening exercises, moist heat, and modification of daily activities to avoid exacerbation

b. Fetal head engagement:

i. Later in the 3rd trimester as the fetus descends

ii. Engagement of the fetal head in the maternal pelvis causes discomfort, pressure, and increased sensation of urgency to urinate.

7. Fatigue:

a. Due to the increased energy demands of pregnancy

b. Encourage mothers to nap when tired and plan to sleep more at night.

c. Eat well and often, and stay hydrated.

d. If extreme and persistent: Consider anemia or thyroid disorders.

8. Anticipatory guidance topics to cover during pregnancy: prenatal nutrition, over-the-counter (OTC) drug options in pregnancy, exercise and sex during pregnancy, anesthesia and birthing options, trial of labor after cesarean section (TOLAC) classes, breastfeeding, newborn care, consent for delivery, maternity leave forms for work, anticipated family planning after delivery

H. **Medical complications of pregnancy**

1. Hypertension in pregnancy:

a. Two blood pressure measurements at least 4 hours apart of >140/90

b. Essential HTN: diagnosis before 20 weeks' gestation

c. Gestational HTN: diagnosis after 20 weeks' gestation

2. Preeclampsia:

a. Risk factors: first pregnancy, prior history, subsequent pregnancy but different father of baby, gestational diabetes

b. Diagnosis after 20 weeks' gestation with HTN plus proteinuria: 24-hour urine protein >300 mg/24 hr; OR > 0.3 mg/dL urine protein/creatinine ratio; OR urine dip protein > +1

c. Diagnosis after 20 weeks with HTN without proteinuria, but platelets <100,000, creatinine > 1.1 or two times the baseline, and/or doubling of aspartate transaminase (AST) or alanine transaminase (ALT)

d. Treatment:

i. Magnesium sulfate in labor and 24 hours postpartum to prevent seizures

ii. Good blood pressure control with methyldopa, labetalol, metoprolol, hydralazine, nifedipine, calcium channel blockers, or hydrochlorothiazide

iii. Complications: HELLP syndrome, fetal/maternal death

3. Gestational diabetes:

a. Affects 6% to 7% of pregnancies

b. Risk factors: obesity, personal history of gestational diabetes, family history of DM2, maternal age >25 years, previous baby weighing >9 lb

c. Pathophysiology: insulin resistance, primarily mediated by secretion of diabetogenic hormones (growth hormone, corticotrophin-releasing hormone, placental lactogen, and progesterone) by the placenta to ensure that the fetus has an adequate nutrient supply

d. Diagnosis

i. See prenatal care section.

ii. High-risk individuals: Fasting blood glucose or A_{1c} may be drawn at the initial prenatal visit.

4. Thyroid disease:

a. Hyperthyroidism: rare, occurring in 0.1% to 0.4% of all pregnancies

b. Hypothyroidism: preexisting disease or Hashimoto thyroiditis

c. Complications: preeclampsia, placental abruption, cognitive impairment of fetus, postpartum hemorrhage

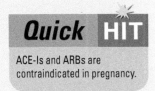

Quick **HIT**

ACE-Is and ARBs are contraindicated in pregnancy.

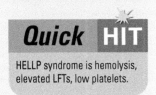

Quick **HIT**

HELLP syndrome is hemolysis, elevated LFTs, low platelets.

5. Asthma:
   a. One of the most common comorbidities, occurring in 3% to 8% of pregnancies
   b. Management goals are prevention of severe exacerbations and optimization of pulmonary function.
   c. Four components of management during pregnancy: monitoring of lung function, avoidance of triggers, patient education, and pharmacologic therapy
      i. Recommended short-acting β-antagonist: albuterol
      ii. Optional inhaled glucocorticoid: budesonide
6. Substance abuse:
   a. Screening all pregnant women for tobacco, alcohol, and illicit drug use is recommended at initial visit and every trimester if self-reporting or positive drug test.
   b. Smoking: the most important modifiable risk factor associated with adverse pregnancy outcomes including growth restriction, placental abruption, placenta previa, preterm premature rupture of the membranes (PPROM), preterm delivery
   c. Opiate substitution treatment is recommended over medical detoxification or no treatment during pregnancy.
   d. Complications of cocaine abuse related to vasoconstriction include spontaneous abortion and placental abruption.
   e. Infants born to substance-abusing mothers are at risk for neonatal abstinence syndrome.
7. Intimate partner violence (IPV) screening:
   a. Up to 20% of pregnant women are victims of physical abuse.
   b. Domestic violence is the most common cause of maternal death in pregnancy in the United States.
   c. Risk factors: previous history, young age, high-risk drug use and sexual behavior, excessive jealousy or possessive behavior by partner, relationships with disparities in education or income between partners
   d. The risk for postpartum depression increases two to three times in women who experienced IPV during pregnancy.
   e. Common screening questions:
      i. "Do you feel safe at home?"
      ii. "Do you feel supported at home?"
      iii. "Do you feel trapped in your current relationship?"

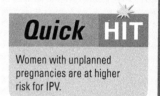

Quick HIT

Women with unplanned pregnancies are at higher risk for IPV.

II. Childbirth
A. **Active labor**
   1. Definition: regular uterine contractions resulting in cervical change in dilation
   2. Can monitor in labor and delivery with fetal heart rate, tocometry, and PE. Encourage the patient to walk and be active while waiting to determine if she is in true labor.
B. **Rule out ruptured membranes**
   1. Pooling: collection of fluid in the vaginal vault indicates rupture
   2. Fern testing: Amniotic fluid creates a fern pattern when dried. Use a sterile swab to collect fluid from the vaginal vault. After a thin film dries on glass slide, fern pattern of salt crystals can be visualized under microscope (Fig. 13-1).
C. **Preterm labor (PTL)**
   1. Definition: labor before 37 weeks' gestation
   2. Risk factors: previous PTL, multiple gestation, uterine anomaly, bacteriuria, GBS colonization/infection, PPROM, placental pathology, substance abuse, depression, anxiety, polyhydramnios, short cervix/cervical incompetence, sexually transmitted diseases (STDs), pyelonephritis, pneumonia, appendicitis, abdominal surgery during pregnancy, African-American race, young or advanced maternal age (AMA) mothers, diabetes, preeclampsia, fetal anomaly

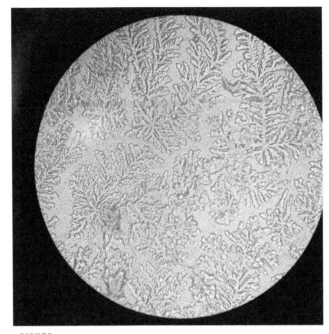

FIGURE
13-1 Positive fern test.

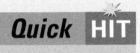

Preterm birth is the leading direct cause of neonatal death.

3. Evaluation
   a. Obtain maternal vital signs, fetal monitoring, review obstetrical history, speculum examination (collect fetal fibronectin and/or swab for fern testing if indicated prior to digital examination).
   b. Labs: GBS, urine culture, GC/chlamydia, and urine drug screen (UDS) in patients with risk factors
4. Women 22 to 34 weeks are hospitalized.
   a. Course of betamethasone or dexamethasone (to reduce neonatal respiratory complications)
   b. Tocolytic drugs for up to 48 hours
   c. Penicillin (PCN) for GBS prophylaxis
   d. Possibly magnesium sulfate (for fetal neuroprotection)
D. **Induction of labor**
   1. Indications: postterm pregnancy, premature rupture of membranes, fetal demise, IUGR, placental abruption, maternal infection, preeclampsia
   2. Bishop score: used to suggest the likelihood of a successful induction (score >5) (Table 13-4)

TABLE **13-4** Bishop Score				
	Score			
Cervix	**0**	**1**	**2**	**3**
Position	Posterior	Mid-Position	Anterior	
Consistency	Firm	Medium	Soft	
Effacement	0%–30%	40%–50%	60%–70%	>70%
Dilation	Closed	1–2 cm	3–4 cm	5–6 cm
Fetal Head Station	−3	−2	−1 to 0	>+1

3. Types of inductions:
   a. Cervical ripening
      i. Recommended for women with a low Bishop score
      ii. Prostaglandins (dinoprostone, misoprostol), foley bulb, and laminaria
   b. Stripping of membranes and amniotomy cause a release of prostaglandins to trigger labor.
   c. Pitocin (synthetic oxytocin): commonly used to stimulate uterine contractions

E. **Stages of labor**
   1. Latent: beginning of labor from closed cervix to 4 to 6 cm dilation
   2. Active: from 4 to 6 cm of cervical dilation through delivery of the placenta
      a. Stage 1: 4 to 6 cm dilation to 10 cm
      b. Stage 2: complete cervical dilation through delivery of the infant
      c. Stage 3: delivery of the placenta, normally in <30 minutes. Active management of the third stage of labor decreases rates of retained placenta and postpartum hemorrhage.

III. Puerperium

A. **In hospital postpartum care**
   1. Patient reports: lochia/vaginal bleeding, abdominal tenderness, bowel movement, breastfeeding, breast tenderness
   2. Examination: lungs, heart, leg tenderness or swelling, abdomen for firm uterus at or under umbilicus, perineum if patient had any tears which required repair
   3. Encourage baby rooming in and breastfeeding.
   4. Follow-up postpartum hemorrhage with CBC.
   5. Early ambulation or pharmacologic deep vein thrombosis (DVT) prophylaxis depending on risk
   6. RhoGam for Rh-negative mothers
   7. MMR vaccination if prenatal testing revealed rubella nonimmune status
   8. Discharge instructions:
      a. Nothing per vagina (no sex, tampons, or douches) until postpartum checkup (6 weeks)
      b. Warning signs: increased vaginal bleeding, tender/swollen/red breasts, fevers, abdominal tenderness, dysuria, leg pain or swelling
   9. Continuation of prenatal vitamins, especially if breastfeeding

B. **Routine postpartum visit**
   1. Usually 6 weeks following any delivery. Cesarean section patients should have a visit within a week of delivery for removal of staples/incision check.
   2. History since delivery: return of menstrual cycle, breastfeeding complications, bonding with infant, resumption of sexual intercourse, domestic violence, persistent vaginal bleeding, fever, or abdominal cramping
   3. Exam: complete exam including breast and pelvic exam
   4. Special cases:
      a. Anemia in pregnancy or around delivery: check Hgb/Hct
      b. Gestational diabetics should have a 2-hour GTT and then yearly screening for diabetes.
      c. Pregnancy-induced hypertension (PIH)/preeclampsia:
         i. Monitor BP for 72 hours inpatient following delivery.
         ii. Follow-up outpatient for BP check in 7 to 10 days.
         iii. Start med if BP still >150/100 in the office.
      d. If prenatal cervical cytology showed atypical squamous cells of undetermined significance (ASCUS) with high-risk human papillomavirus (HR HPV), low-grade squamous intraepithelial lesion (LGSIL), or high-grade cervical dysplasia (HGSIL), patient should have postpartum colposcopy with or without biopsy and follow-up based on results.
   5. Postpartum mental disorders:
      a. Screening for postpartum depression
      b. The EPDS has been validated. A score of greater than 10 indicates additional intervention is necessary.

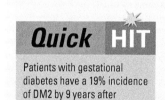

Quick HIT

Patients with gestational diabetes have a 19% incidence of DM2 by 9 years after delivery.

c. Baby blues
  i. Transient period of mild depressive symptoms including irritability, sadness, and crying spells
  ii. Risk factors: prior depression, history of premenstrual syndrome (PMS), family history, stress of childcare
d. Postpartum depression
  i. Depression onset or flare within 1 year of delivery
  ii. Risk factors: personal history of depression, history of abuse, unplanned pregnancy, lack of social support, financial difficulties, uncontrolled hypothyroidism
  iii. Prevalence of 8% to 15% of postpartum women.
  iv. Complications: impaired maternal/infant bonding, impaired child development, suicide, infanticide
  v. Testing: EPDS (see above), TSH
6. Family planning:
  a. The World Health Organization and the United States Agency for International Development recommend interpregnancy interval of 2 to 5 years. This timing reduces risk of anemia, PPROM, premature birth, placental abruption.
  b. Hormonal contraception:
    i. Oral contraception: pills taken daily with combination of estrogen and progesterone or progestin only
    ii. Implantable: intrauterine device (progestin intrauterine device [IUD] lasts 5 years, copper IUD lasts 10 years) or sub-dermal implant (progestin lasts 3 years)
    iii. Others: patch, vaginal ring, depo injection
  c. Natural family planning: combination of body temperature, menstrual calendar, and cervical mucus monitoring to determine fertile periods of a woman's menstrual cycle
  d. Surgical: tubal ligation, vasectomy, essure
  e. Others: condoms, spermicide, and diaphragm
  f. Women and their partners should be counseled on the efficacy, risks/benefits, cost, effects on menstrual cycle, duration of benefit, reversibility, return to fertility, and proper use in a shared decision for the right family planning method for each patient/couple.
  g. Continue daily folic acid 400 mcg while fertile.

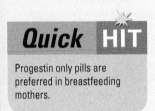

Quick HIT

Progestin only pills are preferred in breastfeeding mothers.

QUESTIONS

1. A 37-year-old G3P1011 presents to your office for an initial prenatal visit. She believes her last menstrual period (LMP) was 13 weeks ago. She has no medical problems. She had a spontaneous abortion at 6 weeks prior to delivery of a full-term male infant. She denies having felt the baby yet move. On exam, you find her fundus to be nearly to the level of her umbilicus. You do not hear fetal heart tones. Her cervix is closed and without any vaginal discharge or bleeding. What is the most appropriate next step in management?

   A. Schedule her routine follow-up appointment in 4 weeks.

   B. Schedule an ultrasound as soon as possible to further evaluate the gestational age and viability of the fetus

   C. Assume her LMP is correct and your fundal height measurement is wrong.

   D. Arrange for a dilation and curettage (D&C) because size > dates without fetal heart tones.

   E. Order maternal serum α-fetoprotein (MSAFP) testing

2. A 28-year-old G1P0 at 38 weeks 4 days presents to labor and delivery after feeling a gush of fluid. She has also been having irregular low abdominal cramps every 8 to 10 minutes. Her pregnancy has been uneventful and she is GBS positive. A fern test was positive. She was found to be dilated to 1 cm. What is the next step in management?

   A. Admit her for penicillin and active management of labor.

   B. Send her home because she is not yet in active labor.

   C. Have her walk the halls of L&D for 2 hours and recheck her cervix to determine if she needs admission.

   D. Observe her in L&D on bed rest until she is 40 weeks.

   E. Perform serial cervical exams every hour to assess change in her cervical dilation.

3. Which of the following increases a woman's risk of developing gestational diabetes?

   A. Maternal grandmother with history of gestational diabetes

   B. Previous diagnosis of hypertension

   C. History of delivering an 8 lb 10 oz infant

   D. Being of African-American descent

   E. Obesity

   F. Different father of the baby for this pregnancy

4. You are meeting a 33-year-old G2P1001 for an initial prenatal visit. Her LMP was 7 weeks ago. She reports she has had morning sickness and mild vaginal spotting for the last week. Her urine pregnancy test was positive. On examination, her uterine fundus is barely palpable outside of pelvis. Her cervix is closed, but dark red blood is seen in the posterior fornix. On bimanual examination, she does not have cervical motion tenderness, but there is tenderness in her right adnexa. What is the most appropriate next step?

   A. Perform a wet prep and KOH prep on vaginal secretions to look for clue cells and yeast. One of these STD is likely causing her vaginal spotting.

   B. Her vaginal spotting is secondary to implantation of the embryo and can be addressed with watchful waiting. She should schedule an appointment in 4 weeks after having routine prenatal labs drawn.

   C. A β-hCG quantitative level and a transvaginal ultrasound should be ordered, in addition to a Blood Type (with Rh) and Hemoglobin/Hematocrit.

   D. Administer RhoGAM if she is Rh+

   E. Administer MMR vaccine, as she is unsure of her immunization status.

   F. The adnexal tenderness suggests an ectopic pregnancy, and she should be offered methotrexate or a D&C.

5. A 26-year-old G2P2 presents for her routine postpartum check-up. She states that breastfeeding is going well but she is anxious about her ability to care for her infant girl. Quietly she mentions she is having difficulty sleeping

and has cried unexpectedly nearly every day since hospital discharge. Her boyfriend has been vocal about questioning whether or not he is really the father of the baby. She also has had decreased appetite and is not interested in activities she normally enjoys. She denies suicidal ideation or wanting to harm or abandon her daughter. Her self-reported EPDS score was 17. Which of the following are true about her diagnosis?

A. More than 20% of women are diagnosed with postpartum depression.

B. If these feelings occurred 6 months after delivery, she would not be diagnosed with postpartum depression.

C. Lack of social support is a documented risk factor.

D. This condition has no impact on maternal–infant bonding.

E. Postpartum depression should only be managed by mental health professionals.

6. A 21-year-old G1P0 at 32 weeks presents to labor and delivery triage with complaints of headache for the past day. Her blood pressure was initially 155/100 and she had 2+ protein on the urine dipstick. Blood work was significant for a transaminitis, hemoglobin of 10.2 g/dL, and a platelet count of 58,000. A repeat blood pressure 2 hours later was 140/95. Her cervical exam showed 2 cm of dilation/50% effacement/-3 station. Which of the following is appropriate management?

A. IV labetalol

B. Oral immediate-release nifedipine

C. Platelet transfusion

D. Monitor serial blood sugars

E. IV magnesium sulfate and plan for delivery

ANSWERS

1. **Answer: B.** The primary goal of an initial prenatal visit is to establish dates as the remainder of her pregnancy care will be guided by her gestational age. A fundus near the level of the umbilicus is consistent with a fetus at 20 weeks' gestational age. Not hearing fetal heart tones at 13 weeks is concerning as they should be present by 10 to 14 weeks. She should be sent for perinatal ultrasound not only to establish dating, but to confirm viability. There is no medical indication for dilation and curettage at this time as viability of the pregnancy has not been established. Dilation and curettage could be an appropriate treatment for a retained embryo or fetus that has no cardiac activity, after serial exams. MSAFP testing is appropriately done at 16 to 21 weeks of gestation, and carries no medical relevance done out of side of that time period.

2. **Answer: A.** There is no evidence that the patient is truly in active labor yet; however, in GBS-positive patients with confirmed rupture of membranes, penicillin must be started to reduce risk of complications in the infant. About 15% to 40% of women are colonized with Group B Strep. Appropriate treatment with two doses of penicillin prior to delivery reduces the risk of an early-onset GBS infection in the newborn. The Centers for Disease Control and Prevention recommendations and standardization of screening and treatment of GBS-positive mothers have resulted in a reduction of incidence of GBS-affected infants from 1.5 per 1,000 live births to 0.24 per 1,000 live births. She should be formally admitted to labor and delivery, and considered for induction of labor if she has no further progress in cervical dilation. With rupture of membranes, she has an increased risk for chorioamnionitis. There is no advantage to waiting for days at a time for labor to progress on its own, as she is already full-term. Minimizing cervical exams will also help reduce the potential risk of further introducing bacteria up into the uterus. There is no point to schedule hourly cervical exams in this scenario.

3. **Answer: E.** The risk factors for gestational diabetes are obesity, personal history of gestational diabetes, family history of DM2, maternal age >25 years, and previous baby weighing >9 lb.

4. **Answer: C.** Any vaginal bleeding early in pregnancy must be investigated. Though there are less concerning causes of bleeding such as implantation of the embryo, sexual intercourse, cervicitis from infection, however, life-threatening causes such as ectopic pregnancy must be ruled out. A transvaginal ultrasound is the best test to evaluate for ectopic pregnancy, and a quantitative β-hCG can be correlated with gestational age as well as be followed serially to assess viability of the pregnancy. While the use of methotrexate can be used to address an ectopic pregnancy, a dilation and curettage (D&C) will not definitively treat an ectopic pregnancy but only allow for sampling of uterine contents. Most bleeding in the first trimester does not portend an adverse outcome. Right adnexal tenderness may also be related to a corpus luteal cyst, which is normal in the first trimester of pregnancy. Obtaining routine prenatal labs can be done during this visit, or held off until the second visit pending the results of the ultrasound and β-hCGs to assess fetal viability. Patients who are Rh- and have a negative antibody titer may need RhoGAM. Clue cells suggest bacterial vaginosis and yeast suggests a candida infection, neither of which are sexually transmitted diseases, but which can cause cervical and/or vaginal spotting of blood. MMR is a live vaccine and should not be administered during pregnancy, but reserved for the postpartum period.

5. **Answer: C.** Patients at risk for postpartum depression generally are younger, primiparous, have a history of depression, an unplanned pregnancy, poor social support, or be involved in an abusive relationship. The diagnosis of postpartum depression can occur at any time in the first year after delivery, and affects 8% to 15% of women. Intervention should be made by any medical professional who suspects the diagnosis. The EPDS is a nonproprietary validated test for this condition, which can be administered in a variety of healthcare settings. Her score of 17 is strongly suggestive of postpartum depression. A score of 10 or less would be considered normal.

6. **Answer: E.** This clinical scenario and the patient's laboratory findings are suspicious for evolving HELLP syndrome and preeclampsia. The treatment of HELLP syndrome is delivery of the infant and placenta. Resolution of the disease process will not happen until delivery is effected, despite this patient being preterm. Magnesium sulfate is used to reduce the risk of maternal seizures during labor and through the first 24 hours of the postpartum period. The decision to induce labor versus proceed to performing a Cesarean section may vary from minute to minute depending on the overall status of mother and fetus, including vital signs, and serial labs. While she does not yet meet the time interval criteria for diagnosing hypertension as part of preeclampsia (elevated blood pressures greater than 140 systolic and/or 90 diastolic on two separate occasions at least 4 hours apart), her overall presentation is strongly suspicious for preeclampsia in evolution and this needs to be monitored and treated appropriately. Oral immediate-release nifedipine may temporarily drop her blood pressure, but will not appropriately address her evolving preeclampsia and HELLP syndrome. Use of this drug in this manner has been associated with stroke and heart attack in older adults. Her blood pressure readings do not require immediate intervention for treatment of her blood pressure, but IV labetalol or hydralazine should be made available to help lower her pressure should it rise above the threshold of 160 systolic and/or 110 diastolic. Glucose monitoring would only be necessary in the face of diabetes, or markedly abnormal glucoses noted on admission labs.

14

DISORDERS OF THE SKIN AND SUBCUTANEOUS TISSUE

Robert V. Ellis • Rick Ricer

I. Terminology

See Table 14.1.

II. Contact Dermatitis

A. Irritant

1. General characteristics:

    a. Exposure to a substance that causes physical or chemical irritation to the skin

    b. Examples: diaper rash, dry skin (xerosis), chemicals, repeated lip-licking, thumb sucking (Figure 14-1)

2. Clinical features:

    a. History of exposure and rash limited to exposed area

    b. Dry, cracked, chapped, or erythematous skin

TABLE 14-1 Terminology	
Primary Lesions	**Secondary Lesions**
Macule: flat, <1.5 cm	Scale: excess dead epidermal cells
Patch: flat, >1.5 cm	Crust: dried serum and cellular debris
Papule: raised, <0.5 cm	Erosion: focal loss of epidermis
Nodule: raised, 0.5–2 cm	Ulcer: focal loss of epidermis and dermis
Tumor: raised, >2 cm	Fissure: linear, defined crack into the epidermis
Plaque: solid elevated area	and dermis
Vesicle: fluid-filled papule	Atrophy: thinning of the epidermis and dermis
Pustule: vesicle filled with leukocytes and fluid	Scar: connective tissue reconnecting the dermis
Bulla: fluid-filled nodule or tumor	Lichenification: thickened epidermis
Wheal: firm, edematous plaque caused by fluid in the dermis	

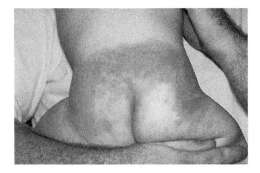

FIGURE
14-1 Diaper rash.

(From Goodheart HP. *Goodheart's Photoguide of Common Skin Disorders.* 2nd ed. Philadelphia, PA: Lippincott Williams & Wilkins; 2003.)

3. Treatment: remove exposure, moisturizers, low-potency topical steroids, barrier creams

B. **Allergic**
1. General characteristics:
   a. Acquired inflammatory reaction of the skin
   b. Caused by the presence of an antigen and previously sensitized T-lymphocytes
2. Clinical features (Figures 14-2 and 14-3):
   a. Pruritic erythematous rash in exposed area
   b. Acute: erythema, edema, papules, may have vesicles or bulla
   c. Chronic: lichenification, erythema, and scaling
   d. Location can give a clue to cause:
      i. Poison ivy: usually on extremities (often linear rash)
      ii. Nickel: around jewelry, snap/button on pants
      iii. Latex: hands or waistband
3. Treatment:
   a. Allergen identification and avoidance
   b. Mild-to-moderate potency topical steroids for localized eruptions
   c. Oral steroids for widespread eruptions
   d. Oral antihistamines
   e. Wet dressings, calamine lotion, and oatmeal baths all can relieve itch.

C. **Atopic dermatitis (eczema)**
1. General characteristics:
   a. Genetic predilection, impaired epidermal barrier function, skin dryness
   b. Common in children
   c. Associated with allergies and asthma

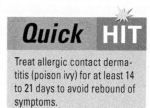

Quick HIT

Treat allergic contact dermatitis (poison ivy) for at least 14 to 21 days to avoid rebound of symptoms.

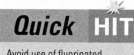

Quick HIT

Avoid use of fluorinated topical steroids on face, groin, and newborns/infants.

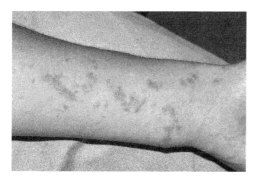

FIGURE
14-2 Allergic contact dermatitis owing to poison ivy.

(From Goodheart HP. *Goodheart's Photoguide of Common Skin Disorders.* 2nd ed. Philadelphia, PA: Lippincott Williams & Wilkins; 2003.)

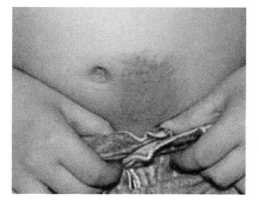

FIGURE
14-3 Allergic contact dermatitis owing to nickel allergy.

(From Goodheart HP. *Goodheart's Photoguide of Common Skin Disorders.* 2nd ed. Philadelphia, PA: Lippincott Williams & Wilkins; 2003.)

Disorders of the Skin and Subcutaneous Tissue

2. Clinical features:
   a. Erythematous macular to papular rash (Figure 14-4)
   b. Face (especially cheeks) with circumoral/paranasal sparing, flexural areas such as antecubital fossa, extensor surfaces
   c. Dry skin with lichenification
   d. Increased palmar markings
3. Treatment.
   a. Topical moisturizers
   b. Cool rather than hot baths
   c. Oatmeal baths
   d. Antihistamines if pruritic
   e. Mild topical steroids
D. **Neurodermatitis (lichen simplex chronicus)**
   1. General characteristics:
      a. Scratching or rubbing leads to lichenification (Figure 14-5).
      b. Only in places people can easily scratch (forearms, shins, upper back and neck, anogenital areas)
      c. Often starts with secondary cause such as dry skin
      d. Associated with psychiatric disorders

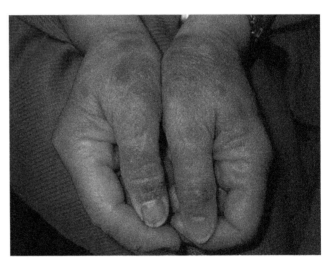

FIGURE
14-4 Atopic dermatitis.

(Image provided by *Stedman's Medical Dictionary*. 28th ed. Philadelphia, PA: Lippincott Williams & Wilkins;2005.)

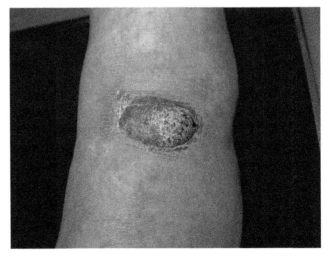

FIGURE
14-5 Neurodermatitis.

(Image provided by *Stedman's Medical Dictionary*. 28th ed. Philadelphia, PA: Lippincott Williams & Wilkins; 2005.)

2. Clinical features:
   a. Multiple excoriated lesions in various stages of healing
   b. Areas that are easily reached
   c. Often present are hyper- or hypopigmented areas from previous lesions.
   d. Biopsy shows chronic nonspecific inflammation.
3. Treatment:
   a. Stop the itch–scratch cycle.
   b. Topical steroid creams
   c. Oral antihistamines

E. **Stasis dermatitis**
1. General characteristics:
   a. Chronic edema occludes lymphatics, which sclerose small vessels.
   b. Most common around ankles and shins
2. Clinical features: hyperpigmented, thickened and scaling areas (Figure 14-6)
3. Treatment:
   a. Prevent and treat lower extremity edema.
   b. Compression stockings
   c. Antibiotics if bacterial superinfection

F. **Xerosis (dry skin)** (Figure 14-7)
1. General characteristics:
   a. Lack of water in the stratus corneum
   b. Very common and often worse in the winter
   c. Any part of the body
2. Clinical features: dry scaly skin, can have mild erythema and/or fissures
3. Treatment: Hydrate and lubricate with moisturizing creams and oils

G. **Dyshidrosis**
1. General characteristics:
   a. Dysfunction of sweat glands
   b. Most common on palms, soles, and between fingers
   c. Differentiate from infectious disease reaction (distant reaction to fungal infection)
   d. Often results from chronic wetness of the area
2. Clinical features: recurrent crops of vesicles that develop into scales and dryness (Figure 14-8)
3. Treatment: topical steroids, keep area dry

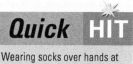

Disorders of the Skin and Subcutaneous Tissue

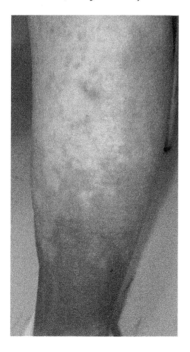

FIGURE 14-6 **Stasis dermatitis.**

(Image provided by *Stedman's Medical Dictionary.* 28th ed. Philadelphia, PA: Lippincott Williams & Wilkins; 2005.)

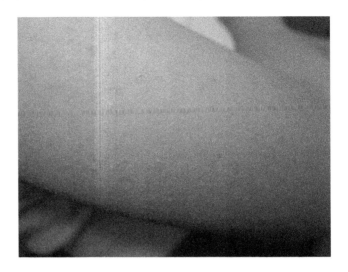

FIGURE
14-7 Xerosis.
(Image provided by *Stedman's Medical Dictionary*. 28th ed. Philadelphia, PA: Lippincott Williams & Wilkins; 2005.)

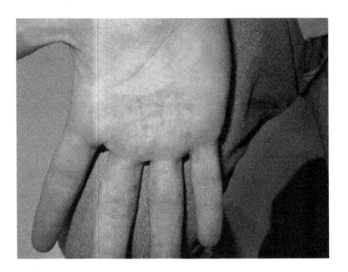

FIGURE
14-8 Dyshidrosis.
(Image provided by *Stedman's Medical Dictionary*. 28th ed. Philadelphia, PA: Lippincott Williams & Wilkins; 2005.)

H. **Nummular eczema**
1. General characteristics: Etiology is unknown.
2. Clinical features:
   a. Coin-shaped patches of pruritic papules that can have scales (Figure 14-9)
   b. Common on trunk and legs, usually not on head
3. Treatment: topical steroids, frequent moisturizers

III. Papulosquamous Lesions
A. **Psoriasis**
1. General characteristics:
   a. Complex immune-mediated hyperproliferation and abnormal differentiation of the epidermis
   b. Risk factors: family history, Caucasian, smoking, obesity, alcohol consumption
   c. Several clinical forms
      i. Plaque psoriasis: most common (80%) (Figure 14-10)
      ii. Psoriatic arthritis
   d. Diagnosis usually clinical based on history and exam

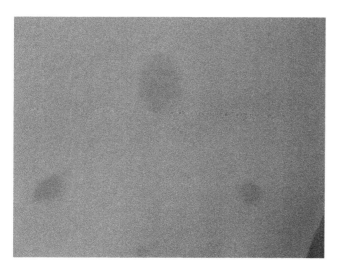

FIGURE
14-9 **Nummular eczema.**
(Image provided by *Stedman's Medical Dictionary.* 28th ed. Philadelphia, PA: Lippincott Williams & Wilkins; 2005.)

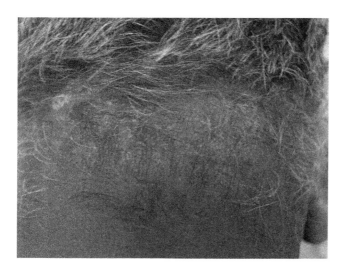

FIGURE
14-10 **Psoriasis.**
(Image provided by *Stedman's Medical Dictionary.* 28th ed. Philadelphia, PA: Lippincott Williams & Wilkins; 2005.)

    e. Biopsy can be performed to confirm diagnosis if needed.
  2. Clinical features:
    a. Sharply defines erythematous plaques with silver scale which easily dislodge
    b. Auspitz sign: pinpoint bleeding when scales are removed
    c. Pitting of the nails
    d. Scalp, extensor surfaces, knees, elbows, external ear canal (classically over elbows and knees)
  3. Treatment:
    a. This is a chronic condition and is not curable.
    b. High-potency topical steroids
    c. Topical tar (this is an over-the-counter salve)
    d. UV light (PUVA: Psoralen + UVA)
    e. Emollients
    f. Topical Vitamin D analogues (calcipotriene)
    g. Topical calcineurin inhibitors (tacrolimus)
    h. Methotrexate
    i. Immunomodulatory drugs for severe cases
B. **Lichen planus**

1. General characteristics:
   a. Unknown etiology
   b. Can happen after trauma to the area (Koebner reaction)
   c. Clinical diagnosis, biopsy if uncertain
2. Clinical features:
   a. Shiny, flat, polygonal papules (Figure 14-11)
   b. White lacy pattern on the surface of the papule or plaque
   c. Flexor surfaces, wrists, thighs
   d. Can have oral lesions
3. Treatment: topical steroids

C. **Pityriasis rosea**
   1. General characteristics:
      a. Self-limited erythematous rash
      b. Viral cause has been hypothesized.
      c. Older children and young adults
      d. May have mild prodrome (headache, malaise, sore throat)
   2. Clinical features:
      a. Begins with a Herald patch (Figure 14-12)
         i. Patch of size 2 to 5 cm, sharply delineated, mildly erythematous, minimally pruritic
         ii. Then starts to scale and clears centrally
      b. Diffuse rash appears 2 to 14 days later.
         i. Smaller lesions, long axis of lesions follow skin cleavage lines
         ii. "Christmas/fir tree" pattern on trunk
      c. Resolves in 6 to 12 weeks.
   3. Treatment: symptomatic treatment only such as antihistamine for pruritic

D. **Seborrheic dermatitis**
   1. General characteristics:
      a. Chronic, relapsing form of dermatitis
      b. Incidence increased during infancy and in adolescence and young adults
      c. Unknown cause
   2. Clinical features:

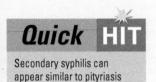

Quick HIT

Secondary syphilis can appear similar to pityriasis rosea and should be ruled out.

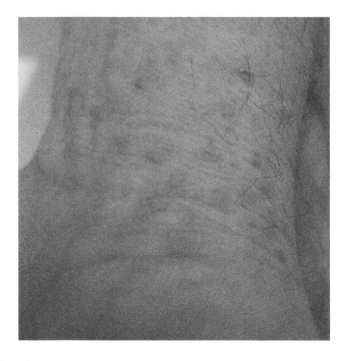

FIGURE
14-11 Lichen planus.

(Image provided by *Stedman's Medical Dictionary*. 28th ed. Philadelphia, PA: Lippincott Williams & Wilkins; 2005.)

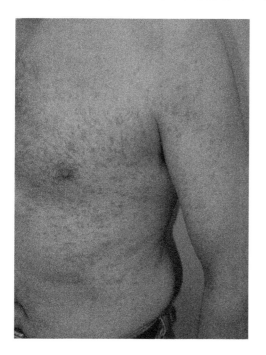

FIGURE
14-12 Pityriasis rosea.

(Image provided by *Stedman's Medical Dictionary.* 28th ed. Philadelphia, PA: Lippincott Williams & Wilkins; 2005.)

   a. Greasy, red, scaling plaque, "bad dandruff" (Figure 14-13)
   b. May involve scalp, cheeks, central chest, back, and eyebrows
 3. Treatment: topical steroids, topical antifungals, anti-dandruff shampoos
E. **Secondary syphilis**
 1. General characteristics:
   a. Sexually transmitted infection caused by *Treponema pallidum*
   b. Appears weeks to a few months after exposure
   c. About 25% of untreated patients will develop secondary syphilis.
   d. Systemic symptoms can include fever, malaise, headache, sore throat, and
      weight loss.
 2. Clinical features:
   a. Diffuse, symmetric, red-to-brown macules (Figure 14-14)
   b. Involves trunk, extremities, palms, and soles
   c. Diffuse lymphadenopathy is common.
 3. Diagnosis: fluorescent treponemal antibody (FTA) and rapid plasma reagin
    (RPR) or venereal disease research laboratory (VDRL) test.

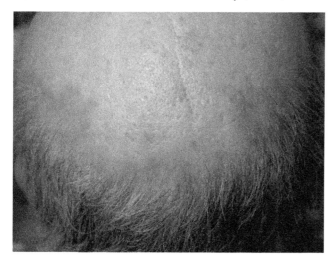

FIGURE
14-13 Seborrheic dermatitis.

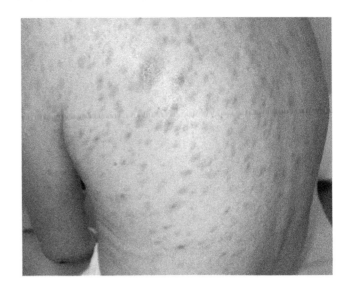

FIGURE
14-14 Secondary syphilis.

(Image provided by *Stedman's Medical Dictionary*, 28th ed. Philadelphia, PA: Lippincott Williams & Wilkins; 2005.)

    4. Treatment: IM **benzathine penicillin G**

IV. Vesiculobullous Lesions

  A. Dermatitis herpetiformis (Figure 14-15):
    1. General characteristics: chronic rash associated with celiac sprue (gluten allergy), IgA mediated
    2. Clinical features:
      a. Small erythematous papules and vesicles in groups, mildly pruritic
      b. Common on elbows and knees, can be widespread
    3. Treatment: gluten-free diet
  B. **Herpes simplex virus**
    1. General characteristics:
      a. Can be caused by HSV-1 or -2
      b. DNA virus
      c. Can break out anywhere on the skin (Table 14-2)
    2. Clinical features:
      a. Crop of erythematous vesicles that progress to ulcers (Figures 14-16 and 14-17)
      b. Itchy, burning, or painful
    3. Diagnosis:

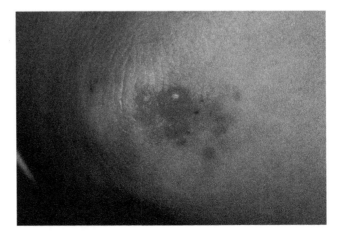

FIGURE
14-15 Dermatitis herpetiformis.

(From Edward S, Yung A. *Essential Dermatopathology*. Philadelphia, PA: Wolters Kluwer Health; 2012.)

TABLE **14-2**	HSV Terminology Based on Location
Terminology	**Location/Definition**
Herpes labialis	Lip, oral
Herpetic whitlow	Finger
Herpes gladitorium	Usually on neck, face, or arm Contact athletes: wrestling, rugby
Eczema herpeticum	Scalp
Genital	Usually HSV-2
Herpetic keratitis	Eye (see Chapter 3)

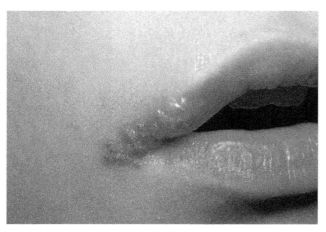

FIGURE
14-16 Herpes labialis.

(Courtesy of Ilona J. Frieden, MD. In Chung EK: *Visual Diagnosis and Treatment in Pediatrics.* 3rd ed. Philadelphia, PA: Wolters Kluwer Health; 2015.)

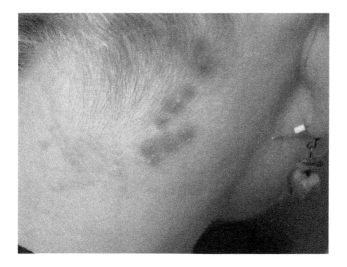

FIGURE
14-17 Herpes gladitorium.

(Image provided by *Stedman's Medical Dictionary.* 28th ed. Philadelphia, PA: Lippincott Williams & Wilkins; 2005.)

    a. Often clinical
    b. Tzanck stain (rarely done) or viral culture if diagnosis in question
    c. High level of false negatives if not done in the first few days
  4. Treatment:
    a. Antivirals (acyclovir, valacyclovir)
    b. Antivirals are of little benefit if not initiated within 72 hours.

c. If untreated, the lesions resolve in 1 to 2 weeks.

d. Can have frequent recurrence in same location

C. **Varicella (chickenpox)**

1. General characteristics:

a. Varicella zoster virus (VZV): DNA herpesvirus

b. Range from mild rash to severe encephalitis

c. Can happen in vaccinated kids, although with less severe symptoms

2. Clinical features:

a. Symptoms within 15 days of exposure

b. Prodrome of fever, malaise, sore throat, poor appetite

c. Rash 24 hours later (Figure 14-18)

    i. Spreads central to peripheral

    ii. Vesicles on an erythematous base ("dew drops on rose petals")

    iii. Lesions at different stages at the same time

3. Diagnosis: based on history and clinical appearance

4. Treatment:

a. Self-limited: resolves in 1 to 2 weeks

b. No longer contagious when all lesions are scabbed over

c. Antivirals such as acyclovir, valacyclovir

d. Antihistamine, oatmeal bath, Burrow's solution for itch

D. **Zoster (shingles)**

1. General characteristics:

a. VZV: DNA herpesvirus

b. Reactivation of latent VZV form sensory ganglia

2. Clinical features:

a. Prodrome of pain can precede rash up to 1 week.

b. Vesicular rash in a dermatomal pattern (usually 1, but occasionally 2 to 3 surrounding dermatomes) (Figure 14-19)

c. Crusts over in 7 to 10 days (no longer contagious)

d. Complications:

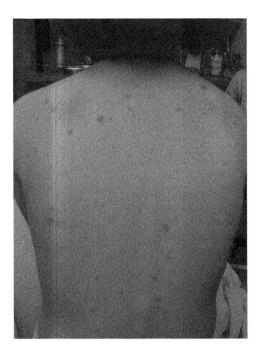

FIGURE
14-18 Varicella.

(Image provided by *Stedman's Medical Dictionary.* 28th ed. Philadelphia, PA: Lippincott Williams & Wilkins; 2005.)

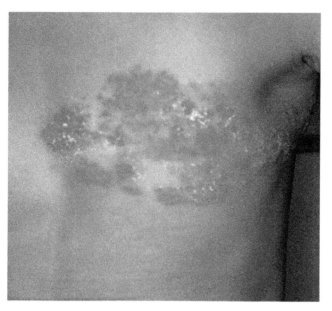

      i. Corneal lesions if affecting the first branch of the trigeminal nerve or the tip of the nose

      ii. Postherpetic neuralgia: chronic pain syndrome following shingles

  3. Diagnosis: based on history and clinical appearance

  4. Treatment:

    a. Most beneficial within 72 hours of developing rash

    b. Antivirals: valacyclovir slightly more effective than acyclovir

    c. Oral steroids: use only in conjunction with antivirals

    d. Pain control: acetaminophen, nonsteroidal anti-inflammatory drugs (NSAIDs), narcotics as needed

    e. Topical capsaicin

    f. Neuropathic pain medications: gabapentin and pregabalin

V. Erythemas

  A. **Urticaria (hives)**

    1. General characteristics:

      a. IgE mediated

      b. Exposure to an allergen: food, chemical, stress, medication, pressure, vibration, solar, cold, heat, dermatographic, infectious (viral or bacterial)

      c. A cause is often not identified (patient diary can help identify a cause if recurrent).

    2. Clinical features: intensely pruritic, circumscribed, blanchable, erythematous plaques that come on quickly and usually resolve in a few hours, and flare in other locations (wheals) (Figure 14-20)

    3. Diagnosis:

      a. Usually clinical

      b. Skin biopsy can be helpful if unsure of the diagnosis.

    4. Treatment:

      a. Avoid trigger.

      b. Antihistamines (H_1 blocker)

      c. Add H_2 blocker if symptoms not improving.

      d. Steroids generally do not help.

  B. **Erythema multiforme**

    1. General characteristics:

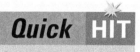

***Quick* HIT**

Shingles is contagious by contact only to a person who is not immune to the VZV (ie., has not been vaccinated for VZV) or previously had the disease.

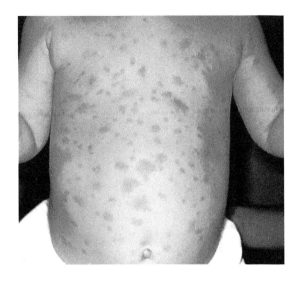

FIGURE
14-20 Urticaria.

(From Hall BJ, Hall JC. *Sauer's Manual of Skin Diseases*. 11th ed. Philadelphia, PA: Wolters Kluwer; 2017.)

> **Quick HIT**
>
> HSV is the most common cause of erythema multiforme.

      a. Acute vascular inflammatory response to infection, medications, chemicals, or other systemic cause.

      b. Infections account for 90% of cases

      c. Medications implicated: antibiotics, NSAIDs, antiepileptics, sulfonamides

   2. Clinical features:

      a. Erythematous target-shaped lesions, usually not painful or pruritic (Figure 14-21)

      b. Mucosal lesions in up to 70% of cases

   3. Treatment:

      a. Treat underlying cause.

      b. Usually self-limited, resolves within 2 weeks

C. Erythema nodosum

   1. General characteristics:

      a. Inflammatory disorder of the subcutaneous fat lobules

      b. Causes include infection, tuberculosis, sarcoidosis, medications, lupus, cat scratch disease

      c. Most cases are idiopathic.

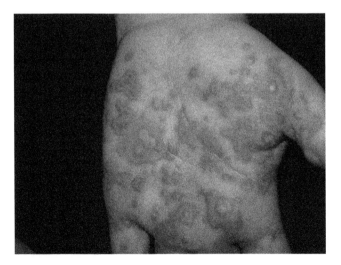

FIGURE
14-21 Erythema multiforme.

(From White AJ. *The Washington Manual of Pediatrics*. 2nd ed. Philadelphia, PA: Wolters Kluwer; 2016.)

2. Clinical features:
   a. Tender erythematous nodules that are firm and progress to spongy over a few weeks
   b. Most frequently on legs (pretibial) (Figure 14-22)
3. Treatment:
   a. Treat underlying cause.
   b. Resolves in 2 to 8 weeks

VI. Infections

A. **Erythrasma**
   1. General characteristics:
      a. Superficial infection of the skin
      b. *Corynebacterium minutissimum*, gram positive, non–spore-forming bacillus
   2. Clinical features:
      a. Interdigital: scaly, macerated lesions usually between toes
      b. Intertriginous: erythematous-to-brown patches in groin and other areas (Figure 14-23)
      c. Mildly pruritic to mildly tender
   3. Diagnosis: "coral red" fluorescence under a Wood's light
   4. Treatment: topical antibiotics such as clindamycin or erythromycin

B. **Erysipelas**
   1. General characteristics:
      a. Infection of the upper dermis and superficial lymphatics
      b. Classically on the face
      c. Most common on the lower extremities
      d. Most often caused by beta-hemolytic streptococci
   2. Clinical features:
      a. Acute onset of painful well-demarcated area of erythema, swelling, and warmth (Figure 14-24)
      b. Can have fever and chills
   3. Treatment:
      a. Oral penicillin or amoxicillin
      b. Alternatives: macrolides, cephalexin, and clindamycin
      c. Toxic patients require IV antibiotics.

Disorders of the Skin and Subcutaneous Tissue

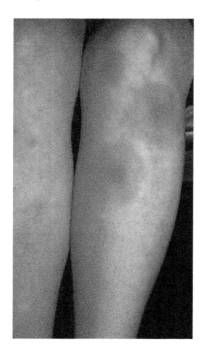

FIGURE 14-22 Erythema nodosum.

(From Ayala C, Spellberg B. *Boards and Wards for USMLE Step 2*. 6th ed. Philadelphia, PA: Wolters Kluwer; 2017.)

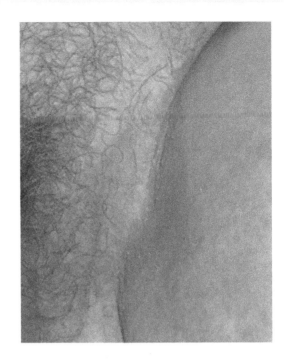

FIGURE
14-23 Erythrasma.

(From Edwards L, Lynch PJ. *Genital Dermatology Atlas*. 2nd ed. Philadelphia, PA: Wolters Kluwer; 2011.)

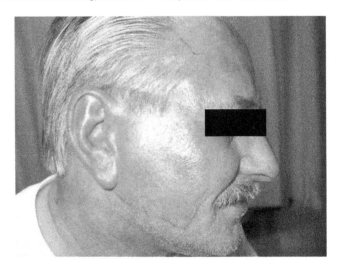

FIGURE
14-24 Erysipelas.

(Image provided by *Stedman's Medical Dictionary*. 28th ed. Philadelphia, PA: Lippincott Williams & Wilkins; 2005.)

C. **Cellulitis**
   1. General characteristics:
      a. Infection that extends through the dermis into the deep subcutaneous tissue
      b. Most common on lower extremities, can be anywhere
      c. Common pathogens: beta-hemolytic streptococci and *Staphylococcus aureus* (methicillin-resistant *Staphylococcus aureus* [MRSA] common even in the community)
      d. Most likely staphylococcus if abscess present
   2. Clinical features:
      a. Warm, tender, swollen, erythematous area, poorly demarcated
      b. Can have systemic symptoms such as fever and malaise
   3. Treatment:
      a. Elevate affected extremity
      b. Purulent/abscess (staph): trimethoprim-sulfamethoxazole, clindamycin, doxycycline, linezolid, tedizolid

c. Nonpurulent (strep or staph): amoxicillin plus trimethoprim-sulfamethoxazole, amoxicillin plus doxycycline, clindamycin, linezolid, tedizolid

d. More severe infections require IV antibiotics

D. **Erythema chronicum migrans (Lyme disease)**

1. General characteristics:

a. Tick-borne illness caused by *Borrelia burgdorferi* or other *Borrelia* species

b. Complications if untreated may include arthritis, encephalopathy, polyneuropathy

2. Clinical features:

a. Skin lesion at site of tick bite usually forms in 7 to 14 days (Figure 14-25).

b. Can have multiple lesions

c. Uniformly red and clears centrally as it expands up to 20 cm or more

d. Warm, not painful, may itch or burn

e. Fatigue, headaches, malaise, joint aches, fever

3. Diagnosis: history of exposure (tick bite), often initially seronegative

4. Treatment:

a. ≥8 years old: doxycycline

b. <8 years old: amoxicillin or cefuroxime

E. **Rocky Mountain spotted fever**

1. General characteristics:

a. Tick-borne disease caused by *Rickettsia rickettsii*

b. Most common in the southeastern and south central states

c. More common in spring and early summer

2. Clinical features:

a. Fever, headache, malaise, joint aches, nausea

b. Rash develops in 3 to 5 days (Figure 14-26).

c. Wrists and ankles, then spreads centrally

d. Rash includes palms and soles.

e. Rash starts maculopapular and becomes petechial.

3. Diagnosis:

a. History and exposure (tick bite)

b. Serology becomes positive in 7 to 10 days.

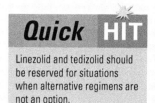

Quick HIT

Linezolid and tedizolid should be reserved for situations when alternative regimens are not an option.

Disorders of the Skin and Subcutaneous Tissue

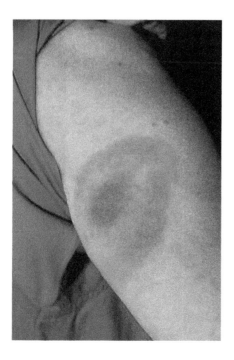

FIGURE 14-25 **Erythema chronicum migrans.**

(Courtesy of James Gathany/CDC. In Schalock PC, Hsu JTS, Arndt KA. *Lippincott's Primary Care Dermatology.* Philadelphia, PA: Lippincott Williams & Wilkins; 2011.)

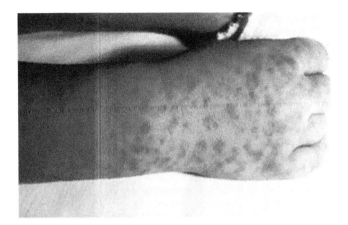

FIGURE
14-26 Rocky Mountain spotted fever.
(From Kline-Tilford AM, Haut C. *Lippincott Certification Review: Pediatric Acute Care Nurse Practitioner.* Philadelphia, PA: Wolters Kluwer; 2016.)

   4. Treatment:
      a. First-line: doxycycline
      b. Alternative: chloramphenicol
      c. Complications: up to 9% fatality rate in certain age groups (<4 and >60)
F. **Dermatomycosis (ringworm)**
   1. General characteristics: fungal infection of the skin and nails (Table 14-3)
   2. Clinical features (Figure 14-27):
      a. Scalp: erythematous scaly patch of alopecia, usually asymptomatic
      b. Body: erythematous annular lesions with scaly raised borders and central clearing
      c. Groin: erythematous patch that is sharply demarcated
      d. Foot: erythematous lesion, often between toes and can have fissures, pruritic and burning
   3. Diagnosis: skin scrape with KOH (spaghetti and meatballs appearance)
   4. Treatment:
      a. Scalp: oral griseofulvin, terbinafine, itraconazole, fluconazole
      b. Other: topical terbinafine, naftifine with oral antifungals reserved for refractory cases
G. **Tinea versicolor**
   1. General characteristics:
      a. Lipid-dependent yeast, malassezia
      b. Worldwide and more common in the tropics
   2. Clinical features (Figure 14-28):
      a. Hypopigmented to hyperpigmented to mildly erythematous, fine scaly lesions
      b. Usually on trunk and upper arms/shoulders
   3. Diagnosis:
      a. Usually clinical
      b. Skin scrape with KOH: hyphae and yeast cells
      c. Wood's lamp can have yellow-green fluorescence.

TABLE 14-3	Ringworm
Terminology	**Location**
Tinea capitis	Scalp
Tinea corporis	Body
Tinea cruris	Groin
Tinea pedis	Feet

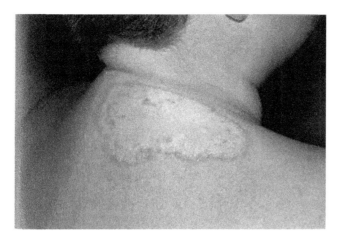

FIGURE
14-27 Ringworm.
(From Acosta WR. *Pharmacology for Health Professionals.* 2nd ed. Philadelphia, PA: Wolters Kluwer Health; 2013.)

4. Treatment:
   a. Easily treated but often recurs
   b. Topical: ketoconazole and selenium sulfide
   c. Oral: ketoconazole, itraconazole, fluconazole
H. **Candida (yeast infection)**
   1. General characteristics:
      a. Common in diaper-wearing children (peaks at 7 to 10 months)
      b. Can happen in intertriginous areas in children and adults
      c. Risk factors: obesity, immunocompromised, antibiotics
   2. Clinical features:
      a. Brightly erythematous area of confluence
      b. Surrounding satellite lesions (Figure 14-29)
   3. Treatment: topical nystatin, miconazole, clotrimazole
I. **Impetigo**
   1. General characteristics:
      a. Superficial bacterial infection
      b. Usually in children (peaks at 2 to 5 years)
      c. Usually *Staphylococcus aureus* (rare MRSA), beta-hemolytic streptococci
      d. Risk factors: poverty, crowding, poor hygiene, scabies infestation

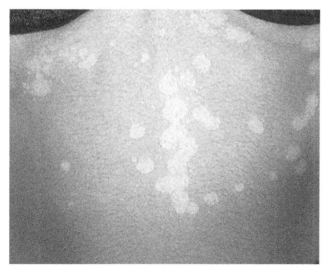

FIGURE
14-28 Tinea versicolor.
(From Aschenbrenner DS, Venable SJ. *Drug Therapy in Nursing.* 4th ed. Philadelphia, PA: Wolters Kluwer Health; 2012.)

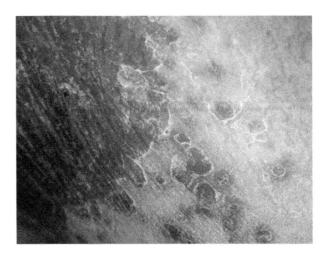

FIGURE
14-29 Candida.

(From Goroll AH, Mulley AG. *Primary Care Medicine: Office Evaluation and Management of the Adult Patient.* 7th ed. Philadelphia, PA: Wolters Kluwer; 2014.)

2. Clinical features: painful superficial erosion with honey-colored crusts (Figure 14-30)
3. Treatment:
   a. Small number of lesions and no bullae: topical mupirocin
   b. More extensive or bullae: oral dicloxacillin, cephalexin, clindamycin
J. **Abscess, furuncle, carbuncle**
1. General characteristics (Table 14-4):
   a. Usually caused by *Staphylococcus aureus* (often MRSA)
   b. Risk factors: diabetes, immunocompromised; often no risk factors
2. Clinical features:
   a. Painful, tender, often fluctuant nodules
   b. Can have purulent drainage and surrounding induration
3. Treatment:
   a. Small lesions: warm, moist compress
   b. Larger lesions if fluctuant: incision and drainage (consider culture)
   c. Consider antibiotics with activity against MRSA if abscess >5 cm, multiple abscesses, extensive cellulitis, immunocompromised patient, systemic symptoms.

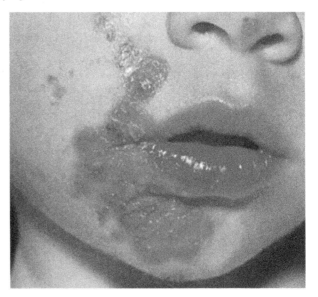

FIGURE
14-30 Impetigo.

(From Whalen K. *Lippincott Illustrated Reviews: Pharmacology.* 6th ed. Philadelphia, PA: Wolters Kluwer; 2015.)

TABLE 14-4	Abscess, Furuncle, Carbuncle
Terminology	**Definition**
Abscess	Collection of pus within the dermis and subcutaneous tissue
Furuncle (boil)	Infected hair follicle with pus extending through the dermis into subcutaneous tissue
Carbuncle	Collection of several infected follicles into one inflamed mass with purulent drainage

K. **Folliculitis**
  1. General characteristics:
     a. Bacterial infection of hair follicles
     b. *S. aureus,* Pseudomonas (associated with hot tubs)
     c. Folliculitis barbae or pseudofolliculitis associated with shaving
  2. Clinical features: multiple erythematous, papular lesions often pruritic to mildly painful (Figure 14-31)
  3. Treatment: usually self-limited, warm compresses
L. **Molluscum contagiosum**
  1. General characteristics: caused by the poxvirus that is contagious by contact
  2. Clinical features: umbilicated pearl-like papules with a cheesy core (Figure 14-32)
  3. Treatment:
     a. Most resolve within a few months without treatment.
     b. Cryotherapy, curettage, cantharidin, or podophyllotoxin
M. **Measles**
  1. General characteristics: caused by the Paramyxovirus
  2. Clinical features:
     a. Prodrome: 1 to 6 days; fever, malaise, headache, conjunctivitis, congestion
     b. Koplik spots (pathognomonic): 1 to 3 mm blue-white spots with red ring on buccal mucosa, precedes rash by 1 to 2 days
     c. Erythematous papules starting on head and spreading downward
     d. Resolves in about 7 days
  3. Treatment
     a. Supportive: antipyretics, hydration, rest
     b. Prevention: immunize at 1 and 4 years old

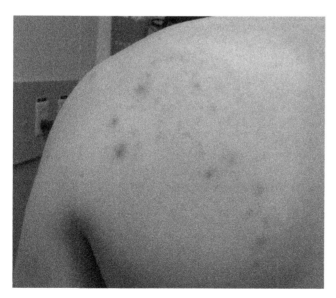

FIGURE 14-31 Folliculitis.
(Image provided by *Stedman's Medical Dictionary.* 28th ed. Philadelphia, PA: Lippincott Williams & Wilkins; 2005.)

Disorders of the Skin and Subcutaneous Tissue

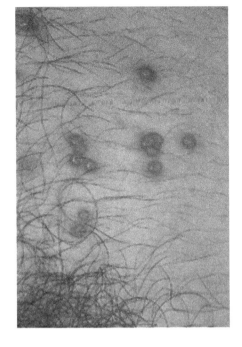

FIGURE
14-32 Molluscum contagiosum.

(From Edwards L, Lynch PJ. *Genital Dermatology Atlas*. 2nd ed. Philadelphia, PA: Wolters Kluwer; 2011.)

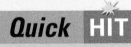

Remember infections that can cause congenital abnormalities using the TORCH mnemonic: Toxoplasmosis, Other (syphilis, varicella-zoster, parvovirus B19), Rubella, Cytomegalovirus (CMV), and Herpes infections.

N. **Rubella**
1. General characteristics:
a. "German measles" or "3-day measles"
b. Caused by the togavirus
c. Infection during pregnancy can cause congenital anomalies.
2. Clinical features:
a. Prodrome: mild, 1 to 5 days; low-grade fever, sore throat, headache, lymphadenopathy
b. Rash starts on face, pink to red
c. Resolves in 3 to 5 days
3. Treatment:
a. Symptomatic
b. Prevention: immunize at 1 and 4 years of age

O. **Roseola infantum**
1. General characteristics:
a. Human herpesvirus 6
b. Usually children <3 years old
2. Clinical features:
a. Prodrome: 3 to 5 days; very high fevers, cervical lymphadenopathy, mild upper respiratory tract infection (URI) symptoms
b. Fever resolves suddenly when rash appears.
c. Rose-pink macules with white halo that starts on the trunk and moves peripherally, then fades in 1 to 2 days
3. Treatment: symptomatic relief

P. **Erythema infectiosum (fifth disease)**
1. General characteristics:
a. Parvovirus B19
b. School-aged children, late winter to early spring
2. Clinical features:
a. Prodrome: 7 to 10 days, low-grade fever, headache, sore throat, malaise, nausea
b. Erythematous plaque on cheeks ("slapped-cheeks"), 1 to 4 days (Figure 14-33)
c. Second rash: lacy, reticular erythema over torso and extensor extremities, lasts 2 to 3 weeks

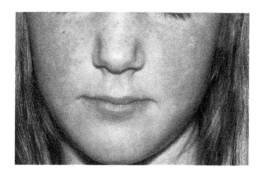

FIGURE
14-33 Fifth disease.

(From Goodheart HP. *Goodheart's Photoguide of Common Skin Disorders*. 2nd ed. Philadelphia, PA: Lippincott Williams & Wilkins; 2003.)

3. Treatment:
    a. Symptomatic relief
    b. No longer contagious once the rash appears
Q. **Coxsackie and ECHO virus (hand, foot, and mouth disease)**
    1. General characteristics:
        a. Caused by coxsackie A16 and enterovirus 71
        b. Usually affects children under 10 years old
        c. Late summer to early fall
        d. Spread oral–oral or fecal–oral
    2. Clinical features:
        a. Prodrome: 12 to 36 hours; low-grade fever, malaise, anorexia, sore throat, cough
        b. Enanthem: 5 to 7 days; red papules that change to yellow-gray ulcers on the hard palate, tongue, and buccal surface
        c. Exanthem: starts just after enanthem, 7 to 10 days; 2 to 8 mm, red elliptical macules to papules with central gray vesicle on hands and feet, can appear on genitals, face, and trunk (Figure 14-34)
    3. Treatment: symptomatic relief

VII. Infestations/Bites
A. Scabies
    1. General characteristics:
        a. Mite infestation, *Sarcoptes scabiei*
        b. Person-to-person transmission, can be zoonotic from dogs and cats
    2. Clinical features:
        a. Extremely pruritic erythematous papules, 2 to 15 mm linear burrows may be present

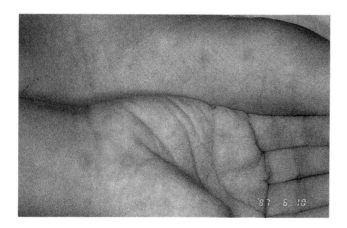

FIGURE
14-34 Hand, foot, and mouth disease.

(From Fleisher GR, Ludwig W, Baskin MN. *Atlas of Pediatric Emergency Medicine*. Philadelphia, PA: Lippincott Williams & Wilkins; 2004.)

Disorders of the Skin and Subcutaneous Tissue

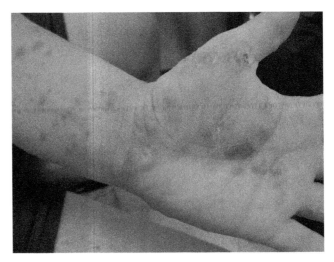

FIGURE
14-35 Scabies.

(Image provided by *Stedman's Medical Dictionary*. 28th ed. Philadelphia, PA: Lippincott Williams & Wilkins; 2005.)

      b. Rash most frequently on sides and webs of fingers, groin, thighs, waist, axilla, elbows, and knees often affected (Figure 14-35)
   3. Diagnosis: usually clinical, skin scrape (<50% sensitivity)
   4. Treatment: topical permethrin, antihistamines, wash clothes and linens
  B. **Bedbugs**
   1. General characteristics: caused by *Cimex lectularius* and *C. hemipterus*
   2. Clinical features:
      a. Painless bites that most have an allergic reaction to in 1 to 10 days.
      b. Pruritic 2 to 5 mm erythematous maculopapular lesions with central hemorrhagic punctum (Figure 14-36)
   3. Treatment: symptomatic relief, antihistamines, professional pest treatment of home
  C. **Dog and cat bites**
   1. General characteristics: Dogs account for >85% of all animal bites.
   2. Treatment:
      a. Clean the skin with iodine-based solution.
      b. Irrigate the wound with saline.
      c. Explore the wound for foreign body, partial tendon ruptures.

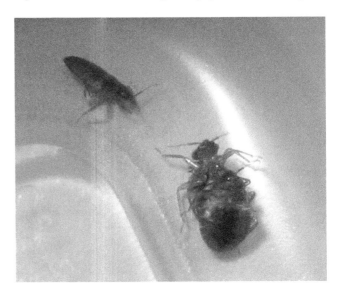

FIGURE
14-36 Bedbugs.

(Image provided by *Stedman's Medical Dictionary*. 28th ed. Philadelphia, PA: Lippincott Williams & Wilkins; 2005.)

TABLE 14-5	Animal Bite Wounds at High Risk for Infection

Crush injuries

Puncture wounds

Involving the hand

Delayed presentation
    Greater than 6–12 hr for arm or leg
    Greater than 12–24 hr for face

Cat or human bites

Immunosuppressed patient

Near or in a prosthetic joint

Extremities with underlying venous and/or lymphatic compromise

Geriatric patient

Diabetic patient

    d. Close the wound with monofilament suture if cosmetically favorable.
    e. Consider antibiotic prophylaxis (amoxicillin/clavulanate) if high risk (Table 14-5)
    f. Report animal bites to local health authorities.
    g. Vaccines: Update tetanus, consider rabies vaccine.

VIII. Other Dermatologic Manifestations

    See Table 14-6.

TABLE 14-6	Other Dermatologic Manifestations		
Condition	**Clinical Features**	**Diagnosis**	**Treatment**
Vitiligo (Figure 14-37)	Well-defined areas of hypopigmentation Autoimmune	Clinical	None needed Bleaching agents like hydroquinone
Melasma "mask of pregnancy" (Figure 14-38)	Associated with pregnancy and oral contraceptive pills (OCP) Hyperpigmented, on face	Clinical	D/C OCP Bleaching agents like hydroquinone
Lentigo (liver spots) (Figure 14-39)	Age and sun exposure Multiple discrete, tan macules on sun-exposed areas	Clinical Punch biopsy if question of malignancy	Topical tretinoin Hydroquinone
Mongolian spots (Figure 14-40)	Congenital Dark, flat spot on buttocks, back, and legs	Clinical	None needed
Rosacea (Figure 14-41)	Middle-aged to older adult Vasodilation of central face Erythema, telangiectasia May have papules, pustules, and nodules	Clinical	Topical metronidazole Topical azelaic acid Benzoyl peroxide
Seborrheic keratosis (Figure 14-42)	"Warty" well, circumscribed, often hyperpigmented, "stuck-on" appearance	Clinical	None needed
Wart (verruca)	Flat, mosaic, or filiform	Clinical	Liquid nitrogen topical
Human papilloma virus (HPV)	Any site		Salicylic acid topical Imiquimod topical

(continued)

TABLE 14-6	Other Dermatologic Manifestations (*continued*)		
Condition	**Clinical Features**	**Diagnosis**	**Treatment**
Skin tag (Figure 14-43)	Areas of high friction: neck, axilla, groin Flesh colored	Clinical	None needed Clip off Cryotherapy
Cherry hemangioma (Figure 14-44)	Benign collection of capillaries Bright red, dome shaped, 1–4 mm	Clinical	None needed
Actinic keratosis (Figure 14-45)	Sun-damaged areas Scaly, poorly defined Easier to feel than see	Clinical	Has potential to form squamous cell carcinoma (SCC) Cryotherapy
Basal cell carcinoma (Figure 14-46)	Predilection for sun-exposed areas Pink- to flesh-colored pearly papule with ulcerated center	Shave, punch, or excisional biopsy	Excision Locally invasive Rarely metastasizes
Squamous cell carcinoma (Figure 14-47)	Presentations vary Often presents as a chronic nonhealing lesion	Shave, punch, or excisional biopsy	Excision Locally invasive 5%–10% metastasize
Melanoma (Figure 14-48)	Usually pigmented, irregular shape and color, poorly defined borders	Punch or excisional biopsy	Excision with wide margins

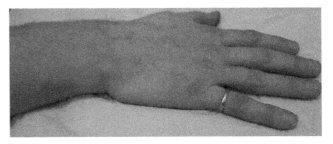

FIGURE
14-37 Vitiligo.
(Image provided by *Stedman's Medical Dictionary*. 28th ed. Philadelphia, PA: Lippincott Williams & Wilkins; 2005.)

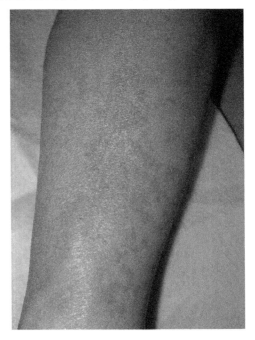

FIGURE
14-38 Melasma.
(Image provided by *Stedman's Medical Dictionary*. 28th ed. Philadelphia, PA: Lippincott Williams & Wilkins; 2005.)

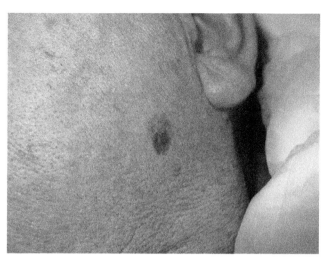

FIGURE
14-39 Lentigo.

(Image provided by *Stedman's Medical Dictionary*. 28th ed. Philadelphia, PA: Lippincott Williams & Wilkins; 2005.)

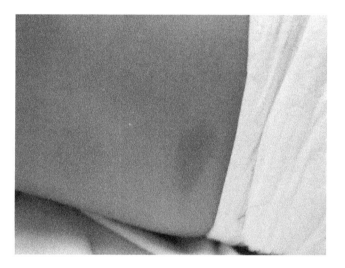

FIGURE
14-40 Mongolian spot.

(Image provided by *Stedman's Medical Dictionary*. 28th ed. Philadelphia, PA: Lippincott Williams & Wilkins; 2005.)

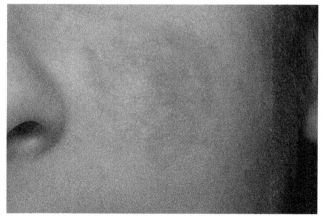

FIGURE
14-41 Rosacea.

(From DeLong L, Burkhart NW. *General and Oral Pathology for the Dental Hygienist*. 2nd ed. Philadelphia, PA: Wolters Kluwer Health; 2013.)

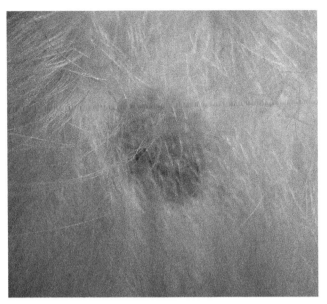

FIGURE
14-42 Seborrheic keratosis.

(Image provided by *Stedman's Medical Dictionary*. 28th ed. Philadelphia, PA: Lippincott Williams & Wilkins; 2005.)

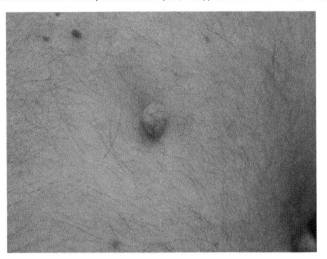

FIGURE
14-43 Skin tag.

(Image provided by *Stedman's Medical Dictionary*. 28th ed. Philadelphia, PA: Lippincott Williams & Wilkins; 2005.)

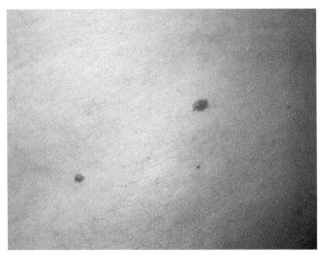

FIGURE
14-44 Cherry hemangioma.

(Image provided by *Stedman's Medical Dictionary*, 28th ed. Philadelphia, PA: Lippincott Williams & Wilkins; 2005.)

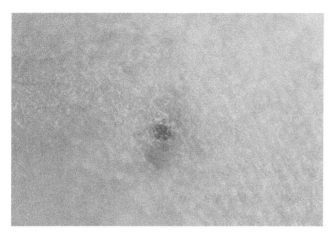

FIGURE
14-45 Actinic keratosis.

(From DeLong L, Burkhart NW. *General and Oral Pathology for the Dental Hygienist.* 2nd ed. Philadelphia, PA: Wolters Kluwer Health; 2013.)

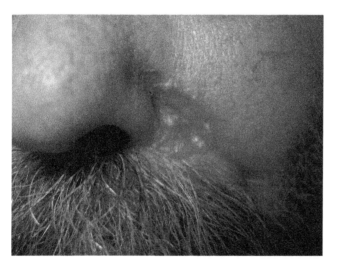

FIGURE
14-46 Basal cell carcinoma.

(Image provided by *Stedman's Medical Dictionary.* 28th ed. Philadelphia, PA: Lippincott Williams & Wilkins; 2005.)

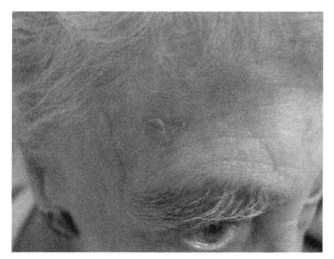

FIGURE
14-47 Squamous cell carcinoma.

(Image provided by *Stedman's Medical Dictionary.* 28th ed. Philadelphia, PA: Lippincott Williams & Wilkins; 2005.)

Disorders of the Skin and Subcutaneous Tissue

Disorders of the Skin and Subcutaneous Tissue

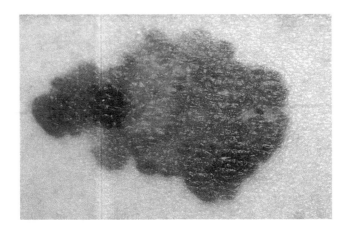

FIGURE
14-48 Melanoma.

(From *Anatomical Chart Company: Understanding Skin Cancer Anatomical Chart*. 2nd ed. Philadelphia, PA: Wolters Kluwer; 2011.)

IX. Common Topical Steroids

See Table 14-7.

Quick **HIT**

Adverse reactions to chronic topical steroid use include skin atrophy, telangiectasia, purpura, striae, ulcers, infection, delayed wound healing, hyper/hypopigmentation, rosacea, acne, and photosensitivity.

TABLE 14-7	Common Topical Steroids		
Medication/Potency	**Forms**	**Size (grams)**	**Use Examples**
Very Low-----------------Class VII			Dermatitis of face and groin
Hydrocortisone 1% (OTC), 2.5%	C, O, L	20, 30, 60, 120	Infants and toddlers
Low-----------------------Class VI			Mild dermatitis
Desonide 0.05%	C, O, G, L, F	15, 30, 60	
Fluocinolone 0.01%	C	15, 60	
Medium--------------------Class V			Atopic dermatitis
Hydrocortisone valerate 0.2%	C, O	14, 45, 60, 120	Nummular eczema
Medium-------------------Class IV			Seborrheic dermatitis
Mometasone furoate 0.1%	C, O, L	15, 30, 45, 60	Severe dermatitis
Triamcinolone acetonide 0.1%	C, O, L	15, 30, 80, 454	
Medium High------------Class III			Lichen planus
Betamethasone dipropionate 0.05%	C	15, 45	Severe contact dermatitis
Fluticasone propionate 0.005%	O	15, 30, 60	Psoriasis
High------------------------Class II			Severe hand eczema
Desoximetasone 0.05%/0.25%	G, C, O	15, 60	
Fluocinonide 0.05%	C, G, O	15, 30, 60	
Ultra High-----------------Class I			
Clobetasol propionate 0.05%	C, G, O, F, S	15, 30, 45, 60	
Halobetasol propionate 0.05%	C, O	15, 50	

C, cream; F, foam; G, gel; L, lotion; O, ointment; S, shampoo.

QUESTIONS

1. A 47-year-old male presents with raised, red plaques covered with multiple small vesicles on both his elbows and both knees. He has not been in any wooded area recently. Which of the following foods should he eliminate from his diet?

   A. Simple carbohydrates
   B. Gluten
   C. Cholesterol
   D. Saturated fats
   E. Medium chain triglycerides

2. A patient has a history of having red, raised plaques with very easily loosened scales over most of his body for almost 20 years. He is complaining of multiple joint pains especially when he plays golf. Which of the following is a classic X-ray finding for this disease process?

   A. A bucket handle tear
   B. Loss of joint space
   C. Subcutaneous nodules
   D. Pencil in a cup deformity
   E. Spiral fracture

3. Which of the following steroid creams are least likely to produce the side effects of long-term steroid use?

   A. Mometasone (Elocon)
   B. Triamcinolone (Kenalog)
   C. Fluocinonide (Lidex)
   D. Betamethasone (Diprolene)
   E. Diflorasone (Florone)

4. A patient presents with a very pruritic wet, weeping rash. Which of the following therapies is most appropriate for this patient?

   A. Moisturizing creams
   B. Bath oils
   C. First-generation antihistamine
   D. Steroid ointment

5. A 5-year-old female has an impressive vascular rash on her face, neck, chest, palms, and soles. She has enlarged lymph nodes, fevers to 103°F, and bright red mucous membranes. Five days after the rash appeared, she had desquamation of the skin of her hands. Which of the following is the most likely diagnosis?

   A. Rocky Mountain spotted fever
   B. Lyme disease
   C. Rubella
   D. Hand, foot, and mouth disease
   E. Kawasaki disease

6. A grandmother babysits her 6-month-old grandson. Grandma developed shingles along her left lower rib cage. Which of the following will the grandson most likely develop?

   A. Zoster
   B. Herpes simplex
   C. Chickenpox
   D. Stevens-Johnson syndrome
   E. Erythema multiforme

ANSWERS

1. **Answer: B.** This patient has the classic appearance and presentation of dermatitis herpetiformis which is associated with celiac sprue and must eliminate gluten from his diet. Reducing simple carbohydrates would be beneficial for patients with DM2. Reducing cholesterol and saturated fats may benefit someone with hypercholesterolemia or xanthomas. A medium chain triglyceride diet is beneficial in patients with hypertriglyceridemia.

2. **Answer: D.** This patient has psoriasis and psoriatic arthritis. The classic X-ray finding of psoriatic arthritis is a "pencil in a cup" deformity on hand films. A bucket handle tear is a finding in a torn meniscus, loss of joint space in osteoarthritis (although this may be present in psoriatic arthritis, it is not a classic finding as it is in osteoarthritis), subcutaneous nodules are classic in rheumatoid arthritis, and a spiral fracture is consistent with child abuse.

3. **Answer: A.** The long-term side effects of topical steroid use include thinning of the skin, discoloration, adult acne, and telangiectasia. Fluorinated (halogenated) steroids are much more likely to produce these side effects. Of the above steroids, only mometasone is a nonfluorinated steroid.

4. **Answer: C.** General treatment for any itching rash is a first-generation antihistamine which has a side effect of making persons somewhat sleepy which helps control the itching. It can also help if the rash is caused by an allergic reaction. Answers a, b, and d could be helpful for itchy, dry problems but are occlusive and are not a treatment for a wet, weeping lesion. The lesion will not dry if occluded.

5. **Answer: E.** This is a classic description of Kawasaki disease (mucocutaneous lymph node disease) with an impressive vascular rash, bright red mucous membrane, and enlarged lymph nodes. It is one of the few vascular rashes that can affect the palms and soles. After the acute disease, peeling of the skin of the hands commonly occurs. The patient is at risk for coronary artery aneurysms. Rocky Mountain spotted fever (RMSF) gives a petechial rash. Lyme disease begins at the tick-bite site, extends peripherally as it clears centrally. Rubella has a nondistinctive rash and many times is a lab diagnosis instead of a clinical diagnosis. Coxsackie (hand, foot, and mouth) presents as shallow ulcerations or small vesicles.

6. **Answer: C.** Grandma has herpes zoster which is the reactivation of the chickenpox virus. The grandson is too young to have had the chicken pox vaccination and may develop chickenpox 7 to 21 days after exposure to grandma's shingles.

15

DISEASES OF THE MUSCULOSKELETAL SYSTEM AND CONNECTIVE TISSUE

Rick Ricer • Robert V. Ellis

I. General Musculoskeletal Conditions

See Table 15-1.

II. Early Childhood

A. **Hip dysplasia**
   1. General characteristics:
      a. Laxity of supporting capsule and poorly developed acetabulum that causes subluxation or dislocation in one or both hips
      b. Occurs in 10 of 1,000 live births with an unknown etiology
      c. Risk factors include large baby or breech presentation.
   2. Clinical features:
      a. Barlow maneuver: adducting hip with knees at 90 degrees, pressure on knees posteriorly, and looking for dislocation of hip
      b. Ortolani maneuver: flex hip, then put anterior pressure on greater trochanters and smoothly abduct legs using thumb with feeling for a click or clunk
      c. Asymmetry of gluteal and thigh fat folds
      d. Galeazzi (Allen sign): Flex knees, ankles to buttocks, and look for knees that are not level.
   3. Diagnosis: ultrasound
   4. Treatment: double diaper, orthopedic referral, harness, cast

B. **Torticollis (wry neck)**
   1. General characteristics:
      a. Tight sternocleidomastoid muscle, possibly from in utero positioning, that can take up to 3 months post birth to develop
      b. Occurs in 1 in 250 live births
   2. Clinical features: head tilted to one side, stiff neck
   3. Treatment: physical therapy, stretching exercises

C. **In-toeing (pigeon toed)**
   1. General characteristics:
      a. Feet pointed inward
      b. Occurs in 2 out of 1,000 children
   2. Causes:
      a. Femoral anteversion (knock knees): usually no treatment necessary
      b. Tibial torsion (bow legs): usually no treatment necessary
      c. Metatarsus adductus (inward curved forefoot or C-shaped): stretching or no treatment necessary

D. **Out-toeing**
   1. Feet pointed outward caused by a rotational problem
   2. Usually no treatment necessary

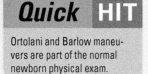

Quick HIT

Ortolani and Barlow maneuvers are part of the normal newborn physical exam.

TABLE 15-1	General Musculoskeletal Conditions		
Condition	**Definition**	**Cause**	**Examples**
Sprain	Ligament of a joint stretched beyond capacity	Trauma	Most common in ankle or wrist
Strain	Muscle stretched beyond capacity	Trauma	Most common in back, legs, and arms
Tendinitis	Inflammatory process involving a tendon	Repetitive motions, incorrect positioning, or acute trauma	Achilles, quadriceps, bicep, supraspinatus
Tenosynovitis	Inflammation of synovial sheath surrounding a tendon	Injury, repetitive motion, arthritis, or infection	DeQuervains, carpal tunnel syndrome
Tendinopathy	Chronic tendon injury with damage at a cellular level	Poor biomechanics, increased traction loads, tensile overload, collagen synthesis disruption, ischemia, overuse with failing of healing response, or microtears	Lateral epicondylitis (tennis elbow), medial epicondylitis (golfer's elbow)
Bursitis	Inflammation of any synovial (bursal) sac	Inflammatory diseases, autoimmune diseases, trauma, or repetitive motions	Trochanteric, olecranon, suprapatellar, infrapatellar
Joint effusion	Abnormal accumulation of fluid in and around a joint	Arthritis, infection, trauma, tear of joint or surrounding structure, gout	Most common in knee, ankle, and shoulder
Fasciitis	Inflammation of connective tissue surrounding muscles, blood vessels, and nerves	Trauma, overuse, infection	Plantar, necrotizing, eosinophilic
Myositis	Inflammation of muscle fibers	Inflammatory condition, infectious, injury, medication side effect (statins, cocaine, alcohol, colchicine, plaquenil)	Autoimmune dermatomyositis, polymyositis, SLE, RA, scleroderma

Diseases of the Musculoskeletal System

E. **Nursemaid elbow**
1. General characteristics:
   a. Subluxation of radial head caused by longitudinal traction of arm with wrist in pronation
   b. Usually occurs in children 1 to 4 years old
2. Clinical features: child keeps arm extended and pronated, will not supinate, stops using arm, often inconsolable
3. Treatment:
   a. Reposition by hyperpronating or supinate and flex
   b. XR if symptoms do not resolve with repositioning maneuvers
F. **Erb palsy**
1. General characteristics:
   a. Loss of sensation of the arm, paralysis and/or atrophy of deltoids, biceps, and brachialis most commonly associated with shoulder dystocia and traction on brachial plexus
   b. Occurs in 1.5 in 1,000 live births

2. Clinical features: Arm hangs limply and is rotated medially (waiter's tip).
3. Treatment: may need physical therapy or neurosurgical referral

G. **Cerebral palsy**
1. General characteristics:
   a. Central motor dysfunction affecting muscle tone, posture, and movement
   b. Affects motor control centers of cerebrum (cognition or speech can be impaired as well)
   c. Occurs in 2 per 1,000 live births with unknown etiology
2. Clinical features: Symptoms are abnormal muscle tone, abnormal reflexes, abnormal coordination, spasticity, spasms, involuntary muscles, balance and gait problems, contractures, scissor walking, and toe walking.
3. Treatment: physical and occupational therapy, may need surgical release procedures or braces

H. **Muscular dystrophy**
1. General characteristics:
   a. Progressive skeletal muscle weakness and atrophy
   b. Duchenne: X-linked, usually diagnosed at 2 to 4 years old, fatal by the late teens or 20s
   c. Becker: later diagnosis, milder symptoms, typically live well into adulthood
2. Clinical features: gives gait problems, muscle atrophy, and weakness
3. Treatment: physical and occupational therapy, patient and caregiver support

III. Later Childhood

A. **Scoliosis**
1. General characteristics: curvature of the spine >10 degrees ("S" shaped spine) that is usually idiopathic
2. Clinical features:
   a. Physical exam shows a unilateral rib hump, uneven musculature, uneven shoulders, uneven hips, leg length discrepancy.
   b. Perform an Adams forward bend to see curve better.
3. Diagnosis: full-length standing X-ray (scoliosis series) and measure Cobb angle
4. Treatment: often just follow with periodic XR, physical therapy, scoliosis brace, shoe lift, and surgery in severe cases

B. **Slipped capital femoral epiphysis**
1. General characteristics:
   a. Fracture through growth plate with slippage of epiphysis
   b. Occurs in 1 in 1,000 to 1 in 10,000 children, usually between 11 and 14 years of age
   c. Risk factors include obesity and male gender.
2. Clinical features: groin, knee, or thigh pain, painful limp, limited internal rotation hip, refusal to walk on the affected leg
3. Diagnosis: XR of pelvis including AP and frog leg
4. Treatment: no weight bearing, urgent referral to orthopedics for surgical pinning

C. **Osgood-Schlatter's**
1. General characteristics:
   a. Apophysitis of tibial tubercle causing irritation and pain of patellar ligament at tibial tubercle
   b. Affects 5% to 15% of population, usually during growth spurt at 9 to 14 years of age, more common in boys
2. Clinical features: painful lump over the anterior/superior tibia
3. Treatment: rest, acetaminophen, NSAIDs, ice, brace/cast in severe cases

D. **Legg-Calvé-Perthes**
1. General characteristics:
   a. Idiopathic avascular osteonecrosis caused by disruption in blood flow to femoral head
   b. Found in 5.5 of 100,000 children ages 3 to 12 years old, with a mean age of 6 years

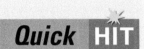

Quick HIT

Children, especially boys, that are not walking by 18 months or have a loss of previously acquired motor function should be evaluated for muscular dystrophy.

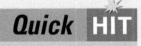

Quick HIT

It is no longer recommended to screen asymptomatic children for scoliosis (USPSTF Category D).

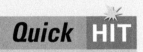

Quick HIT

Like Osgood-Schlatter's, **Sever's** is another type of apophysitis, but of the heel, and affects children 9 to 11 years old.

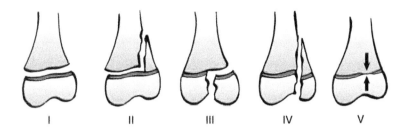

FIGURE 15-1 Salter–Harris fracture types.

(From Flynn JM, Skaggs DL, Waters PM. *Rockwood and Wilkin's Fractures in Children*. 8th ed. Philadelphia, PA: Wolters Kluwer; 2015.)

2. Clinical features: hip, knee, or groin pain especially with internal hip rotation, and limp
3. Diagnose: X-ray
4. Treatment: traction, braces, orthotics, physical therapy (PT), follow for deformity of femoral head, orthopedic referral

E. **Salter-Harris fractures**
   1. General characteristics:
      a. Fractures involving a growth plate (Fig. 15-1)
      b. Up to 30% of fractures in skeletally immature children
   2. Diagnosis: X-ray
   3. Treatment: splint or cast, more complex fractures require orthopedic surgery

IV. Adulthood

A. **Ankle sprain**
   1. General characteristics:
      a. Almost always an inversion (lateral) injury
      b. Injury involves anterior talofibular (most common), calcaneofibular and posterior talofibular ligaments.
   2. Diagnosis and treatment as with any sprain (see above)
   3. Ottawa ankle rules:
      a. Used to determine if an XR is needed in a patient with an ankle injury
      b. 96% to 100% sensitive for a fracture and demonstrated to reduce XRs by 30% to 40%
      c. XR only needed if one or more of the following are positive (Fig. 15-2):
         i. Tenderness of the distal 6 cm posterior edge of tibia (medial malleolus)
         ii. Tenderness of the distal 6 cm posterior edge of fibula (lateral malleolus)
         iii. Tenderness of the navicular
         iv. Tenderness of the proximal 5th metatarsal
         v. Inability to bear weight for four steps immediately after the injury or at examination

B. **Biceps tendinitis**
   1. General characteristics:
      a. Inflammatory process involving a tendon caused by repetitive motions, incorrect positioning, or acute trauma
      b. Most commonly the long head of the proximal biceps
      c. Most common in young and middle-aged patients
   2. Clinical features:
      a. Pain on palpation or motion, restricted motion, rarely swelling and redness
      b. Tenderness over the biceps groove
      c. Positive Speed's test (Table 15-2)

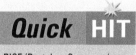

Quick HIT

RICE (Rest, Ice, Compression, Elevation) therapy is a common treatment for musculoskeletal conditions.

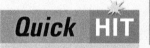

Quick HIT

A **high ankle sprain** is a disruption of the syndesmotic ligaments connecting tibia and fibula just superior to the ankle.

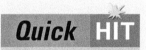

Quick HIT

Always examine one joint above and one joint below area of pain to assess for a referred pain cause.

Diseases of the Musculoskeletal System

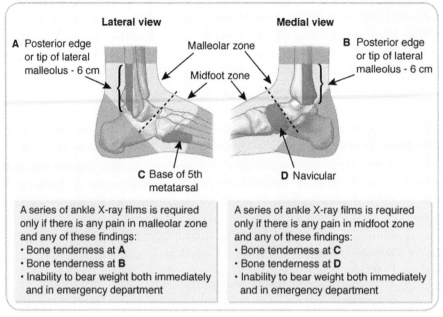

FIGURE
15-2 Ottawa ankle rules.
(From Anderson MK. *Foundations of Athletic Training*. 6th ed. Philadelphia, PA: Wolters Kluwer; 2016.)

TABLE 15-2	Common Musculoskeletal Physical Exam Tests	
Test	**Tests for**	**How to Perform**
ARM		
Finkelstein	De Quervain tenosynovitis	Abductor pollicis longus and extensor pollicis brevis—thumb placed in palm, fingers closed around thumb, wrist maximally ulnar deviated gives pain
Phalen	CTS	Dorsum of hands together with wrists in forced flexion for 30–60 s gives numbness of palmar thumb, index finger, and middle finger
Tinel	CTS	Lightly tapping median nerve at palmar wrist gives "electric jolt" down middle finger
NECK		
Spurling	Cervical nerve root pain	Turn head toward affected side with neck extended, downward pressure on head gives pain, numbness, weakness down arm
SHOULDER		
Speed's	Tendinitis of long head of biceps	Arm supinated, elbow extended, resist forward flexion at shoulder gives pain in biceps groove
Empty can	Supraspinatus tendon	Arms extended at 30 degrees, thumbs pointing down, resist upward motion gives weakness or pain
Drop arm	Supraspinatus tendon tear	Passively hold arm extended at shoulder level and release, allow patient to slowly lower arm to waist gives inability to control maneuver to waist
Lift off	Subscapularis	Dorsum of hands in lumbar area, resist straight lift off gives pain or weakness
External rotation	Infraspinatus and teres minor	Arm against ribs, elbows flexed at 90 degrees, resist external rotation gives pain or weakness

(continued)

Test	Tests for	How to Perform
TABLE 15-2	*Common Musculoskeletal Physical Exam Tests (continued)*	
Neer	Impingement rotator cuff	Arm extended and pronated, examiner passively lifts arm up past head gives pain
Hawkins	Impingement of rotator cuff or labrum	Arm at level of shoulder, elbow at 90 degrees, humerus forcibly internally rotated gives pain
Cross arm	AC joint	Arm at shoulder level, reach over to touch other shoulder gives pain at active AC joint
Apprehension	Subluxation of glenohumeral joint	Arm at shoulder level, elbow at 90 degrees hand toward ceiling, anterior pressure on humerus gives pain or apprehension of joint dislocating
BACK		
Straight leg raise	Lumbar nerve root compression	Leg extended, hip at 90 degrees gives radiating pain or numbness down past knee
FABER	SI joint	Hip in flexion, abduction, and external rotation ("figure 4") gives pain
HIP		
Trendelenburg	Hip abductor weakness	Patient stands on affected leg and lifts other leg gives pelvic drop to contralateral side
KNEE		
Anterior drawer	ACL	Patient supine, knee flexed at 90 degrees, fix foot, pull tibia anteriorly gives displacement of tibia
Lachman	ACL	Patient supine, knee flexed at 30 degrees, stabilize femur, pull tibia anteriorly gives lack of clear endpoint of displacement of tibia
Posterior Drawer	PCL	Same as anterior drawer but push tibia posteriorly gives displacement of tibia
Valgus stress	LCL	Patient supine, leg slightly abducted at hip, knee 30 degrees flexed, stabilize tibia, push knee inward gives laxity
Varus stress	MCL	Same as valgus but push knee out gives laxity
McMurray	Meniscus	Patient supine, thumb and fingers in knee joint line, grasp heel, fully flex and extend knee while exerting valgus stress while externally rotating the knee; repeat with varus stress while internally rotating the knee

3. Diagnosis: usually clinical diagnosis, MRI if unsure, rarely arthroscopic exam
4. Treatment: RICE, NSAIDs, steroid injection, PT, rehab, rarely surgery

C. **Carpal tunnel syndrome (CTS)**
   1. General characteristics:
      a. Inflammation of the median nerve as it runs through the carpal bones caused by injury, repetitive motion, arthritis, or infection
      b. Often worse at night and when awakening
   2. Clinical features:
      a. Pain, numbness, restriction of movement, sometimes weakness
      b. Distribution of symptoms: usually the first three fingers and half of the fourth
      c. Tinel and Phalen test (see Table 15-2)
   3. Diagnosis: physical exam, nerve conduction studies to confirm diagnosis in refractory cases

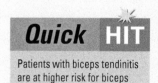

Quick HIT

Patients with biceps tendinitis are at higher risk for biceps rupture.

Diseases of the Musculoskeletal System

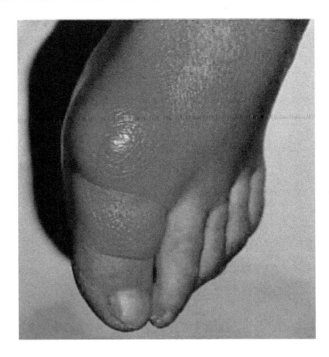

FIGURE 15-3 Gout.

(From Ayala C, Spellberg B. *Boards and Wards for USMLE Step 2.* 6th ed. Philadelphia, PA: Wolters Kluwer; 2017.)

4. Treatment: CTS wrist splint, activity modification, oral steroids, steroid injection, and surgery for refractory cases

D. **De Quervain tenosynovitis**
　1. General characteristics:
　　a. Inflammation of synovial sheath surrounding the abductor pollicis longus and extensor pollicis brevis at the styloid process of the radius
　　b. Caused by injury, repetitive motion, overuse, arthritis, or infection
　　c. Most common in women aged 30 to 50 years, and mothers and daycare workers who routinely carry infants
　2. Clinical features:
　　a. Pain on the radial side of the wrist that radiates to the thumb
　　b. Finkelstein test (see Table 15-2)
　3. Diagnosis: generally a clinical diagnosis
　4. Treatment: activity modification, NSAIDs, thumb spica splint, steroid injection, surgery rarely for refractory cases

E. **Lateral epicondylitis (tennis elbow) and medial epicondylitis (golfer's elbow)**
　1. General characteristics:
　　a. Chronic tendon injury (tendinosis) with damage at a cellular level caused by poor biomechanics, increased traction loads, tensile overload, collagen synthesis disruption, ischemia, overuse with failing of healing response
　　b. Risk factors: smoking, obesity, repetitive activities
　2. Clinical features: tenderness over the lateral or medial epicondyle
　3. Diagnosis: generally a clinical diagnosis
　4. Treatment: RICE, activity modification, PT, counterforce bracing, steroid injection if not improving

F. **Gout**
　1. General characteristics:
　　a. Very painful inflammatory arthritis caused by uric acid crystals
　　b. Usually a single joint but can involve two or more and most often involves the first MTP joint
　2. Clinical features: warm, erythematous, very tender, swollen joint (Fig. 15-3)

3. Diagnosis:
   a. Definitive diagnosis made by microscopy of synovial fluid showing negatively birefringent intracellular uric acid crystals
   b. Serum uric acid level
      i. An elevated level can support the diagnosis but is not diagnostic.
      ii. A third or more of patients with acute gout flare can have a normal or low level.
4. Treatment:
   a. Acute flare: NSAIDs and low-dose colchicine are first-line therapy. Intra-articular or oral steroid for refractory cases or patients with contraindications to first-line medications.
   b. Prevention:
      i. Diet: Avoid/reduce organ meat, shellfish, meat (especially red meats), alcohol, and simple sugars (such as high fructose corn syrup). Dairy products can decrease excretion of uric acid.
      ii. Medications: allopurinol and probenecid
      iii. Target therapy to lower serum uric acid level to <6

G. **Pseudogout**
1. General characteristics: Inflammatory arthritis caused by calcium pyrophosphate crystals that can be acute or chronic.
2. Clinical features:
   a. Painful joint that can be warm red and swollen
   b. Most often in the knee (50%)
3. Diagnosis:
   a. XR can show calcium pyrophosphate deposition.
   b. Aspiration of fluid can show typical crystals (positively birefringent).
4. Treatment:
   a. Glucocorticoid injection
   b. Oral NSAIDs and colchicine

H. **Psoriatic arthritis**
1. General characteristics
   a. Inflammatory arthritis caused by psoriasis
   b. About 4% to 30% of patients with psoriasis
   c. About 30% do not have a history of psoriasis
2. Clinical features:
   a. Pain and stiffness that worsen after periods of immobility
   b. Polyarthritis with multiple patterns
3. Diagnosis:
   a. Rule out other forms of inflammatory arthritis.
   b. HLA-B27 genetic testing may be helpful.
   c. CASPAR criteria (Table 15-3)

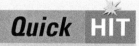

Quick HIT

Xanthine oxidase inhibitors (allopurinol) can precipitate an acute gout attack when initiated. Do not start during an acute attack; concurrent colchicine use decreases this risk.

Diseases of the Musculoskeletal System

TABLE **15-3** CASPAR Criteria for the Diagnosis of Psoriatic Arthritis	
Criteria	**Points**
Psoriasis of the skin	
• Present, **Or**	2 points
• Past history, **Or**	1 point
• Family history	1 point
Nail lesions	1 point
Dactylitis	1 point
Negative RF	1 point
Juxtaarticular bone formation on XR	1 point
3 or more out of a possible 6 points is considered positive.	

TABLE 15-4	European League Against Rheumatism/American College of Rheumatology (EULAR/ACR) Criteria for the Diagnosis of RA

Criterion	Points
1 large joint (shoulder, hip, elbow, knee, ankle)	0
2–10 large joints	1
1–3 small joints (MCP, PIP, 2nd–5th MTP, thumb IP, wrist)	2
4–10 small joints	3
>10 joints (at least one small joint)	5
Duration ≥6 wk	1
Abnormal ESR or CRP	1
Low positive RF or ACPA	2
High positive RF or ACPA	3
≥6 is consistent with RA	

4. Treatment:
   a. Mild disease: NSAIDs
   b. Moderate-to-severe disease or those not responding to NSAIDs: methotrexate, TNF inhibitor. Alternatives include leflunomide, sulfasalazine, and cyclosporine.

I. **Myositis**
   1. General characteristics:
      a. Inflammation of muscle fibers
      b. Causes: inflammatory condition (dermatomyositis, polymyositis, autoimmune [SLE, RA, scleroderma], infectious [usually viral], injury, medication side effect [statins, cocaine, alcohol, colchicine, plaquenil])
   2. Clinical features: pain, weakness, swelling
   3. Diagnosis: creatine phosphokinase (CPK), aldolase, muscle biopsy, erythrocyte sedimentation rate (ESR)
   4. Treatment depends on underlying cause.

J. **Rheumatoid arthritis**
   1. General characteristics: autoimmune inflammatory polyarthritis
   2. Clinical features:
      a. Swelling, erythema, pain, warmth involving several joints
      b. Typically bilateral wrists, metatarsophalangeal joints (MTP), and proximal interphalangeal (PIP) joints
      c. Morning stiffness that lasts over an hour
   3. Diagnosis: European League Against Rheumatism/American College of Rheumatology (EULAR/ACR) criteria (Table 15-4)
   4. Treatment:
      a. Disease-modifying antirheumatic drugs (DMARDs) as soon as diagnosis is made
      b. Methotrexate drug of choice
      c. Second-line either triple therapy or addition of biologic
      d. Treat to remission or low disease activity
      e. Should see a rheumatologist within 1 month of diagnosis

K. **Low back pain**
   1. General characteristics:
      a. Prevalence of almost 100% throughout any one person's life
      b. Back muscles are balanced by weaker abdominal muscles and can easily be strained.

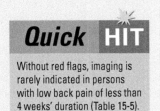

Quick HIT

Without red flags, imaging is rarely indicated in persons with low back pain of less than 4 weeks' duration (Table 15-5).

TABLE 15-5	Red Flags of Back Pain
Past History	Cancer, IV drug use, immunocompromised, recent spinal surgery, recent bacterial infection
History of Present Illness (HPI)	Unexplained weight loss, pain that wakes patient up, fever, trauma, bowel or bladder changes
Age	>50 or <17 yrs old
PE	Saddle anesthesia, anal sphincter laxity, major motor weakness

   c. Causes:
      i. Most episodes caused by injury or overuse of paraspinous muscles
      ii. Pressure on nerve roots can occur with degenerative joint disease (DJD), herniated disc, spinal stenosis, fx vertebrae, arthritis, or spondylolisthesis.
      iii. Other causes—ankylosing spondylitis, infection, tumor, Reiter's
  2. Clinical features:
    a. Symptoms—spasm, cramping, stiffness, pain with movement, sciatica
      i. Sciatica: pain from buttocks into back of thigh to lateral lower leg to foot with tingling, numbness, and weakness of leg or foot (nerve root compression)
      ii. Cauda equine: emergency—saddle anesthesia of skin, urinary retention, fecal incontinence
    b. Physical exam (PE)—tenderness, range of motion (ROM), reflexes, sensation in specific dermatomes, strength of specific muscles testing lumbar nerve roots, straight leg raise (SLR)
  3. Diagnosis: X-ray, CT, MRI, bone scan, electromyography (EMG) depending on suspected cause
  4. Treatment: Nonsteroidal anti-inflammatory drugs (NSAIDs), ice, heat, massage, acetaminophen, opiates, muscle relaxants, PT, abdominal strengthening, stretching exercises, proper sleeping positions, weight loss, acupuncture, epidural steroid injection, surgery

V. Elderly
A. Hip fracture
  1. General characteristics:
    a. Fracture of the proximal femur
    b. Caused by a fall or trauma, usually minor
    c. Higher incidence in women owing to higher incidence of osteoporosis
    d. High morbidity and mortality within 1 year
  2. Clinical features: pain, cannot bear weight, affected leg shorter and externally rotated
  3. Diagnosis: X-ray
  4. Treatment: Surgery, early mobility, occupational therapy (OT)/PT, rehab
B. **Colles fracture**
  1. General characteristics:
    a. Fracture of the distal radius/ulna
    b. Usually from a fall onto the outstretched hand
    c. Osteoporosis increases risk.
  2. Diagnosis: X-ray
  3. Treatment: volar forearm split, cast, open reduction
C. **Vertebral compression fracture**
  1. General characteristics:
    a. Collapse of vertebral body even with minor trauma
    b. Usually associated with osteoporosis, but can be pathologic fracture from cancer

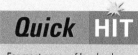

For most cases of low back pain, do not put patient on bed rest as this will worsen the process and delay healing.

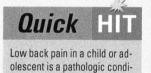

Low back pain in a child or adolescent is a pathologic condition until proven otherwise.

Diseases of the Musculoskeletal System

    2. Clinical features: back pain, shortened height

    3. Diagnosis: X-ray

    4. Treatment:

        a. Pain control: acetaminophen (APAP), NSAIDs, calcitonin, opioids

        b. Severe symptoms: kyphoplasty or vertebroplasty

D. **Trigger finger** (stenosing tenosynovitis)

    1. General characteristics: catching or locking of finger flexor tendon owing to a tendon nodule

    2. Treatment: steroid injection, release procedure by hand surgeon

E. **Polymyalgia rheumatica (PMR)**

    1. General characteristics:

        a. Uncertain etiology

        b. Can be associated with temporal arteritis

    2. Clinical features: pain and stiffness proximal muscle of neck, shoulders, hips and fatigue

    3. Diagnosis: very high ESR

    4. Treatment: oral corticosteroids for at least 1 month, then a slow taper

F. **Swan neck deformity**

    1. General characteristics:

        a. DIP hyperflexion and PIP hyperextension

        b. Causes: rheumatoid arthritis (RA), DJD, trauma—slip of PIP flexor tendons

    2. Treatment: splint, surgery

G. **Boutonniere deformity**

    1. General characteristics:

        a. PIP flexion and DIP hyperextension

        b. Causes: RA, DJD, trauma—slip of PIP extensor tendon

    2. Treatment: Splint, surgery

H. **Frozen shoulder (adhesive capsulitis)**

    1. General characteristics:

        a. Inflamed and stiff glenohumeral joint

        b. Often due to previous trauma or severe osteoarthritis

    2. Clinical features: greatly reduced ROM, pain with motion, progressive loss of active and passive motion

    3. Treatment: PT/OT, NSAIDs, pain meds, manipulation under anesthesia

I. **Osteoarthritis (degenerative joint disease)**

    1. General characteristics:

        a. Degraded joints and cartilage usually from aging

        b. Not an inflammatory process

    2. Clinical features:

        a. Pain, stiffness, loss of mobility, enlarged joints

        b. Affects hands, feet, spine, hips, knees

        c. Bouchard (PIP) and Heberden (DIP) nodes

        d. Bunions, joint effusions

    3. Diagnosis: X-ray

    4. Treatment:

        a. Exercise, weight loss, analgesics, acetaminophen, NSAIDs, opiates, OT/PT

        b. May need joint replacement

QUESTIONS

1. While playing basketball, a 22-year-old male was running down the court, stopped to shoot, and felt a tearing pain in his knee. He was unable to continue playing and his knee swelled within 15 minutes. On exam, he had a knee effusion but no pain over the joint line. Which of the following is the most sensitive physical exam test to diagnose his condition?

   A. Anterior drawer

   B. Lachman

   C. Posterior drawer

   D. McMurray

   E. FABER

2. A 22-year-old female was jogging and slipped off a curb and suffered an inversion injury to her ankle. She presents to the ER requesting an X-ray to rule out a fracture. Which of the following would be an indication for an X-ray?

   A. Bony tenderness of the distal 6 cm of the anterior edge of the tibia

   B. Bony tenderness of the distal 6 cm of the anterior edge of the fibula

   C. Ability to take four steps in the ER

   D. Bony tenderness over the navicular

   E. Bony tenderness at the base of the 4th metatarsal

3. A 55-year-old male presents with acute lower back pain for 2 days without remembered trauma. He denies fever or chills, a history of cancer, any surgery, or any medical problems. He is on no medications, his pain radiates into his buttocks and upper thigh. There are no bowel or bladder problems. His pain is worse with standing or bending and better when lying down. Exam reveals tenderness in the muscles of his lower back, a negative straight leg raise, and no saddle anesthesia. Which of the following is a "red flag" in his presentation?

   A. Age

   B. Gender

   C. No fever or chills

   D. Duration of symptoms

   E. Pain eased when lying down

4. A 45-year-old male presents with a 6-week history of right shoulder pain. He does not recall an injury or trauma but reports that he does lift weights three to four times a week. It has not improved despite occasional use of ibuprofen. He has normal strength and full range of motion of the shoulder. Speed's test is positive. Neer, Hawkins, and O'Brien tests are negative. This patient is at high risk for which of the following complications:

   A. Supraspinatus tear

   B. Infraspinatus tear

   C. Long head biceps tear

   D. Short head biceps tear

   E. Superior labrum anterior to posterior (SLAP) tear

5. A 13-year-old male presents with 2 days of pain in his thigh and knee and a painful limp. Other than obesity, he has no medical problems. He denies trauma. An X-ray confirms the diagnosis. Which of the following is the most appropriate treatment for correcting his problem?

    A. NSAIDs

    B. Acetaminophen

    C. Physical therapy

    D. Brace/cast

    E. Orthopedic surgical procedure

6. A 40-year-old female presents with a 7-week history of swollen and red joints of her hands bilaterally, left shoulder, and right knee. She has fatigue but no fever. Exam reveals red, swollen PIP of all fingers, IP of both thumbs, right knee, and left shoulder. Erythrocyte sedimentation rate (ESR) and anti-cyclic citullinated peptide protein antibody (anti-CCP) are elevated. Which of the following is the most important next step in this patient's treatment?

    A. Referral to see rheumatologist in next 3 months.

    B. Referral to see orthopedist in next 3 months.

    C. Methotrexate

    D. Acetaminophen

    E. NSAIDs

ANSWERS

1. **Answer: B.** The mechanism of injury is a forward displacement of the femur on the stopped tibia. This is the classic mechanism for an ACL injury. The effusion of the knee happened so quickly that the fluid had to be blood and therefore a tear occurred instead of a strain. The Lachman is a more sensitive test for an ACL tear than is the anterior drawer (both are PE test used for ACL tear). The posterior drawer is for a PCL tear, the McMurray for a meniscus tear, and the FABER (flexed, abducted and externally rotated) for sacroiliac pathology. While a meniscus tear could be possible, no rotational force is present in the mechanism of injury and no pain over the joint line makes this less of a possibility.

2. **Answer: D.** According to the Ottawa ankle rules, only her pain over the navicular is an indication for an X-ray. The other positive rules would be bony tenderness of the distal 6 cm of the <u>posterior</u> tibia or fibula, <u>inability</u> to bear weight for four steps, and bony tenderness of the 5th metatarsal.

3. **Answer: A.** Red flags for low back pain includes (among others) age >50 or <17 (He is over 50), pain for >4 to 6 weeks, unexplained fever, and pain at night or at rest. Gender is not a red flag.

4. **Answer: C.** The patient's history and exam are consistent with tendinitis of the long head of the biceps as indicated by a positive Speed's test with a lack of other findings on exam. Patients with long head biceps tendinitis are at a higher risk for rupture. The short head of the biceps is rarely involved in biceps tendinitis. Neer and Hawkins are tests for rotator cuff impingement that is most commonly associated with supraspinatus pathology. O'Brien's is a test for a SLAP tear. TABLE 12-1

5. **Answer: E.** This patient has a classic presentation of a slipped capital femoral epiphysis which is a fracture through the growth plate. This occurs most commonly in early adolescence and is more common in obese males. The pain is usually referred to the groin, thigh, and/or knee and presents as a painful limp. AP and frog leg X-rays of the pelvis confirm the diagnosis. Surgical pinning is the definitive treatment. All the other choices would be inappropriate or incomplete therapies. PT may be utilized, but only after a corrective procedure.

6. **Answer: C.** This patient has definitive RA by EULAR/ACR criteria (>6 points). Five points for >10 joints, at least one small joint, three points for 4-10- small joints, one point for >6 weeks' duration, one point for high-phase reactant, and three points for high anti-CCP or RF. According to EULAR/ACR recommendations, the patient needs treatment with a disease-modifying anti-rheumatic drugs (DMARD) as soon as the diagnosis is made and methotrexate is the DMARD of first choice. The patient should see a rheumatologist within 1 month. Acetaminophen and NSAIDs may be used as an adjunct but are not the primary treatment for RA.

16

ENDOCRINE AND METABOLIC DISORDERS

Rick Ricer • Robert V. Ellis

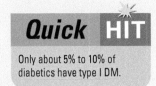

Quick HIT

Only about 5% to 10% of diabetics have type I DM.

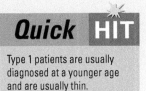

Quick HIT

Type 1 patients are usually diagnosed at a younger age and are usually thin.

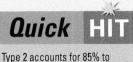

Quick HIT

Type 2 accounts for 85% to 95% of all DM cases.

I. Diabetes Mellitus

A. **Diabetes mellitus type 1 (DM1)**
   1. General characteristics:
      a. The pancreas is unable to produce insulin.
      b. Usually the result of viral illness and immune response producing autoantibodies
         i. Islet cell antibodies (ICA), multiple different subclasses in same patient
         ii. Destroys beta cells in short period of time (weeks to months)
         iii. Unable to produce insulin
         iv. Must get exogenous insulin to prevent death
         v. Prone to diabetic ketoacidosis (DKA)
      c. May occur with any mechanism that destroys the pancreas
         i. Chronic pancreatitis
         ii. Chronic alcoholism
         iii. Acute trauma or hemorrhagic pancreatitis
         iv. "Burnout" of beta cells from chronic DM2
   2. Diagnosis: low or no C-peptide or insulin measured
   3. Treatment: insulin (plus controlled daily activity and diet)

B. **Diabetes mellitus type 2 (DM2)**
   1. General characteristics:
      a. The result of insulin resistance from a combination of genetics and environment (obesity)
         i. Cause is genetics plus weight gain.
         ii. Effect is insulin resistance and hyperinsulinemia.
         iii. Consequences are central obesity, hypertension, DM2, low high-density lipoproteins (HDL), high triglycerides (TG), high uric acid, fatty liver (NASH), obstructive sleep apnea (OSA), polycystic ovarian syndrome (PCOS) in women, and elevated plasminogen activator inhibitor-1 (PAI-1).
         iv. End result is total body atherosclerosis and neuropathy: myocardial infarction (MI), cerebrovascular accident (CVA), renal insufficiency, skin ulcers, sexual dysfunction, autonomic dysfunction, retinopathy, and peripheral vascular disease.
      b. DM2 is one of the components of the insulin resistance syndrome (IRS).
         i. Not all components (1.a.iii) will be present in every patient but will usually develop at some point in their lifetime.
         ii. Old names for this syndrome: syndrome X, dysmetabolic syndrome, metabolic syndrome, deadly quartet
      c. Epidemiology
         i. 21 million Americans diagnosed
         ii. 8 million Americans undiagnosed
         iii. Affects 12% to 14% of the U.S. population
         iv. Another 86 million are "prediabetic."
         v. DM2 and IRS epidemic exactly follows obesity epidemic.
         vi. Globally 387 million diagnosed

d. Risk factors:
  i. "Prediabetes"
     (a) Fasting glucose: 100 to 125
     (b) Postprandial glucose: 140 to 199
     (c) A_{1c}: 5.7–6.4
  ii. First-degree relative with DM
  iii. Race: Native Americans followed by African Americans and then Latinos
  iv. Inactivity
  v. Hypertension
  vi. History of cardiovascular disease
  vii. TG > 250
  viii. HDL < 35
  ix. Woman with gestational DM or baby > 9 lbs
  x. Severe obesity
  xi. Acanthosis nigricans
  xii. PCOS
e. Screening
  i. American Diabetes Association (ADA)
     (a) Any overweight/obese adult with one or more risk factors
     (b) All adults at age 45 and above
     (c) Consider in children and adolescents that are overweight/obese with two or more risk factors.
  ii. U.S. Preventive Services Task Force (USPSTF)
     (a) Adults 40 to 70 who are obese or overweight (B recommendation)
     (b) Consider earlier in patients at increased risk
2. Clinical features:
  a. Symptoms: polyuria, polydipsia, polyphagia, abnormal weight loss, poor healing, sexual dysfunction, paresthesias, autonomic dysfunction, repeated fungal infections, visual changes, 6th nerve palsy, lethargy, hyperosmolar state
  b. Physical exam:
    i. Blood pressure: to evaluate for hypertension (HTN)
    ii. Eye exam: to evaluate for retinopathy yearly
    iii. Foot exam to evaluate for peripheral neuropathy yearly
    iv. Loss of peripheral hair could indicate atherosclerosis.
    v. Decreased pulses could indicate atherosclerosis.
    vi. Bruits could indicate atherosclerosis.
    vii. Body habitus/body mass index (BMI) (obesity)
3. Diagnosis
  a. American Diabetes Association criteria:
    i. Fasting blood sugar ≥ 126 mg/dL
    ii. Random blood sugar ≥ 200 mg/dL with classic symptoms
    iii. A_{1c} ≥ 6.5%
    iv. Results should be repeated unless very high.
  b. Other testing
    i. C-peptide/insulin level if type 1 a possibility
    ii. A_{1c} monitoring every 3 to 6 months
    iii. Blood glucose (fasting/postprandial)
    iv. Lipids
    v. Urine protein (microalbumin) yearly
    vi. Glucose tolerance test (GTT) (mostly just in pregnancy)
    vii. Renal function tests
    viii. Liver function tests
4. Treatment:
  a. ADA goals:
    i. A_{1c} 7.0% (higher in elderly)
    ii. BP < 140/90
    iii. Fasting blood sugar (FBS) 80–130 mg/dL

Endocrine and Metabolic Disorders

iv. Random blood sugar (RBS) < 180
v. Stop smoking
vi. More or less stringent depending on patient
b. Recommendations from American Association of Clinical Endocrinologists/American College of Endocrinology (AACE/ACE):
   i. A_{1c} < 6.5% (unless tight control unwarranted)
   ii. FBS < 90
   iii. RBS < 140
   iv. Low-density lipoprotein (LDL) treated with high-dose statin as high-risk cardiovascular (CV) status
   v. Acetylsalicylic acid (ASA) treatment as high-risk CV status
   vi. Stop smoking.
   vii. F/U q 3 months (or as needed): A_{1c}, self-monitoring glucose results, monitor hypoglycemic episodes, lipids, BP, weight, fluid retention, liver or kidney impairment, medications, psychosocial factors, cardiovascular risk, physical exam
   viii. A_{1c} > 7.5, consider two medications to start
   ix. A_{1c} > 9.0, consider adding insulin
   x. Consider bariatric surgery as weight loss possibility.
   xi. Angiotensin-converting enzyme inhibitor (ACEI)/angiotensin receptor blocker (ARB) preferred treatment for hypertension since they slow progression of nephropathy and retinopathy but, calcium channel blockers, and thiazide diuretics can also be used first line
c. Lifestyle modification: Weight loss with improved diet and increased activity is the most potent therapy.
   i. Reverses cause of IRS
   ii. Bariatric surgery gives highest, most consistent weight loss over time and can reduce DM2 immediately after surgery.
   iii. Diet includes carb counting and low carbohydrates.
d. Medications (Table 16-1)
   i. General
      (a) Insulin is the most potent medication and can be used at any time, even as first-line treatment.
      (b) Metformin is first-line therapy in most situations.
      (c) Any other class of medication can be added as second line and third line and should be individualized based on the patient.
   ii. Metformin (biguanide)
      (a) First-line medication
      (b) Can be used in "prediabetes" but not Food and Drug Administration (FDA) approved for this
      (c) Mechanisms of action: reduces insulin resistance at muscle and fat cell level and reduces gluconeogenesis in liver
      (d) Studies show it provides CV safety.
      (e) Possible lactic acidosis if renal insufficiency or heart failure: do not use if estimated glomerular filtration rate (eGFR) <30
   iii. Glucagon-like peptide 1 (GLP-1) receptor agonist (incretins)
      (a) Increases insulin response to postprandial rise in glucose
      (b) Must have glucose rise in order to work
      (c) Must have pancreas that can produce insulin
      (d) Reduces glucagon secretion
      (e) Lowering of blood pressure
      (f) Slows gastric emptying
      (g) Reduces fluctuations in fasting and postprandial glucoses
      (h) Do not use if multiple endocrine neoplasia type 2 (MEN II) syndrome or medullary thyroid cancer
      (i) Do not use if creatinine clearance <30 mL/minute.
      (j) Caution if history of pancreatitis
      (k) Injection: twice daily, once daily, or once weekly

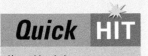

Quick HIT

Home blood glucose monitoring does not improve outcomes in non–insulin-dependent patients and increases patient anxiety.

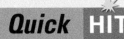

Quick HIT

Base the choice of medication on health beliefs system, patient education, and shared decision making with the patient.

TABLE 16-1 Medications to Treat DM

Class	Examples	Mechanism	Affect on Weight	Risk of Hypoglycemia	A_{1c} Lowering
α-glucosidase inhib	Acarbose, miglitol	Slows gut carbohydrate digestion/absorption	Neutral	Neutral	0.5–0.8
Amylin analog	Pramlintide	Decreases glucagon secretion	Loss	Neutral	0.5
Biguanide	Metformin	Reduces insulin resistance at muscle and fat cell. Reduces gluconeogenesis in liver	Loss	Neutral	1–2
Bile acid sequestrant	Colesevelam	Unknown	Neutral	Neutral	0.5
Dopamine receptor agonist	Bromocriptine	Unknown	Neutral	Neutral	0.2–0.4
Dipeptidyl peptidase IV (DPP IV) inhib	Alogliptin, linagliptin, saxagliptin, sitagliptin	Decreases breakdown of GLP-1	Gain	Neutral	0.5–1
GLP-1	Exenatide, liraglutide	Increases insulin response to postprandial rise in glucose.	Loss	Neutral	1
Insulin	Several	Increases insulin	Gain	High	≥2.5
Sodium-glucose co-transporter 2 inhibitors (SGLT 2i)	Canagliflozin, dapagliflozin, empagliflozin	Blocks reabsorption of glucose in the kidneys	Loss	Neutral	0.5–0.8
Sulfonylureas	Glimepiride, glipizide, glyburide	Increases production of insulin from the pancreas	Gain	High	1–2
TZD	Pioglitazone, rosiglitazone	Decreases insulin resistance at muscle and fat level	Gain	Neutral	1–1.5

Endocrine and Metabolic Disorders

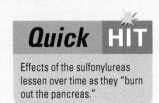

iv. Glitazones (TZDs)
  (a) Decrease insulin resistance at muscle and fat cell level
  (b) Can cause weight gain, fluid retention, heart failure, bone fractures
  (c) Oral: once daily
v. Sulfonylureas (2nd generation)
  (a) Increase production of insulin from pancreas
  (b) High-risk hypoglycemia
  (c) Oral: one to two times daily
vi. Secretagogue glinides (rapid-acting sulfonylurea)
  (a) Increase insulin from pancreas
  (b) Modest A_{1c} reduction
  (c) Shorter half-life than sulfonylureas with less hypoglycemia
  (d) Oral: before meals
vii. Dipeptidyl peptidase 4 (DPP-4) inhibitors
  (a) Decrease breakdown of GLP-1
  (b) Caution with pancreatitis
  (c) Oral: once daily
viii. Sodium glucose cotransporter 2 inhibitor
  (a) Blocks reabsorption of glucose in kidney (glucosuric effect)
  (b) Lowers BP, raises LDL
  (c) Probable decrease in cardiovascular deaths
  (d) Higher-risk fungal genital infections
  (e) Can create dehydration
  (f) Increased risk of limb amputations
  (g) Limited efficiency when eGFR <45
  (h) Oral: once daily
ix. Alpha-glucosidase Inhibitor
  (a) Slows gut carbohydrate digestion/absorption (later in bowel)
  (b) Probable CV benefit
  (c) Causes bloating, gas, diarrhea
  (d) Oral: three times daily
x. Amylin analog
  (a) Decreases glucagon secretion
  (b) Decreases postprandial glucose
  (c) Can cause nausea and vomiting
  (d) Can be used in DM1
  (e) Injection: prior to meals
xi. Bile acid sequestrant
  (a) Unknown mechanism of action
  (b) Lowers LDL, may increase TG
  (c) GI intolerance can be an issue.
  (d) Oral: six tabs daily or one packet daily
xii. Quick-release dopamine receptor agonist
  (a) Unknown mechanism of action
  (b) Side effects: nausea and orthostasis
  (c) Oral: once daily
xiii. Insulin
  (a) Most potent medication to lower A_{1c} short term
  (b) Major anabolic hormone, so creates hunger
  (c) Can give weight gain that worsens the IRS
  (d) Usually injection, one inhaled version available in the United States
  (e) Use in DM2
      (i) Start with single dose basal (10 units or 0.2 u/kg).
      (ii) Increase to target while avoiding hypoglycemia (increase by 1 to 2 units/day until FBS < 110).
      (iii) Add rapid-acting analog to cover largest meal.
      (iv) Add coverage of other meals (5 u/meal or one-third of basal each meal).

(f) Conservative dosing

    (i) Calculate total daily dose as patient's weight in kg × 0.4 units/kg.

    (ii) ½ as basal and ½ divided by 3 per meal

(g) Fixed mixtures of insulins are available but limit flexibility.

(h) Types of insulin

    (i) Rapid acting: aspart, glulisine, lispro, inhaled

    (ii) Short acting: regular

    (iii) Intermediate: neutral protamine Hagedorn (NPH)

    (iv) Long acting: glargine, detemir

  e. Somogyi effect

    i. Caused by increasing insulin too rapidly

    ii. Undetected hypoglycemia followed by rebound hyperglycemia

    iii. Usually happens at night, so undetected

    iv. Next morning, glucose high, so more insulin added when really needs to be reduced

    v. Hypoglycemia releases catechols and cortisol to raise glucose.

    vi. Patient can have vivid nightmares or intense sweating.

  f. Complications: blindness (leading cause), renal failure (leading cause), amputations (leading cause), MI, CVA, skin ulcers, sexual dysfunction, autonomic dysfunction, neuropathy and neuropathic pain, fungal infections, infections

C. Gestational diabetes

1. General characteristics:

  a. Probable DM2 as a result of pregnancy hormones causing insulin resistance

  b. Prone to overt DM2 later in life especially if gains weight

  c. Screen all pregnancies at 24 to 28 weeks' gestation

  d. Screen at-risk women at first visit

  e. Diagnosis of DM in first trimester is DM2, in second or third trimester is gestational

  f. Needs tight control throughout pregnancy

  g. Increases risk of stillborn, delivery complications, "large/dry babies"

2. Diagnosis: Screen with oral GTT.

  a. One-step 75 g

  b. Two-step 50 g and, if positive, 100 g

D. Latent autoimmune diabetes in adults (LADA)

1. General characteristics:

  a. Really slow onset type 1 and not type 2

  b. May have no family history of DM

  c. Only one islet cell antibody (ICA) instead of multiple as in DM1 (rapid onset type 1)

  d. Progressed to no beta cells in pancreas over 2 to 5 years

2. Clinical features: "lean" diabetic without other IRS components (HTN, obesity, low HDL, high TG)

3. Treatment:

  a. Glitazone resistant (not IRS, so reducing insulin resistance does not help)

  b. Will need insulin sooner in course of disease

  c. Can follow downward progression of insulin or C-peptide levels to get estimation of beta-cell population

E. Maturity onset diabetes of the young (MODY)

1. General characteristics:

  a. Hereditary in autosomal dominant fashion

  b. One point mutation on single gene

  c. Multiple types (at least 11) from mutation of several different genes that control insulin production or release

  d. Strong family history

  e. May not be overweight or obese

  f. Early onset (usually before age 30)

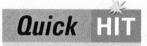

Quick HIT

The USPSTF recommends screening all pregnant women for gestational diabetes after 24 weeks (B recommendation).

Endocrine and Metabolic Disorders

2. Diagnosis: gene typing
3. Treatment: In some types, orals do not work, and in some types, insulin is not necessary.

II. Osteoporosis

A. **Characteristics**

1. Definition/physiology:
   a. Brittle bones
   b. Loss of bone density, mass, and calcium when the creation of bone does not keep pace with the removal of old bone causing bone to become fragile and weak, resulting in a higher risk for fracture

2. Epidemiology:
   a. About 12 million people affected in the United States, making it the most common bone disease
   b. One-half of postmenopausal women will have an osteoporotic fracture in their life.
   c. One of five men will have an osteoporotic fracture in their life.
   d. Common in all racial groups

3. Causes:
   a. Aging
   b. Loss of hormones
   c. Loss of bone mass
   d. Multiple risk factors

4. Risk factors:
   a. Female gender
   b. Loss of estrogen/testosterone
   c. Caucasian or Asian descent
   d. Positive family history (genetics unknown)
   e. Small and/or thin frame
   f. Hyperthyroidism or high thyroxine replacement
   g. Elevated parathyroid hormone (PTH)
   h. Low calcium intake
   i. GI surgery, eating disorder, or malabsorption syndrome
   j. Sedentary
   k. Smoking
   l. Excessive alcohol consumption
   m. Certain medications: corticosteroids, aluminum-containing antacids, gonadotropin-releasing hormones, phenytoin, barbiturates, proton pump inhibitors (PPIs)
   n. Certain disorders: osteogenesis imperfecta, rheumatoid arthritis, multiple myeloma, cancer, celiac

B. **Clinical features**

1. Silent disease, symptoms only late
2. Loss of height
3. Back pain
4. Kyphosis
5. Fracture with minimal trauma
6. Most common fractures—spine, hip, wrist, ribs

C. **Diagnosis** (Table 16-2)

1. Dual energy X-ray absorptiometry (DEXA) scan
   a. Most often used as it gives an accurate and precise measurement of bone mineral density (BMD)
   b. Standard sites measured: total lumbar spine (L1–L4), total hip, and femoral neck (use the lowest of the 3 scores)
   c. T score (risk of fracture)
      i. Amount of bone compared to a young adult of same gender
      ii. Normal: > -1
      iii. Osteopenia: -1 to -2.5
      iv. Osteoporosis: ≤ -2.5
   d. Z score: amount of bone compared to same age and gender

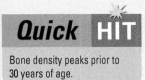

Quick HIT

Bone density peaks prior to 30 years of age.

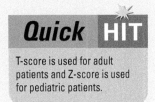

Quick HIT

T-score is used for adult patients and Z-score is used for pediatric patients.

TABLE 16-2	Diagnosing and Treating Low BMD

Diagnosis of osteoporosis can be made with any of the following

One or more fragility type fractures

T-score of ≤ -2.5 on DEXA scan

Pharmacologic treatment is recommended for the following

Individuals diagnosed with osteoporosis

Individuals with T-score -1.0 to -2.5 at high risk for a fracture[a]

[a]Individuals at high risk for a fracture are those with a 10-year probability of hip fracture $\geq 3\%$ or combined major osteoporotic fracture $\geq 20\%$ using the FRAX calculation. http://www.shef.ac.uk/FRAX.

2. Quantitative ultrasound (U/S) usually of heel: not as well studied and evidence not as good as DEXA
3. Quantitative computed tomography (CT): can be used but higher radiation, less reproducible, and more expensive

D. **Preventive screening**
   1. USPSTF recommendations
      a. Women ≥ 65 (B recommendation)
      b. Women < 65 with risk equal or greater than for 65-year-old women (10-year risk $\geq 9.3\%$) (B recommendation)
      c. DEXA of hip and/or lumbar or quantitative ultrasound of the heel
      d. Repeat screening in a person with an initial normal screening has not been shown to be beneficial
      e. Men (I recommendation)

E. **Treatment**
   1. Lifestyle modification
      a. Increase activity/exercise
      b. Stop smoking
      c. Increased dietary calcium and vitamin D
      d. Decrease caffeine
      e. Limit alcohol
      f. Fall prevention
   2. Pharmacologic
      a. Bisphosphonates: alendronate, risedronate, zoledronate (IV)
         i. Usual first-line choice
         ii. Increases bone density and reduces risk of fractures
         iii. Discontinue after 5 years for oral and 3 years for IV.
      b. Calcium and vitamin D supplementation if not getting adequate amounts from diet (1,200 mg and 800 IU)
      c. Estrogen: no longer first-line therapy owing to increased risk of stroke, blood clots, and breast cancer
      d. SERMs (selective estrogen receptor modulator): often used if there is also an independent need for reduction in breast cancer
      e. PTH (teriparatide): not first line; consider in men, intolerate or contraindication to bisphosphonate, postmenopausal women with severe osteoporosis
      f. Denosumab: humanized monoclonal antibody against receptor activator of nuclear factor kappa-B ligand (RANKL) that reduces osteoclastogenesis; not first line; may be useful in those with renal failure
      g. Calcitonin: not as effective; may be useful short term in decreasing pain related to vertebral fractures; long-term use associated with increased cancer rates

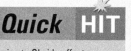

***Quick* HIT**

Owing to GI side effects, patients taking oral bisphosphonates should remain upright for at least 30 minutes after taking the medicine.

Endocrine and Metabolic Disorders

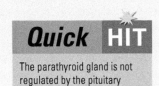

The parathyroid gland is not regulated by the pituitary gland.

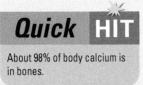

About 98% of body calcium is in bones.

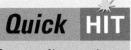

Symptoms of hyperparathyroidism can be remembered by the saying "moans, groans, stones, bones, and psychiatric overtones."

III. Parathyroid Disorders

A. Anatomy/physiology
1. Four pea-sized glands behind each pole of the thyroid comprise the parathyroid.
2. Produces parathyroid hormone
3. Controls regulation of calcium, vitamin D, and phosphorus
4. Low calcium detected by calcium sensing receptor (CaSR) stimulates production of PTH causing:
    a. Decreased renal excretion of calcium
    b. Increased production of calcitriol by kidney (vitamin D)
    c. Increased gut absorption of calcium

B. **Hyperparathyroidism**
1. Characteristics: the most common disorder of the parathyroid, in which too much PTH is secreted
2. Types:
    a. Primary hyperparathyroidism
        i. Causes
            (a) Adenoma: 85% to 90%
            (b) Hypertrophy all glands: 10% to 15%
            (c) Carcinoma: very rare
        ii. Females > males 3:1
        iii. Occurs in ages 50 to 60 years
    b. Secondary hyperparathyroidism
        i. Chronic renal disease (lack of response to PTH)
        ii. Dialysis
        iii. Vitamin D deficiency: dietary or malabsorption (Crohn's, celiac sprue)
3. Symptoms: fatigue (most common), depression, memory problems and confusion, bone aches and pains, fractures/osteoporosis, arrhythmias, kidney stones, hypercalcemia, hypophosphatemia, hypertension, constipation, nausea, vomiting, loss of appetite, peptic ulcer (increased gastrin from hypercalcemia)
4. Diagnosis:
    a. General
        i. Primary hyperparathyroid: elevated Ca with an elevated or high normal PTH (Table 16-3)
        ii. Secondary hyperparathyroid: elevated PTH and low or normal Ca
    b. Locating the problem
        i. Sestamibi scintigraphy scan (technetium): increased uptake in a hypersecreting gland
        ii. U/S: may show an enlarged or abnormal-looking gland

TABLE 16-3 Differential Diagnosis of Elevated Calcium
Causes of Elevated Calcium Levels
Elevated binding (albumin)
Hyperthyroidism
Sarcoid
Tuberculosis
Thiazide diuretics
Excess vitamin D
Prolonged immobilization
Lithium or tamoxifen
Renal transplant
HIV/AIDS

iii. CT: may show an enlarged gland
iv. Fine needle aspiration/biopsy for pathology
c. Other testing
i. Renal function: to rule out kidney disease
ii. Bone density: owing to increased risk of osteoporosis
iii. 24-hour urine calcium will be low in familial hypocalciuric hypercalcemia
iv. 25 hydroxy vitamin D
5. Treatment: may include observation if mild, surgery, or medications such as calcimimetic (cinacalcet) and bisphosphonates
C. **Hypoparathyroidism**
1. General characteristics:
a. Not enough PTH produced causing a low calcium level (Table 16-4)
b. Causes: injury to glands (mostly from surgery) and genetics (extremely rare)
2. Clinical features: tingling lips, toes, fingers (paresthesias), tetany, dry, brittle hair and scalp, fatigue, memory loss, seizures in babies, cataracts
3. Diagnosis:
a. Hypocalcemia with a low or inappropriately low normal PTH
b. Phosphorus: usually high
c. Vitamin D, Mg, and Cr levels usually normal
4. Treatment: calcium and vitamin D (calcitriol) supplementation

IV. Thyroid Diseases
A. **Physiology (feedback loop)** (Figure 16-1)
1. Thyrotropin (TRH)—from hypothalamus and stimulates production of thyroglobulin
2. Thyroid stimulating hormone (TSH)—from anterior pituitary and stimulates production of thyroid hormones
3. Thyroid hormones from thyroid gland (mono- and di- to tetra-iodotyrosine to tri-iodotyrosine)
a. T1 and T2 converted to T4 inside thyroid
b. T4 converted to T3 outside of thyroid
c. T3, T4 (thyroxine) performs thyroid bodily functions and suppresses TRH (and therefore TSH).
d. T3 more active component
e. T4 higher bound to binding globulin
f. In circulation, T4 90%, T3 10% of total thyroid hormones
g. Increases metabolic rate, GI motility, thermogenesis and regulation, cardiac output

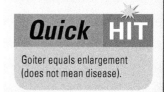

Quick HIT
Goiter equals enlargement (does not mean disease).

TABLE 16-4	Differential Diagnosis of Low Calcium

Causes of Low Calcium Levels

Low albumin
Resistance to PTH
Dietary calcium deficiency (or malabsorption)
Low vitamin D
Low magnesium
Elevated phosphorus
Pancreatitis
Renal failure

Endocrine and Metabolic Disorders

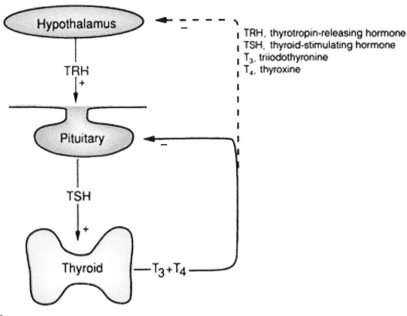

TRH, thyrotropin-releasing hormone
TSH, thyroid-stimulating hormone
T_3, triiodothyronine
T_4, thyroxine

FIGURE 16-1 Thyroid axis.

(From Lawrence PF, Bell RM, Dayton MT, et al. *Essentials of General Surgery.* 5th ed. Lippincott Williams & Wilkins; 2012.)

h. Thyroid only place in body that uses iodine
   i. Allows radioactive iodine (RAI) to be used for treatment of cancer and Graves'
   ii. Struma ovarii (goiter of ovary) teratoma of ovary that contains mostly thyroid tissue and will pick up iodine on scans

B. **Testing**
   1. Blood tests:
      a. T4: direct by radioimmunoassay (RIA)—bound and free
      b. T3: direct—bound and free
      c. TSH: best screening test for both hyper- and hypothyroidism
      d. TRH: rarely used except in case where T3/T4 and TSH all low
      e. Tg: binding—can be checked after thyroid surgery
   2. Thyroid antibodies:
      a. Hashimoto's: antithyroglobulin, antimicrosomal, antithyroperoxidase (TPO)—can also be elevated in Graves'
      b. Graves': antibodies to TSH receptor (TRAb), thyroid-stimulating immunoglobulin (TSI)
   3. Thyroid scans:
      a. Technetium: anatomy only, not function (rarely used anymore)
      b. Iodine 131 thyroid scan: anatomy
      c. Iodine 131 uptake scan: function
      d. U/S: solid versus cystic
   4. Thin needle biopsy: pathologic evaluation for cancer

C. **Hypothyroidism**
   1. Causes:
      a. Hashimoto's (autoimmune): chronic lymphocytic thyroiditis
      b. Iodine deficiency
      c. Status post surgery, radiation, RAI
      d. Medications: propylthiouracil (PTU), tapazole, lithium, amiodarone
      e. Elderly
   2. Clinical features: coarse thin hair, dry skin, brittle nails, goiter, cold intolerance, fatigue, constipation, bradycardia, weight gain, carpal tunnel syndrome, depression, muscle cramps, myxedema

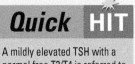

Quick HIT

A mildly elevated TSH with a normal free T3/T4 is referred to as subclinical hypothyroidism.

Quick HIT

Levothyroxine is the preferred treatment. Desiccated thyroid is no longer recommended owing to inconsistent amounts of thyroid hormone.

Endocrine and Metabolic Disorders

3. Diagnosis:
   a. TSH: usually elevated
   b. Free T3/T4: usually low
   c. Antimicrosomal antibodies: positive if autoimmune
4. Treatment: exogenous thyroxine

D. **Hyperthyroidism**
   1. Causes:
      a. Graves' (autoimmune): toxic diffuse goiter
      b. Nodular goiter (hyperfunctioning): "hot" nodule on scan
      c. Medications: too much exogenous thyroxine medication
      d. Burnout phase of Hashimoto's
   2. Clinical features: heat intolerance, sweating, weight loss, tremor, tachycardia, fatigue, irregular menstrual periods, arrhythmias, goiter, exophthalmia, lid lag, hypertension
   3. Diagnosis:
      a. TSH: low
      b. Free T3/T4: high
      c. Autoantibodies: positive if autoimmune
      d. Iodine scan: shows elevated uptake
   4. Treatment:
      a. PTU or tapazole
      b. β blockers for symptoms
      c. RAI
      d. Surgical thyroidectomy

E. **Euthyroid**
   1. Goiter:
      a. Cosmetic, difficulty swallowing, hoarseness
      b. RAI, surgery, replacement thyroxine
   2. Nodule:
      a. Very common, 95% to 99% benign, increases with age
      b. Workup may include iodine 131 scans, U/S, biopsy
      c. Red flags for cancer: male, age <20 years old or >70 years old, hoarse, enlarged regional nodes, history of radiation, irregular, fixed, hard, cold on uptake scan, family history of thyroid cancer, history of MEN II syndrome
   3. Subacute thyroiditis:
      a. Viral
      b. Sore throat, pain with swallowing, pain with palpation, other symptoms of upper respiratory tract infections
      c. Treat with nonsteroidal anti-inflammatory drugs (NSAIDs)

F. **Thyroid cancer**
   1. General characteristics:
      a. About 14 cases/100,000 with a lifetime risk of 1.1%
      b. Female-to-male ratio 3:1 for most types of thyroid cancer
   2. Types:
      a. Papillary: most common (>70%), local spread, low mortality but high recurrence rate
      b. Follicular: about 15%, usually age 40 to 60 years old, often has distant metastasis, does not pick up iodine well on scans
      c. Medullary: C cells (parafollicular)—calcitonin-secreting cells, regional to distant spread, can be part of MEN syndrome
      d. Anaplastic: rare, usually >65 years old, male-to-female ratio 2:1, metastasis to lungs quickly, high death rate
   3. Treatment:
      a. Surgery: subtotal, total, hemi thyroidectomy
      b. RAI
         i. Alpha emitter
         ii. Effects stay local
         iii. Only the thyroid picks up iodine and RAI

Endocrine and Metabolic Disorders

QUESTIONS

1. A 62-year-old patient was admitted to the hospital by the hospitalist and treated for DKA. However, ketones were negative. The patient was discharged on long-acting insulin. You believe the patient may have had hyperosmolar state with lactic acidosis. You are concerned that this patient has Type 2 DM and not Type 1 DM. Which of the following tests would help confirm the diagnosis of Type 2 DM which could affect long-term treatment strategies?
   A. Insulin level
   B. Insulin antibodies
   C. C-reactive protein
   D. Hgb A_{1c}
   E. C-peptide

2. A 62-year-old patient had a fasting blood glucose of 160 and a Hgb A_{1c} of 7.5. Which of the following would this patient be expected to display?
   A. Low blood pressure
   B. Low uric acid level
   C. High PAI-1
   D. High triglycerides
   E. High HDL cholesterol

3. A 62-year-old patient has been diagnosed with DM2. Which of the following is the most potent therapy for patients with Type 2 DM?
   A. Insulin
   B. Metformin
   C. Weight loss
   D. Amylin analog
   E. Sodium glucose cotransporter 2 inhibitor

4. Which U.S. population has the highest prevalence of Type 2 DM?
   A. African Americans
   B. Latinos
   C. Caucasians
   D. Native Americans
   E. Asian Americans

5. According to the USPSTF, which of the following persons should be screened for osteoporosis?
   A. A 62-year-old woman with no risk factors
   B. A 62-year-old man with no risk factors
   C. A 64-year-old woman with risk factors
   D. A repeat test on a 70-year-old woman whose initial screen was negative
   E. A repeat test on a 70-year-old man whose initial screen was negative

6. A patient presents with fatigue, osteoporosis, nausea, and hypertension. Lab studies reveal normal creatinine, normal BUN, high calcium, low phosphorous, and high PTH. Which of the following is most likely to be causing this disorder?

   A. Hypertrophy of all four parathyroid glands
   B. Adenoma of one parathyroid gland
   C. Carcinoma of a parathyroid gland
   D. Chronic renal failure
   E. Secondary hyperparathyroidism

7. A patient presents with tremor, weight loss, heat intolerance, sweating, and tachycardia. Lab results are: T_3 and T4 elevated, TSH elevated, TRH elevated. Which of the following is most likely the cause of this patient's hyperthyroidism?

   A. Hypothalamic tumor
   B. Pituitary tumor
   C. Thyroid tumor
   D. Graves' disease
   E. Hashimoto's thyroiditis
   F. Exogenous thyroid hormone

Questions

ANSWERS

1. **Answer: E.** Since the patient is on insulin, insulin levels would be positive. Insulin antibodies should not exist, but if they did, they would not differentiate Type 1 from Type 2 since they would exist owing to exogenous insulin use. C-reactive protein is a test for inflammation and does not give information about diabetes. Hgb A_{1c} would be the same whether the patient had Type 1 or Type 2. C-peptide is the connecting peptide for the alpha and beta chains of insulin in the proinsulin molecule and remains when endogenous insulin is cleaved from proinsulin. C-peptide would only be present if the patient had the ability to produce their own insulin. If C-peptide was zero, the patient would have Type 1 by definition. If C-peptide is present, the patient would have Type 2.

2. **Answer: D.** The patient has diagnostic criteria of DM2 which is part of the IRS. Other parts of this syndrome can include: central obesity, hypertension, low HDL, high triglycerides, DM2, high uric acid levels, low PAI-1, NASH (fatty liver), PCOS (in females), and OSA.

3. **Answer: C.** Weight loss (lifestyle changes, diet, exercise, bariatric surgery) is the most potent therapy for Type 2 DM. None of the medications are as potent as weight loss. Insulin is the most potent medication, but not the most potent therapy.

4. **Answer: D.** Native Americans have the highest prevalence of DM2 in the United States followed by African Americans, Latinos, Caucasians, and Asian Americans.

5. **Answer: C.** The USPSTF recommends screening women at age 65 with no risk factors or women less than 65 who have risks that equal or are greater than a woman at age 65. Repeat tests after negative screens have never proven to be useful. There is insufficient evidence to recommend screening for men (I recommendation).

6. **Answer: B.** A parathyroid adenoma is the most common cause of hypercalcemia associated with elevated PTH (disorder of parathyroid glands)—85% to 95%. Hypertrophy of all four glands and carcinoma are both rare. Secondary hyperparathyroidism (resistance to PTH) would result in low calcium. A normal BUN and creatinine rule out chronic renal failure.

7. **Answer: A.** Normally, TRH from the hypothalamus stimulates the pituitary to produce TSH which stimulates the thyroid to produce thyroid hormone which feeds back to the hypothalamus to reduce TRH. A pituitary tumor, thyroid tumor, Graves', early Hashimoto's, and exogenous thyroid hormone would all produce excess T3/T4 which would result in a lowering of TRH, but this patient has a high TRH. This combination of labs could only be produced by a hypothalamic tumor producing excess TRH.

Answers

CARE OF THE OLDER ADULT

Susan Schrimpf Davis • Soumya Nadella

17

I. Medicare and Medicaid

A. **Medicare:** federal insurance program run by Centers for Medicare and Medicaid Services (CMS) which pays to provide healthcare for Americans $\geq$ 65 years of age, disabled, or with end-stage renal disease
   1. Part A: covers hospitals, skilled nursing home, home-health, and hospice services. Begins when Social Security starts. Has no premium (Table 17-1)
   2. Part B: covers physicians, nurse practitioners, psychologists, social workers, therapists, lab tests, and durable medical equipment. Optional, has a premium.
   3. Part C: provides benefits offered in parts A and B through Medicare advantage plans which are managed care plans
   4. Part D: covers some of the cost for prescription medications

B. **Medicaid:** joint federal and state program that provides health insurance for people of all ages with low income and limited savings. The exact criteria to qualify for Medicaid and the benefits vary from state to state.

II. Pharmacotherapy in the Elderly

A. **Age-associated pharmacokinetic changes**
   1. Absorption: The *extent* of drug absorption does not change with age, although the *rate* of absorption is slowed.
   2. Distribution: *Hydrophilic* drugs have a *lower* volume of distribution because they have less body water and lean body mass. On the same note, *lipophilic* drugs have a *higher* volume of distribution because older patients have more fat stores than younger patients.
   3. Metabolism: Liver is the most common site of drug metabolism. With aging, there is decrease in liver blood flow and decrease in the size and mass of the liver.
   4. Elimination: Glomerular filtration decreases owing to decrease in renal size and blood flow. Also, there is a decrease in nephron function.

TABLE 17-1 Eligibility and Coverage for Nursing Home Services

Facility	Eligibility	Room and Board	Physician Services	Medication
Subacute	For Medicare beneficiaries requiring skilled care after a 3-d acute hospitalization.	Medicare Part A	Medicare Part B or C	Medicare Part A or C
Nursing care	Activities of daily living (ADL)/instrumental activities of daily living (IADL) needs	Medicaid, long-term care insurance, private pay	Medicare Part B or C	Medicare Part D

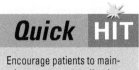

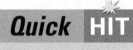

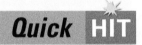

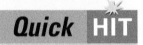

Care of the Older Adult

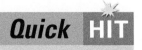

B. **Age-associated pharmacodynamic changes:**
 1. It is less predictable and often altered drug response at usual or a lower drug concentration.
 2. Any drug can cause any side effect at any time in an older patient.

C. **Prescribing pearls**
 1. Review medications regularly and especially when prescribing new medications.
 2. Create dosing regimens based on patient's creatinine clearance not just the creatinine.
 3. Start medications on a low dose and titrate slowly based on the patient's response and tolerability.
 4. Titrate medication to a therapeutic dose before switching to or adding a new medication.
 5. Educate patient and or families regarding each medication and its adverse effects.
 6. Avoid using one medication to treat the adverse events caused by another.
 7. Choose medications that can treat more than one condition to reduce daily pill load and to reduce adverse drug reactions.
 8. Avoid using drugs from the same class or with similar mechanism of action.
 9. When discontinuing medication, taper slowly, one drug at a time.
 10. Refer to American Geriatric Society Beers criteria for list of medications to avoid or use with caution in geriatric population. http://onlinelibrary.wiley.com/doi/10.1111/jgs.13702/full.

III. Delirium

A. **Characteristics**
 1. Acute period of cognitive dysfunction owing to a medical disturbance or condition
 2. Older patients are prone to delirium, approximately one-third of older adults presenting to the emergency department are delirious.
 3. It can persist for weeks to months

B. **Causes**
 1. Drugs: any new drugs, increased dosages or interactions. Also consider over-the-counter (OTC) drugs, postoperative status, and alcohol abuse.
 2. Electrolyte disturbances, endocrine: dehydration, sodium imbalance, thyroid abnormalities
 3. Lack of drugs: withdrawals from chronically used sedative (alcohol and sleeping pills), poorly controlled pain
 4. Infection: urinary and respiratory
 5. Reduced sensory input: poor vision, poor hearing
 6. Intracranial: infection, tumor, stroke, hemorrhage
 7. Urinary retention and fecal impaction
 8. Myocardial and pulmonary: myocardial infarction (MI), arrhythmia, congestive heart failure (CHF) exacerbation, chronic obstructive pulmonary disease (COPD) exacerbation, hypoxia

C. **Clinical features**
 1. Agitation or hyperactive: classical presentation, only 25% of cases
 2. Hypoactive or quiet: more common

D. **Diagnosis**
 1. Detailed history and physical exam
 2. Complete blood count (CBC), electrolytes, renal function tests, urinalysis, urine toxicology, blood alcohol level, liver function tests, serum medication levels, arterial blood gases, chest radiographs, electrocardiogram (ECG), and selected cultures can be helpful.
 3. Bedside tool: confusion assessment method (Figure 17-1)

E. **Treatment**
 1. Modifying the risk factors that are contributing to delirium
 2. Treat the underlying cause.
 3. Managing behavioral problems while ensuring comfort and safety of the patient

4. Prevention measures: providing orientation items like clocks, calendars, a window view, and familiar family or friend interaction
5. Remove or reduce medications that contribute to delirium: anticholinergics, H₂-blockers, benzodiazepines, opioids, antipsychotics.
6. Pharmacologic management may be necessary for symptoms such as delusions or hallucinations (Table 17-2).

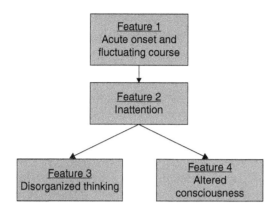

17-1 Confusion assessment method for recognizing delirium provides a model to diagnose delirium. Delirium involves four key features: acute onset and fluctuating course, inattention, disorganized thinking, and altered level of consciousness. Diagnosis of delirium requires features 1 and 2 plus either 3 or 4.

TABLE 17-2 Pharmacologic Management of Agitated Delirium

Agent	Mechanism of Action	Dosage	Benefits	Adverse Events
Haloperidol	Antipsychotic	0.25–1 mg po, IM, or IV q4h prn agitation	Relatively non-sedating; few hemodynamic effects	Extrapyramidal symptoms (EPS), especially if >3 mg/d, avoid in Parkinson's and Lewy-body dementia
Risperidone	Second-generation antipsychotic	0.25–1 mg po q4h prn agitation	Similar to haloperidol	Might have slightly fewer EPS than haloperidol
Olanzapine	Second-generation antipsychotic	2.5–5 mg po or IM q12h, max dosage 20 mg q24h (cannot be given by IV infusion)	Fewer EPS than haloperidol	More sedating than haloperidol
Quetiapine	Second-generation antipsychotic	25–50 mg po q12h	Fewer EPS than haloperidol	More sedating than haloperidol; hypotension
Lorazepam	Benzodiazepine	0.25–1 mg po or IV q8h prn agitation	Use in sedative and alcohol withdrawal; history of neuroleptic malignant syndrome	More paradoxical excitation, respiratory depression than haloperidol

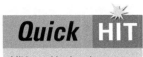

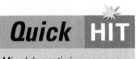

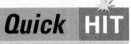

Care of the Older Adult

IV. Dementia

A. Characteristics
1. Dementia is a general term used to describe several disorders that cause significant decline in one or more of cognitive functioning that are severe enough to result in functional decline.
2. Onset usually after 65 years of age
3. Common dementia (Tables 17-3 and 17-4)
   a. Alzheimer disease:
      i. Most common type of dementia, 50% to 80%
      ii. Affecting 6% to 8% of individuals ≥65 years old and 50% or more of those who are ≥85 years old
      iii. Clinically characterized by gradual onset with linear progressive decline in cognitive functioning
      iv. The average time from onset to death is 5 to 10 years (variable).
      v. Memory impairment is the core symptom. Motor and sensory deficits occur in the late stages of the disease.
      vi. Risk factors: age, family history, Down syndrome
   b. Vascular dementia/multi-infract dementia:
      i. Second most common cause of dementia, 20% to 30%
      ii. Clinically characterized by sudden or stepwise decline rather than linear decline in cognitive function
      iii. Risk factors: cerebrovascular accident (CVA) (size of the infract may not matter, what matters is the functional and clinical picture of the patient)

B. Diagnosis
1. Most cases of dementia can be diagnosed on the basis of history from reliable informant, general medical and cognitive testing.
2. Both the patient and the reliable informant should be interviewed regarding patient's current condition, medical, medication history, living arrangements, onset of change, ability to perform activities of daily living.
3. Determination of onset and nature of symptoms can help differentiate between different clinical syndromes and premorbid personality.
4. A comprehensive physical examination should include neurologic and cognitive testing (Table 17-5).
5. Rule out treatable causes with CBC, basic metabolic panel, TSH, vitamin B_{12}.
6. Optional testing based on clinical history and examination: liver function tests (LFTs), HIV, fluorescent treponemal antibody (FTA) to r/o syphilis, urine analysis, cerebrospinal fluid (CSF) analysis, urine tox screen
7. Imaging of the brain:
   a. Not required but can be helpful in certain situations
   b. Computed tomography (CT) without contrast: can show normal pressure hydrocephalus (NPH), cerebral atrophy, chronic subdural hemorrhage

TABLE 17-3	Causes of Chronic Memory Loss	
Potentially Reversible Causes	**Irreversible Causes**
Hypothyroidism	Alzheimer disease
Neurosyphilis	Parkinson's
Vitamin B_{12}	Huntington's
Medications	Vascular dementia
Normal pressure hydrocephalus	Lewy-body dementia
Depression (pseudodementia)	Unresectable brain mass
Subdural hematoma	HIV dementia
	Korsakoff syndrome (alcohol)
	Creutzfeldt–Jakob disease
	Progressive multifocal leukoencephalopathy.
	Chronic traumatic encephalopathy

| TABLE **17-4** Diagnostic Features and Treatment of Dementia Syndromes |||||||
Syndrome	Onset	Cognitive Domains, Symptoms	Motor Symptoms	Progression	Imaging	Pharmacologic Treatment of Cognition
Mild cognitive impairment	Gradual	Primarily memory	Rare	Unknown, 12% per year proceed to Alzheimer disease	Possible global atrophy, small hippocampal volumes	Cholinesterase inhibitors (ChIs) possibly protective for 18 months in subset of patients
Alzheimer disease	Gradual	Memory, language, visuospatial	Rare early, apraxia later	Gradual (over 8–10 yr)	Possible global atrophy, small hippocampal volumes	ChI for mild-to-severe and memantine for moderate-to-severe stages
Vascular dementia	May be sudden or stepwise	Depends on location of ischemia	Correlates with ischemia	Gradual or stepwise with further ischemia	Cortical or subcortical changes on MRI	Consider ChI for memory deficit only; risk factor modifiers
Lewy-body dementia	Gradual	Memory, visuospatial, hallucinations, fluctuating symptoms	Parkinsonism	Gradual but faster than Alzheimer disease	Possible global atrophy	ChI; ± carbidopa/levodopa for movement
Frontotemporal dementia	Gradual; age <60 yr	Executive, disinhibition, apathy, language, ± memory	None	Gradual but faster than Alzheimer disease	Atrophy in frontal and temporal lobes	Not recommended per current evidence

Data from the Geriatric Review Syllabus (8th ed.).

Care of the Older Adult

| TABLE **17-5** | Screening Instruments for Evaluation of Cognition: Examples of Testing |

Instrument Name	Items Scoring	Domains Assessed
Mini-cog	Two items Score = 5 Normal = 3-word recall or 1- or 2-word recall with normal clock drawing	Visuospatial, executive function, recall
St. Louis University Mental Status Examination (SLUMS)	11 items Score = 30 Normal ≥ 27	Orientation, recall, calculation, naming, attention, executive function
Montreal Cognitive Assessment (MoCA)	12 items Score = 30 Normal ≥ 26	Orientation, recall, attention, naming, repletion, verbal fluency, abstraction, executive function, visuospatial
Folstein Mini-Mental Status Examination	19 items Score = 30 Normal ≥ 24	Orientation, registration, attention, recall, naming, repetition, three-step command, language, visuospatial

Scores will reflect cognitive performance, not level of dementia or a "positive/negative" score.

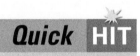

Quick HIT

Primary care doctors can diagnose and treat most cases of dementia without referring to a specialist.

Quick HIT

There is actually better evidence and more significant results in caregiver interventions than any other treatments in dementia.

Quick HIT

Discussion about driving is best started early in treatment. Referral for an independent driving assessment can be useful if there is a question of whether it is safe for the patient to drive.

Quick HIT

Antidepressants play a role in treatment of early dementia patients. Make sure to assess for depressive symptoms such as depressed mood, appetite loss, fatigue, agitation, insomnia.

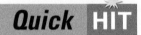

(sidebar) Care of the Older Adult

c. Magnetic resonance imaging (MRI) with contrast: better for vascular disease and tumors
d. Indications for imaging: ≤65 years of age, sudden or rapidly progressive symptoms, and neurological deficits on physical examination, history of trauma or recent fall
e. Neuropsych testing: usually not needed to make a diagnosis; reserve for unusual cases, young patients, or if the diagnosis is questionable

C. **Treatment**
1. The main goals of treatment are to enhance quality of life, maximize functional performance by improving cognition, mood, and behavior.
2. Nonpharmacologic treatment:
   a. Cognitive rehabilitation and supportive therapy
   b. Family and caregiver education and support
   c. Environmental modification and attention to safety
3. Pharmacologic treatment:
   a. Cholinesterase inhibitors: donepezil, rivastigmine, galantamine, and tacrine
      i. Mild-to-moderate Alzheimer disease
      ii. Slows down the breakdown neurotransmitter acetylcholine
      iii. Adverse reactions are common: nausea, diarrhea, insomnia, headaches, dizziness, orthostasis, and nightmares.
   b. N-methyl-D-aspartate antagonist (NMDA antagonist): memantine
      i. Moderate-to-severe Alzheimer disease
      ii. Thought to bind NMDA receptors slowing down the calcium influx and nerve damage
      iii. Adverse reactions: constipation, dizziness, and headache
   c. Other cognitive enhancers
      i. Ginkgo biloba extract: not proven to be beneficial
      ii. High-dose vitamin E (2,000 IU/day): used in the past, but a recent study showed increased mortality and is no longer recommended

V. Palliative Care and Hospice
A. **Palliative care**
1. Characteristics:
   a. Interdisciplinary treatment of symptoms of suffering

b. Goals: improve quality of life outside of curative therapies. This is done by addressing function, managing comorbid symptoms, assisting with complex medical decision making, and helping families cope with advanced stages of illness.

c. WHO definition: "Palliative care is an approach that improves the quality of life of patients and their families facing the problem associated with life-threatening illness, through the prevention and relief of suffering by means of early identification and impeccable assessment and treatment of pain and other problems, physical, psychosocial, and spiritual."

2. Common problems in palliative care

a. Pain
   i. Identify history of pain: acute versus chronic
   ii. Determine type: nocioceptive/neuropathic/functonal/psychogenic-spiritual
   iii. Assess if breakthrough pain or end dose failure of medication
   iv. Use numerical or visual analog scale to determine severity.

b. Constipation
   i. Causes: include antacids, diuretics, iron, antihypertensives, and calcium channel blockers, narcotic pain medications
   ii. Stimulant laxative plus osmotic laxative is first choice for opioid constipation.
   iii. Consider mu receptor antagonists or chloride channel activators as a last choice.

c. Nausea, vomiting
   i. Consider etiology of the nausea first and select antiemetic based on cause.
   ii. Use caution with anticholinergics such as promethazine as they can precipitate delirium in older adults, especially those with dementia.
   iii. Metoclopramide: to treat nausea may also have adverse anticholinergic effects, such as delirium, in older adults, so use caution
   iv. Ondansetron may be useful in the nauseated older adult, owing to lack of anticholinergic effects.

d. Diarrhea
   i. Identify the cause of diarrhea first.
   ii. Rule out infection before using fiber, opioids, or motility agents such as loperamide.

e. Cachexia
   i. Reduced body mass index (BMI) is related to poor prognosis.
   ii. Mirtazapine can be used to stimulate appetite, as well as aid in insomnia and depression in older adults.

f. Delirium
   i. Question staff/caregivers using features of the four areas of the confusion assessment method (CAM) model: inattention, fluctuating course, altered consciousness, and disorganized thinking.
   ii. Also use Single Question in Delirium (SQUiD): "Do you think they are acting differently today compared to yesterday?" This single question test has been shown in the literature to have high sensitivity and specificity for identifying delirium.

g. Dyspnea
   i. Prepare caregivers for dyspnea. Preparation may be the one of the best tools for management.
   ii. Assess etiology; consider morphine, laxatives, benzodiazepines, selective serotonin reuptake inhibitors (SSRIs), repositioning, fan, O_2.

h. Cough
   i. Consider phrenic nerve involvement by tumor.
   ii. Use centrally acting cough suppressants or bronchodilators for symptom management.

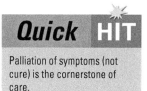

Quick HIT

Palliation of symptoms (not cure) is the cornerstone of care.

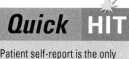

Quick HIT

Patient self-report is the only valid measure of pain.

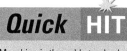

Quick HIT

Morphine is the gold standard for pain in palliative care and hospice.

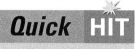

Quick HIT

All patients on routine narcotics should have a bowel regimen in place.

Care of the Older Adult

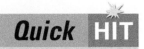

     i. Hiccups/hic-coughs: dextromethorphan cough syrup or benzodiazepines may be helpful

    j. Loud respirations/"death rattle"

      i. Educate family and staff on anticipating oropharyngeal "noise."

      ii. Judicious use of anticholinergics has not been justified in the literature, but some choose to use them to dry excess secretions once the patient is unconscious. Anticholinergics can precipitate delirium in the older adult.

    k. Myoclonus: Benzodiazepines help in treating myoclonus, after reduction of opioids. Phenytoin may be used in prevention.

  3. Evaluation: Be prepared for addressing seemingly "cognitive" questions with empathy. Be mindful of the enormous emotional stress patients and caregivers may be experiencing.

B. **Hospice**

  1. General characteristics:

    a. Hospice care is a comprehensive care system provided to patients nearing the end of life.

    b. Federal government initiated hospice care as U.S. Medicare healthcare benefit in 1982.

    c. The hospice care company (either nonprofit or for-profit) becomes the health maintenance organization (HMO) for the terminal diagnosis.

  2. Access/eligibility:

    a. Determination of prognosis estimated as less than 6 months by a physician

    b. Patient or proxy must elect for the hospice care benefit and agree to the hospice plan of care.

    c. Live discharge from hospice

      i. The patient revokes.

      ii. Patient transfers to another hospice company.

      iii. The patient is discharged because the illness stabilizes and they no longer meet hospice criteria.

  3. Dimensions of end-of-life care that can vary culturally:

    a. Communication of bad news

    b. Locus of decision making

    c. Attitudes and directives at end of life

  4. Evaluation of the hospice patient:

    a. Common diagnoses: cancer, dementia, heart disease, lung disease, stroke, kidney disease, liver disease, amyotrophic lateral sclerosis (ALS) or motor neuron disease, and HIV/AIDS

    b. Functional status and disease state must be determined, and attested to by a physician that if the disease state was left to a natural course, the prognosis would be 6 months or less.

  5. Treatment of the hospice patient

    a. Treatment settings

      i. Most people receive hospice care at home.

      ii. Others receive care in a skilled nursing facility, hospice inpatient unit, or even in the hospital.

    b. Care team

      i. Nurse case manager, a medical director, a spiritual/psychological counselor (chaplain), and a social services coordinator (social worker)

      ii. Palliative services may include music therapy, massage therapy, and any medical therapies determined to be useful to the palliative, not curative, care of the patient.

    c. Special care is given to address the pain and anxiety at the end of life.

    d. Ethical consideration: the rule of "double effect" is especially important in care of patients at end of life. If the intent in offering a treatment is desirable or helpful to the patient and the potential outcome good (such as relief of pain), but a potentially adverse secondary effect is undesired

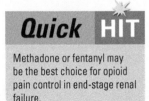

and the potential outcome bad (such as death), then the treatment is considered ethical.

6. Death and bereavement
   a. Grief and bereavement are natural in the dying process.
   b. Anticipatory grief involves looking toward the future without the dying person.
   c. Normal grief is the experience of loss at emotional, cognitive, and physical levels.
   d. Complicated grief is a persistent debilitating phenomenon and has also been referred to as prolonged, traumatic, or pathologic grief. It involves disruptive symptoms that impair functioning over a prolonged period of time. Clinicians should be mindful and anticipate complicated grief if attachment issues or co-dependency exists.

QUESTIONS

1. Which of the following is considered an IADL?:
   A. Ability to dress one's self
   B. Ability to use telephone
   C. Ability to bathe
   D. Ability to ambulate and transfer
   E. Ability to multitask

2. Diagnostic features of dementia include:
   A. Altered level of consciousness
   B. Inattention
   C. Acute onset of symptoms and fluctuating course
   D. Chronic progressive memory impairment
   E. Disorganized thinking

3. A 79-year-old widowed retired school teacher presents to your skilled rehabilitation center for therapy after a 3-day hospitalization. Normally she is independent in all ADLs and IADLS. She had a fall one night at her home when she went up to go to the bathroom and slipped on a rug. Her son found her approximately 5 hours later when he stopped by for breakfast on his way to work. In the hospital, she was diagnosed with a left intertrochanteric femur fracture and a urinary tract infection (*Escherichia coli*). She received open reduction and internal fixation (ORIF) of the hip and antibiotics. She now needs physical therapy, occupational therapy, and skilled nursing. How will this patient's post-acute nursing home stay and rehabilitation be financially covered?
   A. Medicare Part A with secondary insurance
   B. Medicare Part B with secondary insurance
   C. Medicare Part D with secondary insurance
   D. Medicaid

4. An 80-year-old retired electrical engineer presents to your office because of persistent weight loss that he believes is owing to esophageal cancer. He has lost 20 lb in the past 6 months. Past history of cancer screening and workup (upper endoscopy [EGD], CT scan) have been negative. He says he is unable to eat much because of a lump in his throat. He says he "talks" to his deceased wife about his cancer. He does not have suicidal ideation. He has difficulty sleeping, spends much of the day on the couch or in bed, has not been interested in engaging in family activities and is no longer engaged with his hobby of model railways. All laboratory studies, imaging, endoscopy, and swallowing studies are normal. Which of the following is the next best step?
   A. Start quetiapine.
   B. Start sertraline.
   C. Start diazepam.
   D. Start the patient on a BRAT diet.
   E. Start omeprazole.
   F. Refer for a hospice consult.

ANSWERS

1. **Answer: B.** Use of a telephone is an IADL. Dressing one's self, bathing, and ambulating and transferring are ADLs. Ability to multitask is neither an ADL nor an IADL.

2. **Answer: D.** Dementia is disorder that causes significant decline in one or more cognitive functions that are severe enough to result in functional decline. Altered level of consciousness and acute onset of symptoms and fluctuating course are consistent with delirium. Inattention and disorganized thinking are not classic features of dementia.

3. **Answer: A.** Medicare Part A will pay for a rehab stay in a skilled nursing facility following a 3-day or longer hospitalization. Part B pays for outpatient office visits, labs, and some durable medical equipment. Part C is a managed care version of Medicare that combines Parts A, B, and often D and is managed by a private insurance company. Part D covers outpatient prescriptions. Medicaid may pay for this but to qualify, the patient would need to be indigent with minimal assets.

4. **Answer: B.** This patient has depression with psychotic features. The best initial step would be to start an SSRI such as sertraline. Therapy would also be helpful. Referral to a geriatric psychiatrist would be recommended if he worsens or does not really improve. Atypical antipsychotics such as quetiapine are not a first line as they increase mortality rate in the elderly; however, they may be useful in severe and refractory patients. Benzodiazepines such as diazepam should generally be avoided in the elderly. They can cause significant side effects such as worse memory problems and increased fall risk. Restricting a diet in this case would actually be harmful as he is already losing weight. Omeprazole would not be useful. A Hospice referral is not indicated at this time as the patient does not have a terminal disease.

HERBAL MEDICINES AND SUPPLEMENTS

Robert V. Ellis

The 1994 Dietary Supplement Health and Education Act defines dietary supplements and ingredients and classifies them as food. They are regulated by the Food and Drug Administration (FDA) but the rules are not as strict as for prescription or over-the-counter (OTC) medications. Manufacturers of dietary supplements do not have to prove safety or efficacy prior to marketing. The FDA monitors safety and labeling postmarketing and the Federal Trade Commission monitors advertising. Manufacturers are required to follow "Good Manufacturing Practices" and must ensure product consistency and meet quality standards. Dietary supplements are not just single chemicals but multiple compounds that are derived or extracted from "natural" products. As a result, the active ingredient is usually not known and the concentration may vary widely between brands and even production lots. Additional evidenced based information can be found at the National Institutes of Health (NIH) National Center for Complementary and Alternative Medicine web site (http://nccam.nih. gov/health/herbsataglance.htm) or MedlinePlus (http://www.nlm.nih.gov/medlineplus/ druginfo/herb_All.html).

Herbal Medicine or Supplement	Common Use	Dose	Cost per Month	Evidence	Caution	Side Effects
Black cohosh	Hot flashes Vaginal dryness Menopausal symptoms Premenstrual syndrome	20–40 mg twice per day	$5–$10	Studies mixed for menopausal symptoms No evidence for hot flashes	Liver disease Breast cancer No long-term safety studies	GI upset Headache Rash
Calcium	Low bone density Heart disease Acid reflux	500 mg twice per day	$3–$15	May help in low bone density No benefit for heart disease Can buffer in acid reflux	Can be harmful in high doses (>2,500 mg/d) Can have rebound reflux since stimulates acid production	Gas Bloating Constipation
CoQ-10	Muscle aches associated with statins Congestive heart failure (CHF) Angina Parkinson's	100–200 mg daily	$10–$20	Small studies support use in CoQ-10 deficiency and mitochondrial disorders Limited evidence to support other claims	Increase risk of bleeding, avoid perioperatively Decreases affect of warfarin	GI upset Headache
Cranberry	Urinary tract infection (UTI) prevention Helicobacter pylori stomach ulcer prevention	Juice: 10–30 oz daily Capsules: 300–400 mg daily	Capsules $3–$4	Does not treat UTI Some evidence for UTI prevention in high-risk patients	Generally safe Caution with blood thinning medicines Increased risk of nephrolithiasis	GI upset Diarrhea
Dehydroepiandrosterone (DHEA)	Weight loss Increase muscle mass Erectile dysfunction Low bone density	25–50 mg daily	$4–$15	Possibly effective for erectile dysfunction, low bone density, and schizophrenia, but evidence is weak No evidence for other claims	**Banned by NCAA, Olympics, professional sports** May be harmful if used in large amounts or long term Do not use if pregnant or breast feeding, hormone sensitive conditions, liver disease	Acne Hair loss High BP GI upset Menstrual changes Facial hair in women Gynecomastia
Echinacea	Treat and prevent colds, flu, and other infections	250 mg 4 times daily	$8–$10	Mixed results on prevention and treatment of URI	Avoid if allergy to ragweed, daisies, etc. Asthma or atopy	GI Rash

(continued)

Herbal Medicines and Supplements

Herbal Medicine or Supplement	Common Use	Dose	Cost per Month	Evidence	Caution	Side Effects
Ephedra (ma huang)	Weight loss Increase energy Increased athletic performance	N/A	N/A	Risks outweigh benefits	**Banned in the U.S. (2004)** Increase risk of stroke, arrhythmias, MI, death Can still find in Chinese herbal remedies/products	Palpitations Chest pain Weight loss Jitteriness Anxiety
Flaxseed oil	Constipation High cholesterol Hot flashes	600–1,000 mg 1–3 times per day	$7–$12	Fair evidence for constipation Mixed results for cholesterol and hot flashes	Take with plenty of water Do not take with other meds, may lower absorption	Usually well tolerated Diarrhea
Fish oil and omega fatty acids	High cholesterol Heart disease Hypertension Arthritis Many others	1–4 g/d	$6–$30	Most evidence for hypertriglyceridemia and heart disease	High doses increase risk of bleeding, avoid perioperatively	Belching Bad breath Loose stool Heartburn Nausea **Taking with food and freezing caps can reduce side effects**
Garlic	High cholesterol Heart disease Hypertension	Extract: 200–400 mg 3 times/d Fresh: 1 clove daily	$5	May slightly lower cholesterol but evidence mixed May slow atherosclerosis but studies are preliminary May slightly lower BP	Can increase bleeding risk, avoid perioperatively Interacts with saquinavir (HIV med)	Usually well tolerated Breath/body odor Heartburn GI upset
Ginkgo biloba	Dementia Claudication Tinnitus	60–120 2 times/d	$5–$15	Ineffective for prevention or treatment of dementia No significant benefit in claudication Conflicting data for tinnitus	Can increase bleeding risk Discontinue perioperatively Avoid products containing *Ginkgo* seeds	Headache Nausea GI upset Diarrhea Dizziness

Supplement	Uses	Dose	Cost	Evidence	Considerations	Adverse effects
Ginseng	Improve mental and physical performance Lowering blood glucose	200 mg twice per day Glucose: 3 g prior to meals	$5–$10	Some studies show a small lowering of blood glucose No significant evidence for other claims	May lower blood sugars, caution with diabetic meds	Headaches Insomnia GI problems
Glucosamine and chondroitin	Osteoarthritis	G: 1,500 mg daily C: 1,200 mg daily	$15	Large trial showed no benefit except for small subgroup with moderate-to-severe pain (findings preliminary owing to the small size of this subgroup)	Do not take with warfarin Stop perioperatively as it can affect glucose levels	GI symptoms
Kava	Anxiety Insomnia Fatigue	Anxiety: 100–250 mg 1–3 times daily Insomnia: 250–500 mg at bedtime	$8–$15	Some evidence for anxiety No evidence for other claims	**FDA warning: linked to a risk of severe liver damage**	Liver failure Dystonia Drowsiness
Melatonin	Insomnia	1–5 mg 2 hr prior to sleep	$1–$3	May improve sleep latency	Safe for short-term use	Nausea Headache Dizziness Drowsiness
Niacin (B$_3$)	High cholesterol Heart disease prevention Niacin deficiency (pellagra)	1–3 g/d	$10–$15	Good evidence for lowering cholesterol (triglycerides) and deficiency No outcomes-based data for cholesterol	Alcohol can make flushing worse Start with small dose and titrate slowly to reduce side effects Can increase fasting glucose levels in diabetics (<5%)	Flushing of the face, arms, and chest is common **325 mg ASA prior to taking niacin decreases flushing** Headaches GI upset

(continued)

Herbal Medicines and Supplements

Herbal Medicines and Supplements

Herbal Medicine or Supplement	Common Use	Dose	Cost per Month	Evidence	Caution	Side Effects
Probiotics	Diarrhea Prevent UTI IBS Shorten *Clostridium difficile* Vaginosis	Type of probiotic and dose vary	$20–$30	Some data for all of these but effect usually low and more research is needed	Effects of one strain/species not necessarily similar to another or even for different preparations of the same strain	Usually well tolerated Mild GI symptoms
Saw palmetto	Urinary symptoms from BPH	320 mg daily	$5–$10	No evidence for improving BPH symptoms Does not reduce the size of prostate	Does not affect PSA levels	Usually well tolerated Mild stomach discomfort
Soy	High cholesterol HTN Hot flashes Osteoporosis	Extract: 500–1,000 mg daily	$5	May slightly lower LDL May reduce hot flashes but results inconsistent No evidence for other claims	Caution in woman with or at high risk for hormone responsive cancers (breast/ovarian) Safety of long-term use not established	Usually well tolerated Minor GI upset
St. John's wort	Depression Anxiety Sleep disorders	300 mg 3 times/d	$5–$10	May be useful in mild-to-moderate depression Not beneficial in major depressive disorder	Many drug interactions: • Antidepressants • Birth control pills • Warfarin • Antiseizure meds • Digoxin • Cyclosporine • Others	Sunlight sensitivity Anxiety Dry mouth Dizziness GI symptoms Headache Sexual dysfunction
Valerian	Insomnia Anxiety Depression Headaches	400–900 mg 2 h prior to bedtime	$2–$6	May be helpful in insomnia, but studies small and not well designed No evidence for other claims	Safe for short-term use (4–6 wk) Safety of long-term use not established	Headache Dizziness GI upset Morning fatigue ("hangover")

	Uses	Dose	Cost	Evidence	Cautions	Side effects
Vitamin C	Vitamin C deficiency (scurvy) Common cold	Deficiency: 100–250 mg 1–2 times/d URI: 1–2 g daily	$1–$3	Good evidence for preventing and treating deficiency Low-quality studies show it may shorten URI by 1–1.5 d, does not prevent URI	Do not take more than 2 g/d Caution in diabetics, kidney stones, sickle cell, and G6PDD	Headache GI upset
Vitamin D	Low bone density Breastfeeding infants 2–6 mo Rickets	Low bone density: 400–800 IU daily Infant: 400 IU daily	$1–$5	When taken with calcium, may help low bone density AAP recommends for all breast fed infants Prevent rickets No quality evidence for other claims	Do not exceed 4,000 IU/d	Anorexia Palpitations
Vitamin E	Fat-malabsorption disorders Coronary heart disease Macular degeneration Cognitive decline	400 IU daily	$1–$3	Recommended in fat-malabsorption disorders No or conflicting evidence for other claims	High doses increase risk of bleeding, avoid perioperatively Some studies showed increased risk of hemorrhagic stroke and prostate cancer	Dizziness Fatigue Headache Blurred vision GI symptoms
Yohimbe	Erectile dysfunction	15–30 mg of yohimbine alkaloids daily	$10–$25	No good-quality trials	Dangerous in large doses or for long periods of time Do not take in kidney or psychiatric disease, pregnant or breast feeding Do not take with MAOI, BP meds, tricyclic antidepressants, or phenothiazides	High BP Palpitations Headache Dizziness GI upset Tremors Insomnia Priapism

AAP, American Academy of Pediatrics; ASA, acetylsalicylic acid; BP, blood pressure; BPH, benign prostatic hypertrophy; GI, gastrointestinal; G6PDD, glucose-6-phosphate dehydrogenase deficiency; HTN, hypertension; IBS, irritable bowel syndrome; LDL, low-density lipoprotein; MAOI, monoamine oxidase inhibitor; NCAA, National Collegiate Athletic Association; PSA, prostate specific antigen; URI, upper respiratory infection.

Herbal Medicines and Supplements

OVER-THE-COUNTER MEDICATIONS

Robert V. Ellis

 History

- Very popular with patients—biggest reason: don't have to see a doctor
- Can treat over 400 common ailments
- More and more products going Rx to over-the-counter (OTC)
- First drug law—1906—Food, Drug, and Cosmetics Act (T. Roosevelt). Truth in Labeling is purpose.
- 1937—Safety is added after a disaster in Arkansas in which many kids died from a medicine.
- 1951—Food and Drug Administration (FDA) created; public's right to OTC confirmed
- 1963—Efficacy added to truthful labels and safety
- 1972—Review of OTCs to meet standards of efficacy
- 1994—Dietary Supplement Health and Education Act; defines dietary supplements and ingredients and classifies them as food

 Upper Respiratory Infection (URI)

- Over 800 products
- Combination of one or more of the following classes:
  - Decongestants:
    - Mechanism: sympathomimetics: Vasoconstriction leads to shrinking of nasal mucosa which leads to improved air flow.
    - Easy to document efficacy with flow meters; has the most data on efficacy versus other URI medications
    - Side effects—sympathomimetic
      - Increased heart rate (HR), BP, jitteriness, decreased sleep, urinary retention
      - Caution in patients with hypertension (HTN), coronary artery disease (CAD), benign prostatic hyperplasia (BPH)
    - Examples
      - Pseudoephedrine (PSE)
      - Phenylephrine (PE)
      - Afrin (oxymetazoline)—nasal
        - Use more than a few days causes tolerance and rebound congestion. Use for no more than 3 days.
        - Effective for patients with congestion and are going to fly. Use 30 minutes prior to departure.
  - Antihistamines:
    - Mechanism: block histamine release from mast cells
    - Are URIs and symptoms of URI a histamine-driven response? No
    - Are allergies a histamine-driven response? Yes
    - Side effects—drowsiness (used in OTC sleep aids)
    - OK'd for URI owing to an atropine-like drying effect on nasal secretions
      - No role except for drying secretions

- ○ Examples
  - ▪ H_1: sedating: diphenylamine (Benadryl), chlorpheniramine
  Non-sedating: loratadine (Claritin), cetirizine (Zyrtec), fexofenadine (Allegra)
  - ▪ H_2: nonsedating: gastrointestinal (GI) (see GI meds)—also used as 2nd-line tx for urticaria
- Antitussive:
  - ○ Mechanism: opioid analogue, central acting
    - ▪ Gold standard is morphine.
  - ○ Studies are equivocal on efficacy. Cough can be a protective reflex.
  - ○ Can use if cough causing pain, vomiting, sleep disturbance, work difficulty
  - ○ Example: dextromethorphan (DM)
- Expectorant:
  - ○ Mechanism: mucolytic, easier clearance of secretions leads to decrease in cough
  - ○ Studies are old and small numbers: patients only reported that secretions/mucus were thinner.
  - ○ Very safe
  - ○ Example: guaifenesin (Mucinex)
- Saline:
  - ○ Drops (for infants): no real data for this but gives mom and dad something to do
  - ○ Sinus rinse (neti pot):
    - ▪ Cochrane review: no evidence in URI, although no harm; fair evidence in chronic sinusitis
    - ▪ Case reports of amoeba brain abscess but untreated well water was used without the saline packet
- Nasal steroids:
  - ○ Very effective for allergy symptoms
  - ○ OTC: fluticasone (Flonase) and mometasone (Nasonex)
- Peds: No cough meds prior to 4 years old (American Academy of Pediatrics [AAP] recommendation)
- Many combination products contain Tylenol. Warn patients about mixing products.

Analgesics

- Acetaminophen (Tylenol)
  - Adults: Max 4,000 mg/d
  - Peds: 10 to 15 mg/kg every 6 hours
  - Side effects
    - ○ Liver failure: Watch for acute or chronic use.
    - ○ Avoid in patients with liver problems, alcohol
  - Often an additional ingredient in many OTCs; high potential for unintentional overdose
- Nonsteroidal anti-inflammatory drugs (NSAIDs)
  - Ibuprofen (Motrin, Advil)
    - ○ Adults: 200 to 400 mg every 4 to 6 hours
    - ○ Peds: 4 to 10 mg/kg/dose every 6 to 8 hours; max. daily dose: 40 mg/kg/d
  - Naproxen (Aleve): adults: 220 mg tabs, 1 to 2 tabs twice daily
  - Ketoprofen (Orudis): oral version no longer marketed OTC in the U.S.
  - Side effects:
    - ○ Peptic ulcer disease: 50% of NSAID ulcers are from OTCs
    - ○ Renal effects: can worsen renal function
- Acetylsalicylic acid (ASA, aspirin)
  - Discourage use as a pain reliever owing to risk of bleeding and GI ulcers.
  - Use for cardiovascular prophylaxis and treatment.
  - 81 mg daily for most indications
  - Avoid in children (risk of Reye's syndrome).
- Topicals:
  - Oral topical
    - ○ Benzocaine (Orajel): not for children under 2 years old
    - ○ Chloraseptic spray (Phenol)

- Skin
  - NSAIDs (ketoprofen and others)
  - Menthol, camphor: local vasodilation (IcyHot, Tiger Balm, others)
  - Capsaicin: works on nerve ending, depletes them of substance P (pain-inducing peptide), burns when first start using
  - Heating pads
  - Freeze sprays
  - Lidocaine patch

Gastrointestinal tract (GI)

●●● Anti-diarrhea

- Pepto-Bismol (bismuth subsalicylate), also Kaopectate (Kaopectate has gone from pectin to attapulgite to bismuth subsalicylate over the years. Keep the recognized/trusted name, but change the ingredient.)
  - Antibacterial
  - Can be used for traveler's diarrhea prophylaxis
  - Turns stool very dark, can be confused for blood in stool
  - The salicylate component can be a problem for people.
- Loperamide—Imodium AD
  - Slows gut transit
  - Very effective
  - Can cause constipation (caution in children)
  - Caution if suspect a bacterial cause
- Polycarbophil (Fiber—FiberCon)
  - Bulking agent
  - Absorbent—60 times its weight, but takes 3 days to work
  - Used as stool normalizer
- Pectin
  - Was in Kaopectate but no longer
  - Now more of an herbal medicine
  - Diarrhea and constipation
  - From cell wall of many fruits and nuts (apples)

●●● Constipation

- Lifestyle modifications:
  - ↑ fluids, ↑ dietary fiber, ↑ activity
- Two-step process in treatment:
  - Get rid of the hard stool in the rectal vault usually with an enema, suppository, or stimulant.
  - Diagnose and treat the underlying problem that led to this. Chronic daily use of an osmotic or softener may be needed.
- Medications:
  - Most take 1 to 3 days to work (exception: stimulants, enemas, and suppositories)
- Fiber (20 to 35 g/d):
  - Bulking laxatives
    - Metamucil – Psyllium husk
    - Citrucel – methylcellulose
    - Benefiber – hydrolyzed guar gum
    - FiberSure – inulin
    - FiberCon – polycarbophil
  - Stool softeners
    - Mineral oil/others
      - Possible concern of aspiration
    - Colace (docusate sodium)
  - Osmotic laxatives

- Saline agents
  - Milk of magnesia
  - Magnesium sulfate
  - Sodium phosphate
  - Sodium sulfate
  - Sugar alcohols
    - Lactulose, sorbitol (juices)
  - Macrogols
    - Polyethylene glycol (MiraLAX)
      - Gentle for children/elderly
  - Stimulants (oral and suppository forms)
    - Bisacodyl (Dulcolax)
    - Anthraquinones
    - Sennosides (Senokot)
    - Cascara
  - Other suppositories
    - Glycerin
  - Enemas
    - Work by distending colon and inducing evacuation
      - Phosphate (Fleet), tap water, soap suds, mineral oil, others
    - Side effects: mechanical trauma, hyperphosphatemia (Fleet)

Heartburn/Reflux Meds

- Acid buffers
  - Calcium (Tums)
    - Double-edged sword: buffers acid but also stimulates acid production
    - Mg + Ca (Rolaids)
- H_2 blockers
  - Safe for long-term use
  - Examples
    - Ranitidine (Zantac)
    - Famotidine (Pepcid)
      - Comes in combination with calcium (Pepcid-AC)
    - Cimetidine (Tagamet)
      - Advise not to use: frequent drug interactins (P450 inhibitor)
- Proton pump inhibitors (PPIs)
  - Very effective
  - Long-term use
    - Increases risk of pneumonia, *Clostridium difficile*, *Helicobacter pylori*
    - Increases risk of osteoporosis
    - Associated with stomach polyps
    - Can decrease Mg levels
    - Growing evidence for renal damage
  - Examples
    - Omeprazole 20 mg (Prilosec)
    - Esomeprazole 20 mg (Nexium)
    - Lansoprazole 15 mg (Prevacid)

Others

 ### Sunscreen

- Ultraviolet (UV): Both A and B are bad.
  - Ultraviolet A (UVA) – 320 to 400 mm: deeper penetration (ages – cancer)
  - Ultraviolet B – 290 to 320 mm: affects epidermis (burns)
- Sunscreen needs to block both

- UVA and UVA: avobenzone, benzophenones, zinc oxide
- UVB only: PABA (aminobenzoic acid), Salicylates, Cinnamates
- Sun Protection Factor (SPF):
  - SPF is how long an individual can stay in the sun without burning with product × versus nothing. For example, if I burn in 1 minute with nothing, but in 2 minutes with product X, that is SPF 2.
    - SPF 15—93% filtered: if applied in adequate amount; most use ½ recommended amount
    - SPF 30—96.7% filtered
- Apply 20 to 30 minutes before sun exposure.
- Sunscreen and water
  - Water resistant → 40 minutes
  - Waterproof → 80 minutes
  - Wet T-shirt → SPF 3
  - Dry T-shirt → SPF 7

Insect Repellants

- N,N-diethyl-meta-toluamide (DEET) is the best by far.
  - Low toxicity (only approximately 50 cases since 1957)—all were cases of ingestions
  - Higher % not more effective but lasts longer
    - 6.65% lasts about 2 hours
    - 23.8% lasts about 5 hours
    - 10% to 30% safe for children over 2 months old (AAP recommendation)

Acne

- Comedone formation (two causes)
  - Excess sebum production
  - Increased epithelial cell turnover
  - Leads to:
    - open comedones (black heads)
    - closed comedones (white heads)
- Infection of comedones with *Propionibacterium acnes*
- Converts sebum to free fatty acids
- Inflammatory response
- Forms papules, pustules, and cysts
- Treatment:
  - Benzoyl peroxide
    - 2%, 5%, 10% (efficacy not dose related)
    - Mechanism
      - Decreases comedogenesis (improves desquamation)
      - Antibiotic
    - Forms
      - Water base (less drying)
      - Alcohol base (more drying)
    - Warnings
      - Can bleach clothes
      - Can cause allergic dermatitis on some
    - Good for comedonal, popular and mild pustular acne
  - Salicylic acid
    - 0.5% and 2%
    - Mechanism: promotes desquamation
    - Forms:
      - Cream (moisturizes: for dry skin)
      - Lotion (use with dry skin)

- Stick-on discs
- Pads (alcohol based: for oily skin)
  ○ Good for comedonal acne
- With any acne treatment:
  ○ It will take 4 to 6 weeks for improvement.
  ○ Pick delivery vehicle based on skin type.

●●● Plan B

- Plan B Next Choice - 0.75 mg levonorgestrel - 2 pills 12 hours apart
- Plan B One Step – 1.5 mg levonorgestrel - 1 pill
- Reduces a woman's chance of becoming pregnant by 85% to 99% if taken within 72 hours of unprotected intercourse
- Can purchase if ≧16 years old (males or females can purchase)
- Usually covered by insurance plans (if they cover OCPs)
- Not an abortifacient drug
- No contraindications except an established pregnancy (but won't disrupt)
- Advise patients: does not treat or protect against sexually transmitted infections
- Side effects: changes in menses, nausea, lower abdominal pain, fatigue, headache, dizziness, and breast tenderness

Medication Shelf Life

Expiration date:
- By law, 2 to 3 years after manufacture date, prescription drugs 1 year after dispensed (some exceptions)
- Dept. of Defense Study:
  - 90% of meds retained at least 90% potency 5 years past expiration date.
  - Exceptions: insulin, nitroglycerin, reconstituted antibiotics

Over-the-counter Medications

PREVENTIVE MEDICINE GUIDELINES

Robert V. Ellis

Cancer Screening		
Prevention	*USPSTF Recommendation*	*Other Recommendations*
Bladder, urinary cancer	(I)	
Breast cancer testing	Risk in woman based on FHx: Average risk (D) Increased risk (B) Use RST, FHS-7, or other screening tool to assess risk	RST: https://www.breastcancergenescreen.org/providers.aspx
Breast cancer	Mammogram 50–74 every 2 yr (B) Mammogram 40–49 (C) (individualize per patient) Mammogram ≥75 (I) MRI, U/S, 3D or digital mammography (I)	**ACS:** Mammogram 40–44 yearly if patient wants, 45–54 yearly, >54 to as long as in good health and likely to live >10 yr every 1–2 yr; no CBE **ACOG:** Start mammogram at 40, yearly. CBE at 29 every 1–3 yr and yearly at 40. Encourages "breast self-awareness." Consider stopping at 75 depending on the individual
Breast cancer, chemoprevention	Average or low risk (D) High risk (B)	
Cervical cancer	<21 (D) 21–65 have a cervix pap every 3 yr or 30–65 pap with HPV every 5 yr (A) 65+, normal past screening, low risk (D) Total hysterectomy for benign reasons (D) HPV: Alone or with pap <30 (D)	**ACS:** Start at 21 21–29 pap every 3 yr (no HPV) 30–65 pap with HPV every 5 yr; alternative pap alone every 3 yr >65 stop if no abnormal pap, continue for at least 20 yr after abnormal pap **ACOG:** Start at 21 21–29 every 2 yr 30-65 with HPV every 5 yrs, option of every 3 yrs Not needed if status post hysterectomy for benign reasons Stop between 65 and 70 if not abnormal in last 10 yr and not at high risk
Colorectal cancer	**50–75:** (A) **76–85:** (C) **85+:** (D) Colonoscopy q10y FOBT q1y FIT q1y FIT DNA q1-3y Sigmoidoscopy q5y Sigmoidoscopy q10y + FIT q1y Virtual colonoscopy q5y	**ACS:** Start at 50 Colonoscopy every 10 yr Sigmoidoscopy every 5 yr FOBT yearly Virtual colonoscopy every 5 yr Double-contrast barium enema 5 yr FIT yearly Fecal DNA yearly

Cancer Screening

Prevention	USPSTF Recommendation	Other Recommendations
Colorectal cancer, NSAID/ASA for prevention	(D)	
Lung cancer	Low-dose CT yearly in 55–80 with 30+ pack-yr and smoked within last 15 yr (B)	**ACS** and **ACCP**: Low-dose CT yearly in 55–74 with >30 pack-yr and currently smoke or quit <15 yr ago
Oral cancer	(I)	
Ovarian cancer	(D)	
Pancreatic cancer	(D)	
Prostate cancer	(D) for all Drat recommendation: 55–69: (C) = or >69: (D)	**ACS:** Recommend discussing risks and benefits screening, including PSA ± DRE (start at 50 for average risk, 45 for higher risk). http://www.cancer.org/docroot/cri/content/cri_2_4_3x_can_prostate_cancer_be_found_early_36.asp. **AUA:** <40: Do not screen 40–54 average risk: Do not screen 55–69: Discuss risks and benefits of screening and decide based on patient values and preferences ≥70 or life expectancy <10–15 yr: Do not screen
Skin cancer	Behavior counseling ages 10–24 (B) Behavior counseling >24 (I) Clinical exam (I) Patient self-exam (I)	**ACS:** As part of a general cancer prevention check-up
Testicular cancer	Adolescent and adult males (D)	
Thyroid cancer	(D)	

Recommendations are per USPSTF unless otherwise stated. A, strongly recommended; B, recommended; C, selectively recommend; D, not recommended; I, insufficient evidence to make a recommendation.

http://www.ahrq.gov/CLINIC/uspstf/uspstopics.htm.
Updated: February 24, 2017. Compiled by Robert V. Ellis, MD.

3D, three dimensional; ACCP, American College of Chest Physicians; ACOG, American College of Obstetricians and Gynecologists; ACS, American Cancer Society; ASA, acetylsalicylic acid; AUA, American Urological Association; CBE, clinical breast exam; CT, computed tomography; DRE, digital rectal exam; FHS-7, family history screening-7; FHx, family history; FIT, fecal immunochemical test; FOBT, fecal occult blood test; HPV, human papillomavirus; MRI, magnetic resonance imaging; NSAID, nonsteroidal anti-inflammatory drug; PSA, prostate-specific antigen; RST, referral screening tool; U/S, ultrasonography; USPSTF, U.S. Preventive Services Task Force.

Preventive Medicine Guidelines

Non-Cancer Screening

Prevention	USPSTF Recommendation	Other Recommendations
Abdominal aortic aneurysm (U/S)	Males 65–75 who have ever smoked (B) Males 65–75 who have never smoked (C) Woman 65–75 who have ever smoked (I) Women who have never smoked (D)	
Alcohol misuse screening and counseling	Adults 18 and older (B) Adolescents (I)	
ASA (prevent CVD and CRC)	<50 (I) 50–59 if 10-yr CVD risk ≥10% (B) 60–69 if 10-yr CVD risk ≥10% (C) 70+ (I)	10-yr CVD risk calculator http://tools.acc.org/ASCVD-Risk-Estimator
Autism	18–30 mo (I)	
Back pain prevention	Counseling (I)	
Bacterial vaginosis in pregnancy	Low risk for preterm delivery (D) High risk for preterm delivery (I)	
Bacteriuria, asymptomatic	Pregnancy, 12–16 wk or 1st visit (A) Nonpregnant or male (D)	
Breastfeeding counseling	(B)	
Carotid artery stenosis	(D)	
Celiac disease	(I)	
Child abuse	(I)	
Chlamydial infection	Women: Sexually active ≤24 (B) Woman: Sexually active, high risk (B) Men (I)	
Cognitive impairment in older adults	(I)	
COPD, asymptomatic	Spirometry (D)	
Coronary heart disease	ECG, exercise stress test, coronary calcium: Low risk: (D) Intermediate or high risk: (I) Nontraditional risk assessment such as hs-CRP, coronary artery calcification, homocysteine, lipoprotein a: (I) Dietary counseling for high risk (B)	

Non-Cancer Screening		
Prevention	*USPSTF Recommendation*	*Other Recommendations*
Dementia	Older adults (I)	
Dental caries	Fluoride supplementation in preschool children >6 m, whose water does not contain fluoride (B) Fluoride varnish <5 (B) Screening for dental caries birth to 5 yr old (I)	
Depression (assuming adequate f/u)	Adults (B) Adolescents 12–18 (B) Children 11 or younger (I)	
Diabetes mellitus, type 2	Obese 40–70 (B)	
Diet counseling	General population (C) Hyperlipidemia and other diet-related chronic illness (B) Obese (B)	
Drug use, illicit	(I)	
Exercise counseling	(I)	
Fall prevention	65+ Exercise/physical therapy and vitamin D (B) Multifactorial risk assessment (C)	
Family and intimate partner violence	Women of childbearing age (B) Elderly or vulnerable adults (I)	
Folic acid supplementation to prevent neural tube defects	Women planning or capable of pregnancy, 0.4–0.8 mg (A)	
Gestational DM, screening	After 24 wks (B) Before 24 wks (I)	**ACOG:** (at 24–28 wk) **1-hr 50 g glucose challenge**: Positive if ≥130 or 140; if positive, then **3-hr 100 g glucose tolerance test**: Positive if 2 or more values abnormal Fasting: 105 or 95 1-hr: 190 or 180 2-hr: 165 or 155 3-hr: 145 or 140
Glaucoma, screening	(I)	**AAO:** 1. 40–64 should be examined by an ophthalmologist every 2–4 yr 2. 65+ should have an examination performed by an ophthalmologist every 1–2 yr 3. Any individual at higher risk for developing disease, based on ocular and medical history, family history, age, or race, should have periodic examinations determined by the particular risks, even if no symptoms are present. (For young individuals at higher risk for certain diseases, such as African-Americans who are at higher risk for glaucoma, examinations should be considered every 3–5 yr for those aged 20–29 and every 2–4 yr for those aged 30–65, even in the absence of visual or ocular symptoms.)

(continued)

Preventive Medicine Guidelines

Non-Cancer Screening		
Prevention	*USPSTF Recommendation*	*Other Recommendations*
Gonorrhea	Women, sexually active, high risk (B) Women, sexually active, ≤24 (B) Men (I)	
Gonorrhea, newborn	Prophylactic eye medication (A)	
Hearing impairment, older adults	50+ (I)	
Hearing loss, newborns	(B)	
Hip dysplasia, newborns	(I)	
Hemochromatosis	(D)	
Hepatitis B	High risk (B)	**CDC:** Vaccinate all at high risk (including people with multiple partners and anyone presenting for possible STI evaluation)
Hepatitis C	High risk: Hx IV drugs, blood transfusion prior to 1992 (B) Born between 1945 and 1965 (B)	
Genital herpes, serologic screening	Pregnant women (D) (asymptomatic) Asymptomatic adolescents and adults (D)	
Hormone replacement therapy	For preventing chronic conditions (D) (postmenopausal women and women who have had a hysterectomy)	
HIV	All 15–65 (A) Younger or older at increased risk (A) Pregnant women (A)	**CDC:** Screen everyone 13–64
Hyperbilirubinemia	Universal screening in newborns (I)	
Hyperlipidemia and statin use	40–75: Low–moderate dose statin in patient with 1 or more CVD risk factors and ASCVD risk ≥10% (B) 7.5%–10% (C) Under 40 (I) Over 75 (I) http://tools.acc.org ASCVD-Risk-Estimator Dietary counseling for patient with hyperlipidemia (B)	**ATP-3:** All adults 20+, every 5 yr http://www.nhlbi.nih.gov/guidelines/cholesterol/atglance.pdf **ATP-3: 2004 update:** http://www.nhlbi.nih.gov/guidelines/cholesterol/atp3upd04.pdf **AAP and NHLBI:** <2 yr old: No screening 2–17: Screen children at higher risk (obese, HTN, DM, FHx, etc.) Screen all children 9–11 and 17–21
Hypertension	Adults 18+ (A) Children and adolescents (I)	**JNC-7:** Adults 18+, every 2 yr http://www.nhlbi.nih.gov/guidelines/hypertension/phycard.pdf
Hypothyroidism, newborn (congenital)	(A)	**Newborn congenital diseases screening:** Varies by state

Non-Cancer Screening

Prevention	USPSTF Recommendation	Other Recommendations
Iron deficiency anemia	6–24 mo (I) Pregnant women screening or supplementation (I)	
Chronic kidney disease	(I)	**JNC-7:** Screen all with HTN **ADA:** Screen all with DM annually
Lead, blood level	High risk, 1–5 (I) Average risk, 1–5 (D) Pregnant women (D)	**Medicaid:** Continues to require testing on all children at 1 and 3
Motor vehicle restraints	(I)	
Obesity screening and counseling	Adults, using BMI (B) Children 6–18 (B) Refer patients to intense multicomponent behavioral interventions	Children: Overweight = age-/gender-specific BMI at ≥85th–94th percentile Obesity = age-/gender-specific BMI at ≥95th percentile
Osteoporosis	Women, all 65+ (B) Women <65 with ≥ risk as 65 white women with no risk factors (10-yr risk 9.3%, use FRAX score) (B) Men (I) Screen with DXA scan FRAX score: http://www.shef.ac.uk/FRAX Consider meds in postmeno-pausal women and men aged ≥50 based on the following: • A hip or vertebral fracture • T-score ≤ –2.5 at the femoral neck or spine after appropri-ate evaluation to exclude secondary causes • Low bone mass (T-score between –1.0 and –2.5 at the femoral neck or spine) and a 10-yr probability of a hip fracture ≥3% or a 10-yr probability of a major osteoporosis-related fracture ≥20% based on the US-adapted WHO algorithm • Clinicians judgment and/or pa-tient preferences may indicate treatment for people with 10-yr fracture probabilities above or below these levels	**ACR:** • All women aged 65 and older • All men aged 70 and older • Postmenopausal women under age 65 with risk factors • Premenopausal women with oligo- or amenorrhea • Vertebral abnormalities or X-ray evidence of osteopenia • History of fragility fracture • 1st-degree relative with an osteoporotic fracture • Chronic medications: Glucocorticoids, phe-nytoin, heparin, anti-androgens, and gonado-tropin-releasing hormone agonists • Males with hypogonadism • Patients with chronic inflammatory arthritis • Individuals with GI diseases associated with calcium or vitamin D malabsorption (celiac) • Individuals with any other disease associated with osteoporosis or low bone mass
Peripheral artery disease	With ankle brachial index (I)	
PKU	Newborns (A)	**Newborn congenital diseases screening:** Varies by state

(continued)

Non-Cancer Screening		
Prevention	*USPSTF Recommendation*	*Other Recommendations*
Preeclampsia	ASA 81 mg/d after 12-wk gestation for high risk (B) Screening with BP measurement throughout pregnancy (B)	
Rh (D) incompatibility	All pregnant women at 1st visit (A) Repeat testing of all unsensitized Rh D–negative women at 24–28 wks gestation unless dad is Rh⁻	
Scoliosis	*Draft: (I)* Adolescence (D)	
Sickle cell disease	Newborns (A)	**Newborn congenital diseases screening:** Varies by state
STI counseling	Sexually active adolescents and adults (B)	
Smoking screening and counseling	Adults (A) Pregnant women (A) Children and adolescents (B) Pharmacotherapy in pregnant woman (I) E-cigarettes in adults (I)	
Speech and language delay	Children up to 5 (I)	
Suicide risk	General population (I)	
Syphilis	Increased risk (A) Pregnant women (A) Low risk (D)	
Thyroid disease	(I)	**AACE:** Do not screen asymptomatic patients http://www.aace.com/pub/positionstatements/subclinical.php
Tuberculosis screening	Latent TB in high risk: (B)	**CDC:** Does not recommend screening general population http://www.cdcnpin.org/scripts/tb/cdc.asp
Visual impairment	<3 yr old (I) 3–5 yr old (B) (once) 65+ (I)	
Vitamin supplementation for cancer and CVD prevention	Multivitamins (I) Single or paired nutrients (I) Beta-carotene and vitamin E (D)	

Non-Cancer Screening		
Prevention	*USPSTF Recommendation*	*Other Recommendations*
Vitamin D	Screening asymptomatic adults (I) Fall prevention 65+ at increased risk (B) W/Ca primary prevention of fractures in premenopausal women (I) >400 IU w/>1,000 mg Ca for primary prevention of fractures in postmenopausal women (I) ≤400 IU w/≤1,000 mg Ca for primary prevention of fractures in postmenopausal women (D) w/Ca in men (I)	

Recommendations are per USPSTF unless otherwise stated. A, strongly recommended; B, recommended; C, selectively recommend; D, not recommended; I, insufficient evidence to make a recommendation.

http://www.ahrq.gov/CLINIC/uspstf/uspstopics.htm.
Updated: August 16, 2017. Compiled by Robert Ellis, MD.

AACE, American Association of Clinical Endocrinologists; AAO, American Academy of Ophthalmology; AAP, American Academy of Pediatrics; ACOG, American College of Obstetricians and Gynecologists; ACR, American College of Rheumatology; ADA, American Diabetes Association; ASA, aspirin; ASCVD, atherosclerotic cardiovascular disease risk calculator; ATP, adult treatment panel; BMI, body mass index; Ca, calcium; CDC, Centers for Disease Control and Prevention; COPD, chronic obstructive pulmonary disease; CRC, colorectal cancer; CVD, cardiovascular disease; DM, diabetes mellitus; DXA, dual-energy X-ray absorptiometry; ECG, electrocardiogram; FHx, family history; FRAX, fracture risk assessment tool; GI, gastrointestinal tract; HIV, human immunodeficiency virus; hs-CRP, highly sensitive C-reactive protein; HTN, hypertension; JNC, Joint Nation Committee; JNC-7, the seventh report of the Joint National Committee on Prevention, Detection, Evaluation, and Treatment of High Blood Pressure; NHLBI, National Heart, Lung, and Blood Institute; PKU, phenylketonuria; STI, sexually transmitted infections; TB, tuberculosis; U/S, ultrasonography; WHO, World Health Organization.

INDEX

Note: Page numbers followed by *f* and *t* denotes figure and table respectively

Index

Index

Index